ADVANCING WITH THE ARMY

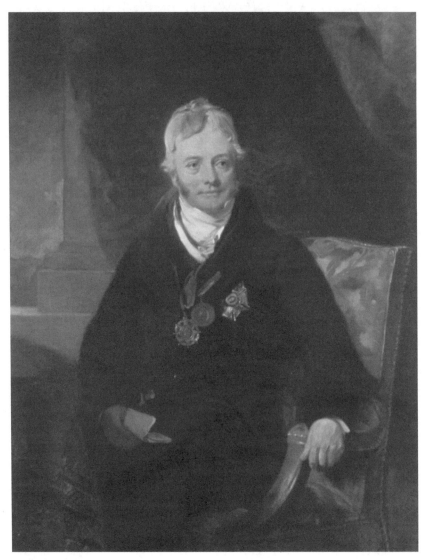

Andrew Geddes, *Sir James McGrigor* (n.d) [Oil Painting: By courtesy of the Aberdeen Medico-Chirurgical Society].

Advancing with the Army

Medicine, the Professions, and Social Mobility
in the British Isles, 1790–1850

MARCUS ACKROYD
LAURENCE BROCKLISS
MICHAEL MOSS
KATE RETFORD
and
JOHN STEVENSON

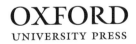

OXFORD
UNIVERSITY PRESS

OXFORD

UNIVERSITY PRESS

Great Clarendon Street, Oxford OX2 6DP

Oxford University Press is a department of the University of Oxford.
It furthers the University's objective of excellence in research, scholarship,
and education by publishing worldwide in

Oxford New York

Auckland Cape Town Dar es Salaam Hong Kong Karachi
Kuala Lumpur Madrid Melbourne Mexico City Nairobi
New Delhi Shanghai Taipei Toronto

With offices in

Argentina Austria Brazil Chile Czech Republic France Greece
Guatemala Hungary Italy Japan Poland Portugal Singapore
South Korea Switzerland Thailand Turkey Ukraine Vietnam

Oxford is a registered trade mark of Oxford University Press
in the UK and in certain other countries

Published in the United States
by Oxford University Press Inc., New York

British Library Cataloguing in Publication Data

Data available

Library of Congress Cataloging in Publication Data

Data available

Typeset by Newgen Imaging Systems (P) Ltd., Chennai, India
Printed in Great Britain
on acid-free paper by
Biddles Ltd., King's Lynn, Norfolk

ISBN 0-19-926706-5   978-0-19-926706-4

1 3 5 7 9 10 8 6 4 2

Preface and Acknowledgements

This book is a study of the small section of the medical community of Britain and Ireland in the first half of the nineteenth century who joined the army medical service during the long war against France from 1793 to 1815. It is not an account of their medical work as army doctors. For those who wish to read about the horrors of battlefield surgery and the appalling mortality which resulted from the many epidemic diseases to which armies on all sides fell victim during these years, there are already several works to which they may turn, most recently Martin Howard's *Wellington's Doctors*.[1] Rather, this is a study of the army medical officers of the Revolutionary and Napoleonic wars as a social group.[2] What it aims to shed light on is their collective biography: their background, education, military career, eventual civilian life, wives and children, wealth, contribution to the wider community, and so on. In consequence, the book is primarily not a history of medicine (although social historians of medicine should find it illuminating) but a contribution to our understanding of the development of the professions and social mobility in the era of the classic industrial revolution.

The material for the study has been chiefly drawn from an ongoing prosopographical database of 454 medical officers which the authors have been constructing over the past five or six years. The book is meant to provide a solid and reliable statistical analysis of the lives of its chosen subject: it is not a concatenation of random vignettes culled from a handful of surviving memoirs or contemporary correspondence. The authors are well aware, however, that even the most sympathetic reader might wilt under the welter of tables and figures and find a bare statistical survey dry and unrewarding. As much as possible, therefore, the statistical conclusions have been enlivened and enhanced with information penned by the doctors themselves or their relatives. As a result, a small percentage of the cohort—perhaps 15 per cent—will appear so frequently and in such detail in the course of the study that by its end they should have ceased entirely to be statistical ciphers and become flesh-and-blood human beings. This is important: too often quantitative history, especially as pursued in France by the Annales school, has led to the charge that its authors are 'historians in white coats', uninterested in the foibles, peculiarities, and unique potentiality of individual agents.[3] We are anxious to escape such censure, all the more that our doctors were for the most

---

[1] Martin Howard, *Wellington's Doctors: The British Army Medical Services in the Napoleonic Wars* (Staplehurst, 2002). The work, 242 ff., has some valuable statistical appendices and a good bibliography of relevant primary and secondary material.

[2] Every member of the army medical service gradually acquired officer rank over the period: see p. 47.

[3] Richard Cobb, 'Historians in White Coats', *Times Literary Supplement*, 3 Dec. 1971.

part brave men with astonishing powers of endurance, of whom it is difficult not to be in awe at the beginning of the twenty-first century. All the same, it is the collective statistical skeleton which determines the argument. The qualitative information puts flesh on the bones; it does not provide the wherewithal for the collective statistical skeleton to stand.

We hope then to have written a readable and humane book as well as an informative one. We hope too that the tone is even. The work is the product of five individuals who have been responsible for uncovering source material, collecting and inputting the data, making sense of the information, and ultimately writing it up. Once we had decided on the framework of the book and the general thrust of its argument, each of the five was entrusted with writing specific chapters. Given the difference in writing styles, age, and research background of the five authors, some unevenness of tone was inevitable, however much common consent there was over the interpretation of the data and material presented. In completing the book for publication, considerable attention was paid to the ironing out of any discord between the authorial voices. The intention was not to make the style bland and colourless, but to make the book a seamless web, so that the reader can move from one chapter to the next without that disconcerting feeling that he or she is encountering a new mind. The need to reach a consensus on the argument, write and rewrite drafts in the light of colleagues' criticisms, and continually hone the style in search of a single authorial voice inevitably makes preparing a collective book a long-drawn-out task. In many ways, it has more in common with producing a film than writing a normal historical work. Indeed, the fact that the authorial team never succeeded in working to a common timetable makes the film analogy particularly apt. Later chapters were completed before earlier ones, much in consequence had to be rewritten or jettisoned, and many of the best lines seemed to end on the cutting-room floor. Nevertheless, collaboration has many benefits. Besides the close friendships which develop across time, the continual discussion and reworking of drafts ultimately produces a much more rigorous and limpid narrative. Moreover, given the revolution that the new digital technology is beginning to wreak on historical research, collaboration may well be the future.[4]

Like all history books, this could not have been written without the assistance of many other people. First, mention must be made of the bevy of individuals with no connection to the academic profession who supplied us with many precious nuggets of information concerning members of our cohort in whose lives they had taken a personal interest. We are particularly grateful in this regard to Sir Anthony Montague-Browne, Mr E. H. D. Este, Bride Rose of New Ross, County Wexford, Mrs Susan Sharp of the Alderson Family History Society, Mr David Hurst of Knaresborough, Mrs Gill Lawley of Fernhill Heath, Worcestershire, and the late Michael and Mrs Maclagan of Oxford and their daughter Ianthe. Next, our thanks

---

[4] See the comments in Ch. 8.

are due to the ever-increasing number of librarians and archivists in Britain, Ireland, and the Commonwealth who allowed us to peruse their collections, often at the shortest of notice, and answered our many petty queries by post or telephone with continual courtesy and speed. Their number is legion and they cannot all be personally named, but Dr Elizabeth Hallam Smith of The National Archives, Arnott Wilson of the University of Edinburgh, Iain Bevan of the University of Aberdeen, Ian Milne of the Royal College of Physicians of Edinburgh, Julia Shepard of the Wellcome Library, Alison Fraser of Orkney Archives, Murdo Macdonald of Argyll & Bute Archives, Steve Due of the Medical Pioneers Database, Michael Barfoot of the Lothian Health Board Archives (Edinburgh University), and the staff of the Bristol Record Office, deserve special mention for the considerable amounts of time they have devoted to our cause. Third, we must thank several of our friends and relatives who acted from time to time as data collectors and pushed our research along at a faster pace than would have been otherwise possible, especially William Brockliss, William Gordon, Charlotte and Philippa Moss, and John Cardwell (the last the researcher's researcher).

Fourth, we must express how deeply we are in the debt of Karl Calckstein, former IT officer of the Oxford Modern History Faculty, and the staff of Oxford University's Computing Service. Without Karl's assistance in particular in devising the database according to our complicated instructions, the project could never have got off the ground. Fifth, our warmest thanks must be given to the three institutions who largely funded this research. It became possible in the first place thanks to a start-up grant from Oxford University which allowed Kate Retford to be employed for six months as a research assistant. The project then continued to be subsidized by Glasgow University and Magdalen College, Oxford, until the Wellcome Trust kindly awarded us a grant to complete the study. This permitted Marcus Ackroyd to act as a freelance researcher for a year and ensured we could pillage the treasures in the many personal papers left by our doctors in libraries around the British Isles. Last, but not least, we must register our appreciation of the sterling work done by Anne Gelling and her team in getting the proposal for this book accepted by the Delegates of Oxford University Press and then seeing the eventual manuscript through production. Commissioning a book by five authors must always be something of a gamble. We thank Anne and her team for so willingly investing their faith in our project and we earnestly hope that the following pages are sufficient proof that their trust has not been misplaced.

Marcus Ackroyd
Laurence Brockliss
Michael Moss
Kate Retford
John Stevenson

Magdalen College,
September 2005

Note

The dates of all medical practitioners not in the authors' prosopographical database are given in the text, if known, when an individual is first mentioned. The dates of surgeons in the database, where known, are given in Appendix 2.

Contents

List of Illustrations

Frontispiece and Cover: Andrew Geddes, *Sir James McGrigor* (n.d.) [Oil painting: By courtesy of the Aberdeen Medico-Chirurgical Society]

List of Figures

List of Tables

List of Abbreviations

Add MSS	Additional Manuscripts (BL)
ADM	Admiralty series (TNA)
AMB	Army Medical Board
BD	Bachelor of Divinity
BL	British Library (London)
BRO	Bristol Record Office
Burtchaell	G. D. Burtchaell, *Alumni Dublineses: A Register of the Students, Graduates, Professors and Provosts of Trinity College in the University of Dublin (1593–1860)* (Dublin, 1935)
c.-in-c.	commander-in-chief
C. of E.	Church of England
C. of I.	Church of Ireland
CO	commanding officer
DID	doctor's identity number (in database)
DNB	*Oxford Dictionary of National Biography*
Drew	Sir R. Drew, *Commissioned Officers in the Medical Services of the British Army, 1660–1960*, 2 vols. (London, 1968)
EMJ	*Edinburgh Medical and Surgical Journal*
EUL	Edinburgh University Library
Foster	Joseph Foster, *Alumni Oxoniensis, 1715–1886*, 4 vols. (Oxford, 1888–92)
FRS	Fellow of the Royal Society
Gibney	William Gibney, *Eighty Years Ago, or the Recollections of an Old Army Doctor; his Adventures on the Field of Quatre Bras and during the Occupation of Paris in 1815*, ed. by his son Major R. D. Gibney (London, 1896)
IGI	International Genealogical Index (on-line resource) *www.familysearch.org*
IR	Inland Revenue series (TNA)
McGrigor	Mary McGrigor (ed.), *Sir James McGrigor, The Scalpel and the Sword: The Autobiography of the Father of Army Medicine* (Dalkeith, 2000)
MD	doctor of medicine

NAI	National Archives of Ireland (Dublin)
NAS	National Archives of Scotland (Edinburgh)
NASA	National Archives of South Africa
NLS	National Library of Scotland
PP	Parliamentary Papers
Prob	Probate Court Canterbury (TNA)
q	quire
RAMC	Royal Army Medical Corp series (WL)
RC	Roman Catholic
RCSE	Royal College of Surgeons England (London)
RCSI	Royal College of Surgeons Ireland (Dublin)
RCSS	Royal College of Surgeons Scotland (Edinburgh)
RE	Royal Engineers
RO	Record Office
Rosner	Lisa Rosner, *The Most Beautiful Man in Existence: The Scandalous Life of Alexander Lesassier* (Philadelphia, 1999)
SC	Sheriff Court series (NAS)
TCD	Trinity College Dublin
TNA	The National Archive (formerly the PRO), Kew
TWA	Tyne and Wear Archives (Sunderland)
Venn	J. A. Venn, *Alumni Cantabrigienses*, Part 2: *From 1752 to 1900*, 6 vols. (Cambridge, 1922–54)
WL	Wellcome Library (London)
WO	War Office series (TNA)

Introduction: The French Wars, Industrialization, and the Professions

THE CONTEXT

The social history of the professions has attracted considerable attention in recent years, moving on from the narrative and institutional history of individual professions common in the past to a wider appreciation of the place of the professions in the broader historical and social context. Echoing the perspective taken by some of the first generation of sociologists, notably Weber, Harold Perkin in particular has argued that *professionalization*—the process whereby the professions became autonomous institutions controlling a field of knowledge or expertise and entered through competitive examination—is a key factor in the emergence of what we think of as 'modern' society.[1] The century 1750 to 1850 was a crucial period in the development of the modern British profession. Over the century, the professions underwent both numerical expansion (almost certainly at a faster rate than the population), as well as significant changes in their organization and their relationship with society at large. At one level, specialized subprofessions emerged from the traditional 'learned professions' of the law, the Church, and medicine. On another, the period witnessed the emergence of completely new professions, such as engineering, accountancy, and architecture. Further, within some professions, but not all, there was an early development of greater internal organization that paved the way to the rise of the self-regulating profession which was to become regarded as the norm by the twentieth century.[2]

The development of the professions during this era can be seen as a consequence of both an expanding and increasingly complex mercantile and industrial society and the concomitant development of a more powerful state apparatus. The late eighteenth and early nineteenth centuries in Britain were dominated by two

---

[1] H. J. Perkin, *The Rise of Professional Society: England since 1880* (London, 1989).

[2] G. Holmes, *Augustan England: Professions, State and Society, 1680–1730* (London, 1982); W. Prest (ed.), *The Professions in Early Modern England* (London, 1987); P. J. Corfield, *Power and the Professions in Britain, 1700–1850* (London, 1995); R. O. Day, *The Professions in Early Modern England, 1450–1800: Servants of the Commonwealth* (Harlow, 2000). Developments on the continent were similar but there the state played a greater role: see G. Geison (ed.), *Professions and the French State, 1700–1900* (Philadelphia, 1984); C. E. McClelland, *The German Experience of Professionalisation: Modern Learned Professions and their Organizations from the Early Nineteenth Century to the Hitler Era* (Cambridge, 1991); M. Burrage and R. Thorstendahl (eds.), *Professions in Theory and History: Rethinking the Study of the Professions* (London, 1990); eid., *The Formation of the Professions: Knowledge, State and Strategy* (London, 1990).

major features which distinguished them from what had gone before, although both had antecedents. One was the highly complex phenomenon of economic growth in all its aspects and ramifications. This was an era of expansion in trade, agriculture, manufacturing, and services which by the late eighteenth century had begun to manifest qualities distinctive from expansion earlier in the century, principally in the breakthroughs in transport, technology, and power which has led the period from about 1770 to 1830, though with caveats outlined below, to be taken as the classic locale of the 'first industrial revolution'. The other was war. The series of conflicts with France which began in the 1690s and ended with the final defeat of Napoleon at Waterloo have been dubbed the 'Second Hundred Years War'. They were to reach a culmination with the wars fought against Revolutionary and Napoleonic France, with Britain committed to warfare on an unprecedented scale on both land and sea from 1793. Indeed, of all the combatants of the Revolution Militant and the ensuing Napoleonic Imperium, Britain was the most persistently engaged and, as a result, was to face twenty-two years of warfare with only two short interruptions. At its peak, in the latter phases of the struggle against Napoleon, participation ratios have been compared with the 'total wars' of the twentieth century. Similarly, public expenditure as a percentage of the gross domestic product was to reach levels by the end of the Napoleonic wars not approached again until the Edwardian era under the pressure of rearmament and the beginnings of the welfare state.[3]

Economic growth in its various forms and Britain's huge involvement in the Revolutionary and Napoleonic wars could not but have significant social repercussions. For the founding fathers of sociology, economic growth was seen as part of the process of 'modernization', taken as breaking free from traditional agrarian based societies and the creation of a more highly differentiated and complex urban and industrial society. In terms of social organization 'modern society' has been seen as moving away from structures based upon family and kinship, face to face community, and non-market orientated economic relations to those characterized by associational organizations, bureaucracy, and the operation of the market. Traditionally, 'modernization' was identified with the growth of commercial society and its culmination in the 'industrial revolution' for which Great Britain provided the prototype 'first industrial revolution'. According to the early generation of economic historians such as Paul Mantoux, the Hammonds, or T. S. Ashton, the industrial revolution with all its societal repercussions was born in the eighteenth century. In their view, there was a relatively short period of 'transition' in which the major technological breakthroughs occurred and the foundations of the new society were laid. For the young Engels, writing in the early 1840s in Manchester, this new society was already taken as a fact of life. At its crudest, then, but sustained by the critique of enough historians, sociologists, and

---

[3] For a recent summary of these two developments, see W. Prest, *Albion Ascendant: English History, 1660–1815* (Oxford, 1998), chs. 5, 10, 14, 16, and 18.

contemporaries to give it robustness, the commonplace view has been that 'modern society' was in large part born out of the industrial revolution and that in Britain this process was occurring from the second half of the eighteenth century.[4]

But, however sustainable as a broad generalization, there has latterly emerged a much more nuanced view of the economic changes which were taking place from the late eighteenth century and which has attempted to put the undoubtedly far-reaching effects of the breakthroughs in technology and economic organization into the more balanced perspective of economic growth throughout the economy as a whole. Historians are now far more likely to see the classic form of industrialization—large factories, mechanized production, and the application of steam power—as the exception rather than the rule in the period up to 1815 and even beyond. Small but significant details illustrate a larger conclusion. The average 'factory' as late as the 1840s still employed only twenty people and new water-powered mills were still being installed in the West Riding during the same decade. A large percentage of the increase in output of manufactured goods up to the middle of the nineteenth century was being produced by totally 'unrevolutionized' methods of production and often little change in organization. Economic historians today would look more to the Victorian period for the transformation of the economy to one dominated by industry and perhaps even later for one dominated by the factory system and predominantly mechanized production. As a result, the classic period of the 'first industrial revolution' in the late eighteenth and early nineteenth centuries has increasingly been put into a broader context of economic growth in general and integrated within a more widespread set of contemporaneous developments, including for example urbanization and consumerism and the dissemination of the 'this-worldly' values of the European enlightenment.[5]

Yet, revisionism notwithstanding, no historian would disagree that British economic growth in the eighteenth and early nineteenth centuries had many facets and that its repercussions on society were complex, spawning a more widely differentiated social structure than the traditional hierarchies, without entirely destroying or displacing them. In particular, economic development in all its aspects had repercussions upon the growth of the professional classes. The expansion of trade and commerce, especially from the late seventeenth century, influenced the growth of a large mercantile sector, ranging from the fabulously wealthy London merchant elite to the burgeoning shopkeeper class which met the needs of an

---

[4] This, the 'classic' view of the industrial revolution, is discussed in J. Stevenson, 'Social Aspects of the Industrial Revolution', in P. K. O'Brien and R. Quinault (eds.), *The Industrial Revolution and British Society* (Oxford, 1993), and in Deane's essay on Great Britain in Roy Porter and M. Teich (eds.), *The Industrial Revolution in National Context* (Cambridge, 1996), ch. 2.

[5] See Prest, *Albion Ascendant*, ch. 10, esp. 239–41; D. S. Landes, 'The Fable of the Dead Horse; or the Industrial Revolution Revisited', in J. Mokyr (ed.), *The British Industrial Revolution: An Economic Perspective* (London, 1993); Roy Porter, *Enlightenment: Britain and the Creation of the Modern World* (London, 2000), esp. ch. 16. The most recent study of eighteenth-century consumerism is Maxine Berg, *Luxury and Pleasure in Eighteenth-Century Britain* (Oxford, 2005).

ever-expanding consumer revolution. Wealth, property, contracts, and insurance all provided in turn custom for professional services of every kind, but especially those of the law. The development of a highly capitalized and increasingly product-ive agriculture offered opportunities for the advancement of a wealthy class of tenant farmers and the service professions which were essential to the conduct of agricultural activities and business, such as lawyers, surveyors, and vets. Early industrialization would bring a growing demand for engineers, architects, and corporate lawyers. Medicine, like the Church, occupied more the position of an ancillary provider of services, benefiting from a growing segment of the popula-tion that was able to spend increasing amounts money on its own medical welfare and anxious to do so in an age that placed a new emphasis on health and beauty.[6]

While the stimulus to the professions from an expanding economy was a persistent and pervasive feature of the long eighteenth century, the impact of war was more episodic. The British civil service grew steadily from 1688 but the complement of the army and navy officer corps on active service see-sawed up and down according to the international situation.[7] Traditionally geared to a small standing army in times of peace, the land forces of the crown underwent rapid expansion in time of war. In the 'great wars' of the eighteenth century, the army establishment mushroomed. For example, the army establishment voted by parliament numbered under 30,000 on the eve of the Seven Years War (1756–63). By its end, its had risen to 120,000. Reduced to a rump of 45,000 after the Peace of Paris, the wars of the late eighteenth and early nineteenth century swelled the payroll enormously, the army rising to almost a quarter of a million regular troops by the end of the Napoleonic wars, over twice the size of the force mobilized for the American War of Independence. The navy followed a similar pattern of rapid expan-sion and demobilization: a half-pay officer corps in times of peace and a tiny cadre of full-time seamen could be rapidly expanded as occasion arose by means of the press-gang and the prospect of prize-money and glory. At its peak, at the end of the Napoleonic wars, the Royal Navy included over 1,000 ships and 142,000 sailors.[8]

Two observations are important here. The standing military forces of the Crown were puny compared to those of major continental powers like France, Prussia, and Austria-Hungary, all of whom maintained standing armies of over 150,000 men. Even Britain's reliance on the navy did not commit it to the scale of full-time professional forces in peacetime equivalent to those found on the continent. Second, although the long eighteenth century saw a gradual increase in the size of the residual military establishment, parliamentary impatience with military

---

[6] See J. Rule, *Albion's People: English Society, 1714–1815* (Harlow, 1992), 55–84; Laurence Brockliss, 'The Professions and National Identity', in Laurence Brockliss and David Eastwood (eds.), *A Union of Multiple Identities: The British Isles c.1750–c.1850* (Manchester, 1997), 9–11; Roy Porter, *Health for Sale: Quackery in England, 1660–1850* (Manchester, 1989).

[7] There were 16,000 civil servants in 1780 and 54,000 in 1870: Eric J. Evans, *The Forging of the Modern State: Early Industrial Britain 1783–1870* (London, 1983), 285.

[8] For the effects of war, see J. Brewer, *The Sinews of Power: War, Money and the English State, 1688–1783* (London, 1989), and L. Stone (ed.), *An Imperial State at War: Britain from 1689 to 1815* (London, 1994).

expenditure saw a rapid reduction in all the armed forces after 1815. Britain returned substantially to its low-key military establishment. The achievements of the 'fiscal-military' state in appropriating increasing revenues from a rising national income to pay for its wars and its subsequent debt servicing should not blind us to the unwillingness of parliament in the early and mid-nineteenth century to sanction further expenditure of this kind.[9]

The professions have normally been treated as an adjunct to the growth of the middle classes and, like them, embraced a wide range of incomes and circumstances. John Rule, in his survey of eighteenth-century English society, like many others, treats the professions as part of the heterogeneous 'middling people', along with farmers, yeomen, manufacturers, and merchants, lying between the labouring poor and the substantial landowners and nobility. In a more dynamic scenario, echoing Asa Briggs's analysis many years ago that the early nineteenth century saw the emergence of both the terminology and self-identity of the 'middle class', Davidoff and Hall argue that the growing urban middle class of provincial England 'took shape' during the 'turbulent decades' of the late eighteenth and early nineteenth centuries:

It was the crises of these decades which brought out common interests and drew its disparate membership together; the vicissitudes of war and trade cycles, the near breakdown of the old Poor Law, the pressure from the growing body of wage labourers. Although the eighteenth-century middling groups had many affinities with aristocracy and gentry, the basis of their property and their value system and, not least the nonconformity of many in their ranks, set them apart. These differences coalesced in the growing desire for independence from the clientage of landed wealth and power.

It was not a simple or unilinear process. Davidoff and Hall note the initial attraction to many professional men and merchants, especially nonconformists, of the liberal, early stages of the French Revolution, while recognizing that the subsequent growth of jacobinical radicalism at home and abroad produced a backlash which temporarily drew all men of property together. But the interests of different kinds of property could diverge and Briggs emphasized the importance of divisive issues towards the latter years of the Napoleonic wars, such as the Orders in Council and the Corn Law of 1815 in defining specifically urban and commercial middle-class interests against those of the landed classes. It was out of these circumstances that a raft of legislation in the period after 1829 consolidated middle-class interests in national and municipal government.[10]

---

[9] For the recruitment practices of the European states in the eighteenth century see J. Black, *Eighteenth Century Europe: 1700–1789* (London, 1990), 315–21. After 1815, for an illustration, the effective strength of the British army even in the Crimean War was under 100,000 men; France put 310,000 in the field, Turkey 230,000, and Russia over 500,000.

[10] Rule, *Albion's People*, 55, 60–1; L. Davidoff and C. Hall, *Family Fortunes: Men and Women of the English Middle Class, 1780–1850* (rev. edn., London, 2002), 18–19, 260; A. Briggs, 'Middle Class Consciousness in English Politics, 1780–1846', *Past and Present*, 9 (1956), 65–74. For the emergence of a middle-class discourse, see Dror Wahrman, *Imagining the Middle Class: The Political Representation of Class in Britain, c.1700–1840* (Cambridge, 1995).

However, within this rise of the middle class there were distinctions to be drawn. Davidoff and Hall record the tendency during this period for the professions, dependent as they were on the sale of services which involved the deployment of expert knowledge, to become more formal and to establish their own entry requirements, period of training, code of conduct, fixed scale of fees, and even certification. Thus unlike merchants or manufacturers the professions have been seen as beginning to develop the particular attributes of autonomy and control over an area of special expertise and the ability to draw boundaries around the group and defend its standards. This trend has been confirmed both on an empirical basis and by sociologists studying the behaviour of professional organizations.[11] For a considerable period before the twentieth century, the situation of much of the rest of the mercantile and manufacturing classes was quite different. After the breakdown of the tightly controlled merchant corporations of the medieval and early modern periods, the expansion of the merchant and manufacturing classes made it difficult to establish firm criteria of what particular expertise was involved in these areas. Men, and sometimes women, might be 'apprenticed to a business' and inducted into its activities and expertise, but until the age of professional management recruitment and qualifications, these processes were carried on through informal social and cultural networks. No distinctive qualification or recognized professional grouping linked the huge variety of people engaged in buying and selling, in retailing, or in manufacturing. Even though highly specialized groupings might emerge within particular branches of trade and industry, one of the characteristics of the age of economic expansion was the openness of trades and industries to new recruits. While survivals of older corporate structures certainly remained, such as the City Companies and provincial bodies like the Sheffield Cutlers' Company, they were becoming increasingly honorific by the eighteenth century, no longer providing any distinctive identity for those engaged in the activities concerned.[12]

The professions were different. As Larson has written within the larger context of economic modernization:

In all walks of life, the industrial revolution was separating work and training from the household and from the community. Professional work was becoming a *full-time* means of earning a livelihood, subject to the dictates of capitalist competition for income and profit. To insure their livelihood, the rising professionals had to unify the corresponding areas of the social division of labor around homogeneous guarantees of competence. The unifying principles could be homogeneous only to the extent that they were universalistic—that is,

[11] For a sociological overview see K. M. Macdonald, *The Sociology of the Professions* (London, 1995), especially ch. 1; for more historically informed perspectives, see Corfield, *Power and the Professions*, esp. chs. 1 and 2, and Day, *The Professions in Early Modern England*, ch. 1; also Davidoff and Hall, *Family Fortunes*, 260–1.

[12] See Rule, *Albion's People*, 72–84, and R. Sweet, *The English Town, 1680–1840: Government, Society and Culture* (Harlow, 1999), 185–90, for general accounts of the 'middling sort' and their associational culture. For the Sheffield Cutlers see C. Binfield and D. Hey (eds.), *Mesters to Masters: A History of the Company of Cutlers in Hallamshire* (Oxford, 1997).

autonomously defined by the professionals and independent, at least in appearance, from the traditional and external guarantees of status stratification. Thus, the modern reorganization of professional work and professional markets tended to found credibility on a different, and much enlarged, monopolistic base—the claim to sole control of superior expertise.[13]

The essentials then of professionalization were the development of tests of competence and standards, what has been called by Freidson 'a credential system', defined either by law or by legally sanctioned recognized custom, controlled by the profession itself.[14] The development of professional organizations to establish and maintain these 'tests' has been seen as the hallmark of professional development from the eighteenth century. But these developed erratically and unevenly over the course of the period from the eighteenth century and earlier. In many instances, well into the nineteenth and even the twentieth century, professional 'training' consisted to a considerable extent—and sometimes even exclusively—in a form of apprenticeship, learning the profession on the job and, in some cases, providing the sole evidence of professional expertise. The legal profession has been seen as one of the earliest to develop the kind of autonomy over its own affairs that has been seen as the characteristic of the professions in the modern era. Macdonald regards the legal profession as 'the epitome of that telling seventeenth-century legal phrase "lesser governments" '. This meant that its members obtained control over their own affairs in every respect and extensive power over the functioning of the legal and judicial system. Even so, apprenticeship to an attorney provided the bulk of the practising lawyers in the eighteenth century.[15]

In Britain, moreover, the ancient professions, law, Church, and medicine, retained strong links to the gentry, particularly the class of younger sons for which they provided alternative careers to the land, and in which formal qualifications mattered less than a little money and influence for making a start in life. This inevitably militated against the early emergence of professions which were clearly differentiated from the 'traditional and external' categories of social stratification, according to Larson one of the marks of successful professionalization.[16] An interest in defining membership of a profession in terms of a set of qualifications was only likely to grow once they could be seen as offering a clearer mark of social status than the vaguer categories of 'gentleman' and 'Esq.' which comprised some of the most amorphous of the status terms used in the eighteenth century. That this happened eventually, particularly after 1850, is testimony to the growing democratization of the terms customarily associated with a respectable standing in the world. Younger sons of real gentlemen must have increasingly come to value the

---

[13] M. S. Larson, *The Rise of Professionalism: A Sociological Analysis* (Berkeley, Calif., 1977), 13.

[14] E. Freidson, *Professional Powers: A Study of the Institutionalization of Formal Knowledge* (Chicago, 1986), 209.

[15] Macdonald, *Sociology of the Professions*, 75–7. Attorneys or solicitors far outweighed barristers (usually university educated) in 1851. The best study is H. Kirk, *Portrait of a Profession: A History of the Solicitors' Profession, 1100 to the Present Day* (London, 1976).

[16] Larson, *Rise of Professionalism*, 13.

distinctive status which sprang from being the accredited and properly examined member of a specific profession in a nineteenth-century world where any member of the middle classes would call himself a gentleman.[17]

One of the essential characteristics of the period 1750–1850 is that this process was only just beginning. In practice there was considerable diversity of status, income, and expertise both within what would later be called the professions and between the professions and sections of those who could be considered as part of the 'middling sort'. On the face of it, the diversity amongst some groups was so great as to stretch them almost beyond the possibility of considering them as a single, distinctive body. Just as the poor curate had little in common with the wealthy bishop, so the country sawbones had little in common with the London medical elite, ministering to fashionable, wealthy clients. But the reality was complex. The clergy, at least the Anglican clergy, provide an interesting example. While commonly by the eighteenth century all possessed a degree and the basic requirements of ordination and subscription to the Thirty-Nine Articles of the Church of England, even an Oxford-educated parson with a reasonable living, Parson Woodforde, was conscious when dining with the bishop in Norwich that he was mixing with social superiors.[18] On the other hand, the challenge of Methodism and its use of lay and even women preachers, reviving fears of the sectaries of the seventeenth century, re-emphasized the special nature of Anglican orders, an issue which was to bedevil attempts to reconcile the Anglican and Methodist ministries from the eighteenth century through to the twentieth.[19] An Anglican parson could still cling to some degree of social respect, even if increasingly vulnerable to religious pluralism and growing secularization.

In the medical sphere there was not, for much of the eighteenth and early nineteenth centuries, even the precarious exclusivity of the Anglican parson. The medical 'profession' in 1750 was informally organized. In the capital cities of London, Edinburgh, and Dublin, there was a small university-educated elite of graduate physicians and surgeons and apothecaries who carried out their instructions. The majority of medical men, however, had simply completed an apprenticeship with an apothecary or surgeon before setting up as general practitioners in their locality. Others spent some years learning the job at a London hospital or acquiring a smattering of knowledge by attending courses at a university, by the late eighteenth century usually in Scotland. The situation was further complicated by the rise of untrained but often highly paid 'quacks' in the eighteenth century, ministering to the wealthy in the largest cities, notably London, and

[17] The evidence of status inflation is most graphically evinced in the matriculation registers of Oxford and Cambridge where virtually every nineteenth-century student described his father as a gent.

[18] J. Woodforde, *The Diary of a Country Parson, 1758–1802*, ed. J. Beresford (Oxford, 1967), 211–13, 215–16.

[19] Robert Currie, *Methodism Divided: A Study of the Sociology of Ecumenicalism* (London, 1968).

fashionable resorts such as Bath.[20] Nonetheless, over the course of the century after 1750, the structure of the medical profession saw substantial developments in medical training and organization, although never sufficiently tightly drawn to exclude the untrained and part-timers. The number of graduate physicians expanded, and training became heavily dominated by the Scottish medical faculties and London hospitals, where most British medical practitioners would have spent some time. In England, licensing examinations for surgeon-apothecaries became compulsory from 1815, and thereafter anyone who wished to dispense medicine had to be examined by the London Society of Apothecaries. As a result, all English general practitioners thereafter had to come up to London to be examined and, usually, obtain a degree of formal instruction in order to pass. The London teaching hospitals and the Scottish medical faculties became the principal common elements in medical training, while still falling far below levels of professionalization found later, notably after the Act of 1858.[21]

If 'modern' qualifications were still largely absent to mark out clearly the status of many professionals, other features need to be borne in mind in defining the professions in this formative period. In practice, the increasingly urban character of the professional classes contrasted with the rural character of the landed sections of the middling sort below the aristocracy and the gentry—the substantial tenant farmers and the middling yeomen. Although the 'country doctor' still plied his trade, often combining his practice with farming, nonconformist preaching, or animal dealing, there were tremendous pressures on doctors to site themselves near the growing and increasingly affluent sections of the middle-class town-dwellers. But the battle to maintain status and a decent income was not always easy. Rule cites a letter of 1808 from Cornwall complaining that hardly any of the local doctors had 'provided against what is termed a rainy day'. He warned that one of the problems was the need to keep up appearances for 'a medical man must always look and appear to live genteely or he is a *nobody* . . .'[22] Many an aspiring young doctor in a county town must have stared financial ruin in the face, as George Eliot's over-indulgent husband, Tertius Lydgate, was to do in 1830s Coventry.[23]

With the merchants and early industrialists, therefore, the professional classes formed an inchoate, but largely urban class whose boundaries are not easy to define. An income of £50 a year has been estimated as the minimum in the middle of the eighteenth century at which it was possible to aspire to membership of the middling rank, a figure that would embrace one in five families in England, equally divided between town and country. As this was a sum which skilled

[20] Irvine Loudon, *Medical Care and the General Practitioner, 1750–1850* (Oxford, 1986), chs. 1 and 2. An elite pre-1750 trained at Leiden, Europe's leading Protestant medical school.

[21] Lisa Rosner, *Medical Education in the Age of Improvement: Edinburgh Students and Apprentices 1760–1828* (Edinburgh, 1991); Susan C. Lawrence, *Charitable Knowledge: Hospital Pupils and Practitioners in Eighteenth-Century London* (Cambridge, 1996), esp. chs. 4–5; Brockliss, 'Professions' (n. 6 above), 19–21; Loudun, *Medical Care*, chs. 7–8.   [22] Cited in Rule, *Albion's People*, 65.

[23] In *Middlemarch* (1871–2), Lydgate was an outsider brought in to run the new hospital.

workmen, particularly those in the capital, might earn in favourable circumstances, it was the marks of status in education, clothes, and style of life which
were more secure barometers of social standing. Paul Langford notes that use of
the term 'Esquire' expanded considerably in the eighteenth century but continued
to be restricted to men of property or professional standing. 'Mr' and 'Mrs', on the
other hand, was beginning to encroach on an even wider spectrum of the social
scale, 'widely accepted in towns, and increasingly in the countryside, as the automatic entitlement of anyone who owned property, hired labour, or simply laid
claim to a degree of rank and respectability'.[24] In effect the late eighteenth century
was a time of uncertain status for many in the professions, especially medical practitioners. In a world where only some men without income from land qualified as
gentlemen, most medical men would be given nominal gentlemanly status, though
some, particularly the barber-surgeons and apothecaries, could only precariously
lay claim to the title. In a sense professional status rubbed off, in that professionals
of however humble status might have to deal with the elite and were expected to
conduct themselves as gentlemen.

Professional insecurity in the period was arguably increased further in that the
professions only ever represented a small proportion of the total workforce, albeit
one that was growing, but almost certainly less fast than the mercantile sector as a
whole. Although long-term comparisons are at best tentative, the estimates of
Gregory King suggest that at least 2.1 per cent of English and Welshmen in 1688
were engaged in the professions, while by 1851 the figure had risen to 2.6 per cent.
Penelope Corfield has noted that these figures stand comparison with anything
before very modern times (after 1945) when professional occupations have risen
to over 10 per cent of the workforce, and eighteenth-century figures certainly
stand comparison with the Victorian period in this respect.[25]

Nonetheless, even if overshadowed by the more prominent rise of the merchant
class in the eighteenth century and by the industrialists in the nineteenth, the
professional classes overlapped with and often dominated them in their wider role
in local government, especially urban government. Indeed Langford has suggested
that in many small places in the eighteenth century, such as market towns, the
learned professions constituted the elite. The 'rule of three'—Lawyer Claw, Parson
Thrift, and Doctor Lopp, with 'best house, best living, and best pay'—formed
the centre of polite society 'around which shopkeepers and their wives, retired
officers, ambitious schoolmasters, neighbouring "gentlemen farmers", and all the
numerous tribe of the marginally middle class might cluster'.[26] Rosemary Sweet,
in greater detail, has supported this view, showing that it was not unknown for
some professional families, though more usually lawyers than doctors, to become
petty oligarchs in local politics. In most urban communities of the late eighteenth
and early nineteenth centuries, she argues, the 'professions' were ranked above

[24] Paul Langford, *A Polite and Commercial People: England, 1727–1783* (Oxford, 1989), 62–5.
[25] Corfield, *Power and the Professions*, 33. The second figure is based on the 1851 census which
recorded occupation for the first time.   [26] Langford, *Polite and Commercial People*, 73.

shopkeepers and generally on a par with the merchant elite. Generally, they could mix with the country gentry with greater ease than the shopkeeping class, and the emergence of the 'professions' as an urban elite has come to be regarded as an eighteenth-century phenomenon. This can be demonstrated by the changing composition of the governing bodies of many incorporated towns, especially those where traditional trades had ceased to play an important part. A striking example was Exeter, where the Chamber of Twenty-Four, once dominated by cloth merchants, had become dominated by members of the medical profession by 1831; in Oxford, it was attorneys and bankers who dominated the scene by the same year, displacing the traditional food retailers. In the burgeoning industrial cities, doctors were simply becoming part of the fabric of civic life. In 1843, Birmingham listed 200 medical men, had its own medical institute from 1828, and by mid-century had eight hospitals. The last were vital as places where doctors could gain experience and enhance their reputations in order to attract apprentices and pupils, paying premiums of up to £200 a year.[27]

The professions of late eighteenth-century and early nineteenth-century Britain operated within what Pat Thane has described as 'a distinctive type of *Ancien Regime* state', in which a strong, but undespotic central government was associated with an unusual range of free institutions, official and voluntary, enabling local communities, corporate bodies, and new institutions to deploy considerable delegated power and freedom of action. The time has long passed when historians contrasted a moribund, corrupt eighteenth century with a vigorous reforming Victorian 'age of progress'. At the governmental level, emphasis has increasingly been placed upon the eighteenth-century state's ability to win a succession of wars, become the major imperial power by 1815, accommodate the enormous forces of demographic and economic expansion, and survive them without major political upheaval. At the local level, it has been recognized that the locally based, unpaid justices of the peace provided a system of enormous flexibility for carrying out the increasingly complex tasks demanded of them by a rapidly changing society. The framework of a national poor law, at least in England and Wales, financed by local rates and administered very largely according to local needs and conditions proved capable of adaptation and renewal. Also striking was the growth in civic and municipal amenities—'the urban renaissance'—which took place in response to the first phases of urban growth in the eighteenth and early nineteenth centuries. Improvements to paving, lighting, and water supply, as well as the gamut of urban maintenance which the eighteenth century understood by the term 'policing', were already under way before the 'age of reform'. The provision of assembly rooms, fashionable promenades, theatres, spas, and racecourses in large numbers of provincial towns, not just the fashionable resorts, was testimony to the vigour of urban society, much of it designed to capitalize upon consumer demand for leisure and pleasure from local gentry, as well as the indigenous urban inhabitants.

[27] Sweet, *The English Town*, 181.

Although significant problems were beginning to affect this system by the early Victorian period, modern scholarship has questioned how sharp a break there was between 'unreformed' and 'reformed' England.[28]

Part of the explanation for this transformation in the view of late Hanoverian England is the undoubted evidence of a response from the last quarter of the eighteenth century, largely in reaction to the pressures of demography, economic growth, and war, to make central government more professional and more efficient. As Thane notes:

Steps were taken to reduce the role and influence of patronage in the civil service. The Treasury was reorganised, sinecures reduced, a new career structure initiated. The first moves were made towards a new conception of 'service' which gave salience to responsibility and efficiency. Government placed more reliance upon expertise and greater specialisation of work in departments . . . The period of the French wars, from 1793, demonstrated the effectiveness of the central state apparatus in its successful conduct of the war administration and of war finance, the costs of war, its organisational demands and, not least, the fear in elite circles of the spread of the revolutionary contagion from France brought about changes in the structure and activities of government.[29]

Although the extent to which changes in the ethos of central government were transmitted into the professions or vice-versa is difficult to assess with precision, something of the same mixture of older traditions of amateurism and patronage which existed in the late Hanoverian state and the moves towards a more professional and bureaucratic outlook were reflected in the professions. The traditional professions were expanding and, as we have seen, the processes of state building, agricultural improvement, industrialization, and urbanization developed new professions, such as engineering and architecture, and enhanced others like the civil service. The assault on 'old corruption' and the rise of the middle-class values of thrift, sobriety, and respectability enhanced the status of the professions and gave them a dominant part in the ethos of the new society. All the same, the professions did not uniformly or immediately adopt 'rational' structures and bureaucratic organization. The new professions may have gained 'a semantic existence' and obtained identities in the public mind, but they remained largely structureless in national terms until the second half of the nineteenth century. This remained true for the most obvious beneficiaries of the impact of change, new professions, such as engineering, the civil service, accountancy, journalism, and architecture. Only the small actuarial profession had its own London institute, founded in 1848, and had its entry conditional on examinations from 1850.[30] Although moving in the direction of greater professionalization and regularity of training,

---

[28] P. Thane, 'Government and Society in England and Wales, 1750–1914', in F. M. L. Thompson (ed.), *The Cambridge Social History of Britain, 1750–1950*, vol. iii (Cambridge, 1990), 2–5; for the urban renaissance, see P. Borsay, *The English Urban Renaissance: Culture and Society in the Provincial Town, 1660–1770* (Oxford, 1989), and Sweet, *The English Town*, esp. ch. 6.

[29] Thane, 'Government and Society' (n. 28 above), 8–9.

[30] Brockliss, 'The Professions' (n. 6 above), 10.

the medical profession was not untypical of British professions in only gradually acquiring what would be regarded in the twentieth century as the essentials of a profession, a uniform system of formal training and licensing and the establishment of a single, respected policing authority with the passage of the Medical Act in 1858.[31]

As we have seen, the professions have traditionally been viewed as part of the growing middle class of Hanoverian Britain. In a sense, the professions had two different roles in the development of British society. On the one hand, the placing of younger sons in the professions connected the landed classes to the middling sort perhaps even more directly than was the case with the increasingly self-sustaining merchant oligarchies and the newly emerging industrialists. On the other hand, the slow but steady sophistication of the professions gradually encouraged the development of a separate professional class along the lines outlined by Perkin with its own mores and influence upon society at large.[32] In spite of their former role, however, there remained significant distinctions between the landed classes and the 'middling sort', primarily because of the different basis of their property. Although the landed classes and the middling sort might find it relatively easy to mix in the social milieu of the spa, pleasure garden, or assembly room, access to landed property was a different matter. Thus, in spite of its reputation as an 'open society', there were significant barriers to advance into or, in some cases, back into, the ranks of landed society. As Lewis and Maude noted some years ago:

> though the land-owning aristocracy had intermarried with the upper middle class, and was largely middle-class in origin, inasmuch as few titled families could trace their lineage further than the fifteenth century, a determined exclusiveness was practised. Though everyone could rise, and rising in social scale for the first time became a general ambition, the land-owning interests were supreme. For a time, perhaps nearly two centuries, it was difficult to break into that society whose resources, invested in land and capitalistic agriculture, were overwhelmingly great; only the most successful merchants and bankers, the 'nabobs' returning from India gorged with spoil, and the slave-owning West Indian planters, did break in.[33]

Such views have been subjected to closer investigation in the work of Lawrence and Jeanne Stone, in establishing the composition and change of the landed elite over the period 1540 to 1880. Their overall finding is that there was remarkable continuity within the landed elite over this period and that the number of new purchasers even in the Home Counties were never large enough to swamp the older elite families. Moreover, they have identified a significant variance between the conventional wisdom that most newcomers were men of business and industry and the reality. In practice they have found that such influx into land as took

---

[31] Loudon, *Medical Care*, 296–301.
[32] R. Lewis and A. Maude, *The English Middle Classes*, 2nd edn. (London, 1953), 33.
[33] Ibid. 33–4.

place was mainly of professionals and office holders rather than of merchants or bankers (industrialists being almost entirely absent). In their view 'the unity of English elite society was a unity of the land and the professions, only marginally of land and industry'.[34]

If these suggestions of upward social mobility—of a new middle class including professional people, pushing its way ever onward and upward, including thrusting itself into landed society—receives some support, there is a certain circularity in the argument. It was not only upward social mobility which has been identified in this period but also what might be called potential downward or at least lateral mobility.

Although the aristocracy and sections of polite society still sometimes affected contempt for 'trade' and the professions, younger sons were directed to the established professions in which gentlemen did not lose caste—law, the Church, medicine, the civil administration, and the army and the navy. 'Here aristocracy met middle classes; for the middle classes put their sons into these professions to acquire gentility and rub shoulders with the nobility'.[35] It has been suggested that trade too, by the late eighteenth century, was no longer too menial an occupation. As the Stones have suggested, 'Generation after generation, younger sons were left to trickle downwards through the social system with only some education, some money, and influential patronage to give them a head start in life.'[36] They have, however, also suggested that although fortunes could be made by younger sons and thereby obtain the means of buying their way back into landed society, few in fact did so on the basis of the samples they used. Over 340 years in the three counties they examined, only forty-two younger sons bought their way back into landed society, two-thirds of them office holders or lawyers.[37] Further, John Rule has suggested that funding, education, and 'friendship' networks of younger sons could be put to more effective use in the traditional outlets of the armed forces, the Church, and the established professions than in commerce or industry.[38]

The aspirations of younger sons to return to the fold helps to explain the point made by Rule about the peculiar ambiguities of some aspects of professional life in the eighteenth century. There remained a dichotomous character to aspects of public service, the armed forces, and the Church. 'Young Esqrs.' coexisted with hard-working professionals in many walks of life. Public service could be both a profession for young bloods and a means of advancement for middle-class entrants. He cites the example of the late eighteenth-century Stamp Office where a quarter of all tasks were in the hands of deputies paid from the emoluments of the nominal office holders.[39] Britain in this period was still only partly on the way to the situation described by Harold Perkin in the mid-Victorian era when the

---

[34] L. Stone and J. C. Fawtier Stone, *An Open Elite? England, 1540–1880*, abridged edn. (Oxford, 1986), 184.   [35] Ibid. 34.
[36] Stone and Stone, *An Open Elite?*, 5.   [37] Ibid. 185   [38] Rule, *Albion's People*, 60–1.
[39] Ibid. 61.

professions constituted a kind of fourth class, but one whose mores increasingly pervaded the rest of society.[40]

THE PROJECT

The picture of the complex social role of the professions in the century 1750 to 1850 outlined above is primarily based on qualitative evidence. No one to date has undertaken a statistical examination of a particular profession or one of its subgroups to put solid flesh on this skeletal framework. This has been scarcely surprising. Before the invention of the relational database, the labour involved in compiling a prosopography of a representative sample of members of a profession and manipulating the information collected was a lifetime's work. Since the mid-1990s, however, the development of easy-to-use database management systems and the ever-expanding resources of the World Wide Web have changed for ever the research landscape and made such a statistical study realizable. The present study demonstrates for the first time the potential of the new technology for the social history of the professions by looking in detail at the membership of a subgroup of the medical profession—the surgeons who joined the army medical service during the French wars, 1793–1815. Its aim is to examine both the nature of the professional development of the service during and after the long conflict and the position of army doctors in relation to the expanding and increasingly complex economy and society of the first industrial revolution.

Army surgeons were chosen as the point of entry for several reasons. In the first place, they had a foot in both the state and private professions. On the one hand, as a cadre they expanded in response to the increasing demands of the wars of the 'long eighteenth century', growing in numbers and organizational sophistication. But, although called into being by war, they were also the beneficiaries of an expanding economy and an increasingly consumer-orientated society. Frequently forced out of army service or simply choosing to return to civilian life on the cessation of hostilities, they were often able to take advantage of the general level of economic growth and of the opportunities offered by a wealthy society with growing demands for medical care. Indeed, even as the army progressively expanded in the wars of the eighteenth and early nineteenth centuries and the number of army doctors with it, the flow into civilian life became all the greater. The rapid dismantling of the huge military apparatus built by the end of the Revolutionary and Napoleonic wars and the almost breakneck demobilization after 1815 did not merely affect humble soldiers and sailors, but the whole of the military establishment.[41] Army doctors in Britain could never look forward to being part of the large peacetime professional military corps found on the

---

[40] H. J. Perkin, *The Origins of Modern English Society 1780–1880* (London, 1969), esp. 319–39.
[41] See pp. 195–7.

continent both under the Ancien Régime or in the nineteenth-century European states with their large professional armies and increasingly bureaucratic support structures. As a result, many who started their careers as army doctors were to pass into non-service life as civilian practitioners.

In the second place, the Army Medical Service was precociously professional-ized compared with the wider British medical community before 1858. At no time across the century 1750 to 1850 did army surgeons have to be graduate physicians, but they always had to pass an entrance examination in surgery and eventually another in physic, while from 1816 quite stringent entry demands were laid down relating to education and character.[42] The service was also hierarch-ically organized into regimental, staff, and general appointments with different levels of pay. By the end of the French wars there was a definite career ladder and promotion was supposed to be based on experience and competence.[43] The service therefore is an ideal institution with which to gauge the competing claims of jobbery and merit in early nineteenth-century professional life and test the extent to which even the most 'modern-looking' of careers was still an Ancien Régime world.

The life of the army surgeon, furthermore, was scarcely glamorous. Dangerous—especially if posted to the West Indies—and unremittingly uncomfortable on campaign, it was not the obvious choice of the young medical practitioner who generally looked to set up his plaque in his local town. At the turn of the nineteenth century, the army believed it could only gain the recruits that it needed in the long war with France by raising pay and giving all ranks in the service officer status and a chance to mess with the sons of the well-to-do. Potentially, then, the army medical service offered a window of opportunity for medical practitioners who lacked the family and patronage contacts to move straight into a lucrative practice, particularly in the years 1793 to 1815 when the service was usually taking on 100–200 surgeons a year.[44] The army offered good pay and the chance to meet the right kind of people. A study of the origins of army surgeons and their eventual careers ought to throw interesting light on the role of the professions *tout court* as vehicles of social mobility.

Admittedly, surgeons attached to the navy could equally have been chosen as a point of departure. They too belonged to a particularly professionalized subgroup of the medical community and naval service was even more unglamorous: again recruits were hardly likely to be found in large numbers among young medical practitioners with easy openings in civilian life. The army, however, has the edge for the first study of this type because of the surviving documentation. Thanks to the *Navy List*, there is no problem in isolating a random sample of navy surgeons who served during the French wars.[45] However, the doctors' service records for

---

[42] See pp. 23, 28, 39–40.   [43] See pp. 31, 34, 38 and Table 1.1.   [44] See Table 1.2.
[45] The official *Navy List* was first published in 1814 but its predecessor, *Steel's Original and Correct List of the Royal Navy* was published privately from 1782: the latter only contains names of naval surgeons, not their mates or assistants.

this period in the Admiralty series of the National Archive were only compiled by officials in 1835 and provide no information about their lives before they entered the navy.[46] The War Office series, on the other hand, has a collection of pro-forma questionnaires filled in by army surgeons in the French wars in the years following Waterloo which offer invaluable details about an individual's background. If they do not reveal parental occupation, they do usually give a surgeon's date and place of birth (sometimes only by country) and the facts of his medical education: the details of his apprenticeship, the medical courses that he had followed, his experience in civilian hospitals, and his medical qualifications. In addition, the pro-forma documents his military career in varying degrees of detail up to the moment the questionnaire was completed, then in a different, obviously later, official hand, briefly notes his subsequent history of service and sometimes date of death.[47]

No reference to the existence of the pro formas can be found in the papers of the Army Medical Board that ran the service. However, according to the autobiography of the then director-general of the service, Sir James McGrigor, they were issued so that he might better inform himself of the qualifications and experience of the men under his command and ensure that henceforth the sick soldier could be guaranteed first-rate attention.

I gradually collected full statements of the education and services of every individual medical officer in the army which were drawn up and individually signed by each. Having thus come to the full knowledge of the education and qualification of each individual, I intimated to everyone who was deficient that he was not to expect any further promotion in the service until he had completed his medical education according to a scale which, in conjunction with my colleagues at the Board, I had established.[48]

It would seem that a pro forma was sent to everyone then thought to be in the service, either active or on half-pay, probably in 1815. Inevitably, given the deficiencies of early nineteenth-century bureaucracy some were sent to surgeons already dead, such as the Scot David Hutcheon from Arbroath, who had died at Berbice in British Guiana in 1805. In such cases, relatives or friends seem to have returned the questionnaire blank.[49] Presumably, too, many questionnaires were not returned or have got lost over the years. Some 2,850 surgeons were recruited during the French wars, of whom about a quarter died before 1815.[50] The collection,

---

[46] TNA, ADM 104/12–14, 20: service records of surgeons by date of entry 1774–1815 and records of assistant surgeons 1795–1823. Because of the late date of compilation, the source only contains the records of those who served in the French wars and survived to middle age and beyond.

[47] TNA, WO 25/3904–11. Some surgeons gave the barest of details about their career; others even copied out testimonials they had received from grateful commanding officers. Official additions to the pro formas are usually incomplete, which suggests that they were not seen as service records as such.

[48] McGrigor, 81. McGrigor took over the service in June 1815 and remained in control until 1851. For his career as director-general, including the qualification rules he introduced, see Ch. 1.

[49] TNA, WO 25/3909, fo. 66.

[50] See Table 1.4. The information is based on Drew. Drew used the WO 25 series in constructing his service biographies but did not include any of the information relating to background or education.

however, only contains 1,350 returns, including a small proportion—3 per cent—from surgeons who joined the service many years before 1793.

The forms were gradually returned in the years 1816–18 and at some later juncture filed in eight registers. The returns in each register are usually in alphabetical order but there is no reason why a particular surgeon should appear in a particular register: the registers have not been constructed according to date of entry into the army. By and large, the forms seem to have been honestly filled in. When the information relating to courses attended and qualifications obtained has been checked against the relevant university, college, and hospital records, no evidence of fabricating an educational cursus has been discovered. McGrigor too must have judged the exercise a success for all future entrants to the service seem to have been automatically required to fill out a similar questionnaire on entry that grew more formal over the years. Post-1825, these have been catalogued in a separate War Office series but a number of returns for entrants after 1815, especially in the second half of the 1820s and early 1830s, have been included with the original pro formas, making up some 16 per cent of the total.[51] The number of returns from surgeons actually joining the service during the French wars is thus only some 1,100.

Whatever the purpose of the questionnaires, their value to the historian is self-evident. One single source supplies answers to many of the obvious questions about the army surgeon's life and career. Above all, then, the existence of this source explains why it was decided to make the army medical corps the subject of the first quantitative study of professionalization in the late eighteenth and first part of the nineteenth century. The prosopographical database, which has been slowly constructed over the last six years and on which this study is based, consists of information on 454 army surgeons, every third returnee. No decision was initially taken to exclude surgeons who entered the service after 1815, so the database contains doctors who joined the army from 1772 to 1833, although the large majority—over 80 per cent—were recruited during the wars. As a result, the interval of time is enough for one father and son pairing to appear in the cohort—John Hennen (1779–1828), born Castlebar, Co. Mayo, and John Hennen Jnr (1800–71), born Deal, Kent. The father entered the service in the year his son was born, John Hennen Jnr in 1824.[52] The information in the questionnaires was first transferred to the database in a machine readable format as far as was possible. Answers to other crucial biographical questions were next obtained by searching other series in the National Archive and other libraries and archives throughout Great Britain and Ireland, and making use of the growing number of on-line sources. Of particular use were the list of estate valuations in the Inland Revenue series of the National Archive, the wills and inventory series of the National

[51] TNA, WO 25/3923–43: candidates for commission in surgery 1825–75. By the register covering 1847–9, the pro forma is printed.

[52] Nos. 28 and 380. Individuals in the database are numbered 3 to 451 according to the order that they appear in the WO series. For the full alphabetical list, see Appendix 2.

Archives of Scotland, the on-line International Genealogical Index (Family Search), and the National Archives' on-line catalogue of wills proved in the court of Canterbury. In consequence, it has been possible to construct a series of individual biographies, which at their fullest contain information about origin (in its widest sense), education and qualifications, army and civilian medical careers, wife and children, honours and civic positions, publications, and wealth on death.[53] In addition, in a small but significant number of cases, a much more rounded sense of the individual surgeon has been realized thanks to the survival of personal memoirs and letters.

The information in the database is presented and analysed in the following chapters, which except for the last on the cohort's contribution to the arts and science, broadly follows the surgeons' life cycle. This is not the place to reveal the contents of individual chapters, even briefly. Suffice it to say that they fully confirm the supposition that the army medical service was a window of social opportunity for those from relatively humble backgrounds. Director-General McGrigor is a prime example. Born in 1771 to a tacksman in Strathspey, Inverness-shire, with a surname which a few years before was still proscribed, he died a baronet worth £25,000. He put his two sons through Eton and the eldest, a banker and army agent, left the staggering fortune of £191,772 in 1890.[54] But successful self-promotion in the service was always a bit of a lottery: it required a strong constitution, talent (and not always at medicine), luck, and an ability to network in an age where patronage and meritocracy rubbed shoulders without apparent mutual discomfort. In consequence, some surgeons who had given stolid service but lacked patrons died in penury, such as another Scot, John Williamson, who spent more than twenty years in the West Indies, was court-martialled for petty embezzlement in 1824, and died a year later leaving a wife and paralysed daughter: Mrs Williamson was forced to become a servant.[55]

As the names of the surgeons in the database already referred to clearly suggest, army service was particularly a window of opportunity for medical practitioners from the Celtic fringe. Englishmen were very under-represented in the corps.[56] This book is therefore more than a study of professionalization and social mobility. It is also a contribution to the construction of Britishness. This is a subject upon which as much ink has been spilt as upon the social history of the professions in the last two decades, and one that continues to fuel debate.[57] The role of the

---

[53] The database is held on the mainframe of Oxford University and the personal computers of the authors. Access at present is only through Professor Brockliss and Moss's machines. The authors would like to construct entries for the remaining two-thirds returnees and make the database publicly available. So far, though, they have been unable to raise funds to do this.

[54] No. 320 in the database.

[55] No. 231 in the database. His place of birth is unknown but he was apprenticed in Edinburgh so almost certainly came from Scotland: see comments on cohorts' place of origin in Ch. 2 under 'Geographical Origin' and Ch. 3 under 'Apprenticeship'.   [56] See Table 2.1.

[57] E.g Keith Robbins, *Nineteenth-Century Britain: England, Scotland and Wales: The Making of a Nation* (Oxford, 1988); Linda Colley, *Britons: Forging the Nation, 1707–1837* (London, 1992); Brockliss and Eastwood, *Union of Multiple Identities.*

professions in creating a non-confessional sense of British identity in the nineteenth century, however, has not yet been properly commented on.[58] The conclusion of the book will suggest that this is fruitful area for future consideration. The army surgeons—just like the army officers more widely—formed a distinctive all British elite in which Englishmen were a minority. Moreover, most Irish and Scottish doctors eventually settled outside their homeland. What this meant culturally, however, is much more difficult to say. Typical was William Gibney of County Meath, who claimed a distant kinship to another Anglo-Irishman, the duke of Wellington.[59] Gibney, on leaving the army after Waterloo, built up his civilian career in Cheltenham, married a Warwickshire lady with West Indian planter connections, and put his son in the army. In later life, was he Irish, English, or British? His son possibly despised his Irish roots, for he changed his surname to Dwarris, his mother's maiden name.[60]

Finally, the book, especially Chapter 6, will throw interesting comparative light on the naval medical corps as an agent of social mobility. Although, as has been noted, constructing a prosopography of naval surgeons during the French wars is a much more difficult task, two of the authors—Brockliss and Moss—have begun to do so, using as their initial source the service registers dating from the early 1830s. In this case, given that there are only about 900 records, material relating to every second naval surgeon has been entered into the new database in order to create a cohort of an equivalent size.[61] This research is still ongoing, but enough information, especially about wealth on death, has been collected to permit its use in the present study.[62]

---

[58] It is touched upon in Brockliss, 'Professions' (n. 6 above), esp. 23–4.

[59] No. 24 in the database.

[60] It was as Major Dwarris that his estate was registered for probate in 1905.

[61] The same restrictions to access apply as for the army database: see above, n. 53.

[62] The naval database has also been used to ground Laurence Brockliss, John Cardwell, and Michael Moss, *Nelson's Surgeon: William Beatty, Naval Medicine and Trafalgar* (Oxford, 2005), ch. 1.

1

The Army Medical Service

EARLY HISTORY[1]

At the outbreak of the French wars, the army medical service was already 150 years old. From the inception of Parliament's New Model Army in 1645, an embryonic medical corps was created to support it and ten years later its organization was stabilized with the decision that henceforth there was to be one surgeon and surgeon's mate per regiment of foot and one surgeon per regiment of horse. At the same time, a small contingent of medical staff officers was established attached to the commander-in-chief, while overall supervision of the medical service was loosely placed in the hands of a troika comprising a physician, surgeon, and apothecary-general. Although Cromwell's army of 30,000 men was completely disbanded at the Restoration fifteen years later, the small standing force that initially replaced it and the much bigger British army of the eighteenth century largely replicated its institutions. The army medical corps in 1793 therefore was still in essence the service of the Protectorate.

The developments in the interim had been minor and reflected the growing size, activity, and sophistication of the army, which increased from some 75,000 men in the Williamite wars at the end of the seventeenth century (1688–97) to some 110,000 in the American War of Independence (1776–83).[2] From the time of the Williamite wars, it became customary to establish field hospitals when the army was on campaign on the continent, where the large numbers of men suffering from the ravages of disease and the smaller number of wounded could be sent to recover. This necessitated the speedy recruitment of an ad hoc medical and administrative staff, which could accompany the invading army and be stood down at the end of the war, and it greatly enhanced the powers and

---

[1] This section is chiefly based on the following sources: Neil Cantlie, *A History of the Army Medical Department*, 2 vols. (Edinburgh, 1974), i, chs. 1–6; Paul E. Kopperman, 'Medical Services in the British Army, 1742–1783', *Journal of the History of Medicine*, 34 (1979), 428–55.
[2] J. Brewer, *The Sinews of Power: War, Money and the English State, 1688–1783* (London, 1989), 30–2. In peacetime the army was reduced to less than 40,000 men. Both in war and peace, it was always considerably smaller than its French rival: see Paul Kennedy, *The Rise and Decline of the Great Powers: Economic Change and Military Conflict from 1500–2000* (London, 1988), 128 (table).

business of the small number of permanent general medical officers, who had to find the physicians, surgeons, apothecaries, hospital mates, and purveyors and ensure their provision. The office of surgeon-general became particularly import-ant since it fell to his lot to organize the medical support for all overseas expedi-tions, although the graduate physicians who headed the temporary staff and directed the field hospitals were always the appointees of his physician colleague. Both general officers normally found the senior medical staff among London practitioners. Surgeons were drawn from members of the Corporation (from 1800 the Royal College) of Surgeons, while physicians were graduates of Oxford and Cambridge and were either Fellows or Licentiates of the Royal College of Physicians.[3]

The Williamite wars, too, saw the establishment of the first permanent military hospital in England with the opening of the veterans' home at Chelsea in 1691, modelled on Louis XIV's earlier foundation of Les Invalides in Paris in 1670 and, like it, designated to hold 10 per cent of the standing army.[4] The maintenance of a regular peacetime army of some 30,000–40,000 men in the eighteenth century led in turn to the creation of a number of permanent barracks' hospitals in Ireland, where most of the soldiers were stationed, in Edinburgh, and in London and Windsor, where the prestigious guards regiments were based. It would be the War of American Independence, however, before permanent hospitals for troops involved in foreign campaigns were founded at Portsmouth (later Gosport), Chatham, and Carisbrooke (later Newport, Isle of Wight), thereby ensuring there were army doctors available to treat sick soldiers at the chief points of embarkation and disembarkation. Prior to this, local civilian surgeons seem to have been commandeered as needed to deal with the sick and wounded as they struggled off the ships.

In time of conflict, therefore, there was always a dramatic expansion in the number of medical staff officers, but throughout the eighteenth century—in peace or war—the lynchpin of the army medical service remained, as it had been in Cromwell's day, the regimental surgeon and his mate (the latter from the War of Spanish Succession of 1702 to 1713 attached to cavalry regiments, too, where he often doubled as a veterinarian). Whatever had been the case in the mid-seventeenth century, the regimental medical team was largely out of the control of the three general medical officers. The appointment of

---

[3] Sir George Clark, *A History of the Royal College of Physicians of London*, 2 vols. (London, 1964); Cecil Wall, *History of the Surgeons' Company 1745–1800* (London, 1937). Both corpora-tions were exclusive. The fellows of the Royal College of Physicians formed its governing body and had to be Anglicans and Oxbridge graduates. Licentiates of the college, who could hold an MD from another university, were only its certificated practitioners. For the two corporations' authority, see below, n. 6.

[4] C. J. T. Dean, *The Royal Hospital Chelsea* (London, 1950); *Les Invalides: trois siècles d'histoire* (Paris, 1974). Chelsea's establishment was preceded by the foundation in Dublin of the Royal Hospital, Kilmainham, built in 1680–4 to house Irish veterans and later extended to provide general medical facilities for the army in Ireland.

regimental surgeons had to be approved by the surgeon-general, but the position was in the gift of the colonel and often openly bought and sold, although an attempt was made to put a stop to the practice in 1783. The apothecary-general had even less authority at regimental level, since until 1796 the regimental surgeon was responsible for purchasing the medicines he needed in return for an annual allowance docked from soldiers' pay.[5] However, from 1756, an attempt was made to bring the regimental surgeon under closer central supervision when a new general officer was appointed, the inspector of regimental infirmaries, bringing the number to four. Wherever a regiment was based, in peace or war, the surgeon was expected to set up a regimental hospital by hiring a suitable building. The new inspector's job was to ensure that such hospitals, be they temporary or permanent, were properly run, both medically and financially.

At some time, too, in the second half of the eighteenth century, it became a requirement that regimental surgeons or surgeons' mates, however nominated, had to have passed an army surgical examination. In the eighteenth century, few medical practitioners in the British Isles had formal qualifications. Separate corporations of physicians, surgeons, and apothecaries existed in the three capital cities of London, Edinburgh, and Dublin, while Glasgow boasted a combined faculty of physicians and surgeons. Their power to control medical practice, even in their immediate vicinity, however, was strictly limited, and only those who wanted to belong to these august bodies needed a medical degree or had to submit to their examination to become a fellow or licentiate. Most doctors, whatever the extent of their training, had never had their competence assayed before setting up in practice.[6] The insistence, therefore, that army doctors give some proof of their skill before entering the service immediately set the group apart from the majority of their peers. In the first instance, the examination was solely administered by the London Corporation of Surgeons, but from 1788 the right was extended to her sister colleges in Edinburgh and Dublin.[7]

---

[5] The allowance came to about £80 p.a. in wartime: see Robert Hamilton, *The Duties of a Regimental Surgeon Considered*, 2 vols. (London, 1787), i. 7–9.

[6] Irvine Loudon, *Medical Care and the General Practitioner, 1750–1850* (Oxford, 1986), esp. ch. 2; Susan Lawrence, *Charitable Knowledge: Hospital Pupils and Practitioners in Eighteenth-Century London* (Cambridge, 1996), esp. ch. 3. In theory the corporations had a monopoly over medical practice in the four cities and the Irish colleges claimed the right to license practice throughout Ireland, but in the eighteenth century they were unable to prevent unlicensed practitioners (both educated and uneducated) undermining their rights. Medical practice in the British Isles was peculiarly under-policed in the eighteenth century: see L. W. B. Brockliss, 'Organization, Training and the Medical Marketplace in the Eighteenth Century', in Peter Elmer (ed.), *The Healing Arts: Health, Society and Disease in Europe 1500–1800* (Manchester, 2004), 346–71. For a detailed study of the position in France: see id. and Colin Jones, *The Medical World of Early Modern France* (Oxford, 1997), chs. 3 and 8. For medical training in the British Isles in the period 1750–1850, see Ch. 3.

[7] The colleges also supplied certificates for naval surgeons and recruits to the medical service of the East India Company.

THE FRENCH WARS, 1793–1815

The army medical service of the eighteenth century was a classic Ancien Régime institution.[8] Not only were the key posts at regimental level filled through non-medical patronage, but there was little opportunity for regimental surgeons to obtain staff appointments. The general medical officers themselves, appointed by the commander-in-chief, frequently had no military service and, even when they had, treated their position as a part-time one, which they fitted around their more prestigious London hospital posts and private practice and training.[9] Moreover, they had no secretarial assistance or bureaucratic support, so had little way of enforcing their will. This did not mean that army medical officers were incompetents— a service which included Sir John Pringle (1707–82), John Hunter (1738–93), and Sir Jeremiah Fitzpatrick (1740–1810) in its roll of honour could scarcely be dismissed as lacking in talent.[10] Nor is there any evidence that contemporaries found anything amiss with its performance in the field (although expectations cannot have been high). Nonetheless, to modern eyes, the eighteenth-century army medical service was not a professional organization: it lacked a single-point of entry, had no obvious career structure, and suffered from an amateur leadership. In this respect, it was no different from the army as a whole.[11]

The war that broke out in 1793, and dragged on incessantly except for two short breaks in 1802–3 and 1814–15, was the longest, most intense, and most expensive that the British state had yet been called upon to fight.[12] In order to ensure even the most rudimentary medical cover for the 266,000 men under arms by 1805, the general officers ultimately in charge had to entice an unprecedented number of doctors into the service, keep them there, and ensure that they were

[8] On the eve of the French Revolution, it was less professional than its French counterpart. The much larger French service mirrored the British one in many respects, but its permanent hospitals, dotted around the frontier, were already centres of medical research and a number became official training schools in 1772: see J. des Cilleuls et al., *Le Service de santé militaire dès ses origines à nos jours* (Paris, 1961); D. Voldman, *Les Hôpitaux militaires dans l'espace sanitaire français, 1708–1789* (Paris, 1980); Brockliss and Jones, *Medical World*, 689–700.

[9] The eighteenth century saw the foundation of a number of new London hospitals, and the capital after 1750 became a flourishing centre of medical teaching: see Lawrence, *Charitable Knowledge, passim*.

[10] Pringle was physician in charge of His Majesty's forces overseas at the time of the War of Austrian Succession and was the author of *Observations on the Diseases of the Army* (1753). He was a leading member of the mid-century Republic of Letters: see *John Pringle's Correspondence with Albrecht von Haller*, ed. Otto Sontag (Studia Halleriana, IV: Basel, 1999). For Hunter and Fitzpatrick, see: George Quist, *John Hunter 1728–93* (London, 1981); Wendy More, *The Knife Man* (London, 2005), esp.125–50; Oliver Macdonagh, *The Inspector General: Sir Jeremiah Fitzpatrick and the Problems of Social Reform, 1783–1802* (London, 1981).

[11] No institutionalized professional training was provided for army officers in the eighteenth century, except for officers in the artillery and engineers who were trained at the Woolwich Academy, opened in 1741. 'Sandhurst' was founded at Great Marlow, Bucks., in 1802, but it initially educated only a sprinkling of officers. The engineers had their separate school at Chatham from 1812.

[12] It was more than thirty times as expensive as the Williamite wars: see Kennedy, *Great Powers*, 105.

in the right place at the right time and properly equipped.[13] An account of their recruitment and retention will be given later in this chapter. The present section examines the effect of this unprecedented pressure on the central administration. Not surprisingly, given its rudimentary organization and unprofessional ethos, it often spectacularly failed, and soon became the butt of criticism, both from within and outside the service, in some ways carrying the can for the general lack of success in the war until Wellington's Peninsular campaign. A first salvo was fired against the general medical officers as early as 1794, but their most virulent critic was the army surgeon and Leiden MD, Robert Jackson (1750–1827) who in the years 1803–8 published a number of works attacking the organization of the medical service after he resigned in disgust in 1802.[14] Not surprisingly, too, the army command and the government, increasingly irritated by the appalling losses from disease on the campaigns in the West Indies and Europe, were moved on several occasions to try to improve the general officers' efficiency.[15] Although it took most of the war to establish a formula that commanded confidence—and even in the Waterloo campaign the central administration of the medical service did not cover itself in glory[16]—the period witnessed the gradual appearance of an organizing authority which really had teeth. In consequence, in the years following the end of the war, as the army itself began to professionalize, the Ancien Régime medical service was gradually transformed into a professional modern-looking army department with a *raison d'être* which extended beyond simple care of soldiers to what may be termed scientific enquiry.[17]

[13] Some sort of medical service had also to be organized for the 385,000 volunteers. Figures in John Cookson, *The British Armed Nation, 1793–1815* (Oxford, 1997), 95.

[14] Robert Jackson, *Remarks on the Constitution of the the British Army with a Detail of Hospital Management* (London, 1803); id., *A System of Arrangements and Discipline for the Medical Departments of Armies* (London, 1805); id., *A Letter to Mr Keate, Surgeon General to the Forces* (London, 1808); id., *A Letter to the Commissioners of Military Enquiry Containing a Refutation of Some Statements Made by Mr Keate…* (London, 1808); id., *A Letter to the Commissioners of Military Enquiry Explaining the True Constitution of a Medical Staff, the Best Form of Economy for Hospitals, etc* (London, 1808). Other critical works included: H. Moises, *An Inquiry into the Abuses of the Medical Department in the Militia of Great Britain with Some Amendments Proposed* (London, 1794); Nathaniel Sinnott, *Observations Tending to Show the Management of the Medical Department of the Army* (London, 1796); John Bell, *Memorial Concerning the Present State of Military and Naval Surgery* (Edinburgh, 1800); Dr Charles Maclean, *An Analytical View of the Medical Department of the British Army* (London, 1810). Bell thoughtfully dedicated his excoriating pamphlet to the army minister, Earl Spencer. Jackson defended himself against insubordination by claiming he had only gone public when he had received no response from his personal approaches to Pitt and other government ministers on the need for reform: see *System of Arrangements*, pp. xx–xxi. For Jackson's continual conflict with the general medical officers, see [Borland], 'The Life of Robert Jackson MD. Inspector General of Army Hospitals', in Robert Jackson, *A View of the Formation, Discipline and Economy of Armies*, 3rd edn (London, 1845), pp. lxxix–lxxx. Jackson is not one of the surgeons in the authors' database. For his career details, see Drew, no. 1190. He gained his MD in 1785: see 'Life of Robert Jackson', lxxxii.

[15] As in earlier wars, losses from disease were always higher than losses in battle: see figures in Cantlie, *Army Medical Department*, ii, *passim*.

[16] Medical support in the battle was woeful: see Richard L. Blanco, *Wellington's Surgeon-General: Sir James McGrigor* (Durham, N.C., 1974), ch. 8.

[17] For developments in the army generally, see Hew Strachan, *Wellington's Legacy: The Reform of the British Army, 1830–1854* (Manchester, 1984).

At the beginning of the French wars the army medical service was effectively run by one man—the surgeon-general, the choleric John Hunter—because the other general officers of the day were too old to play an active role. But Hunter himself died suddenly of apoplexy after organizing the first Flanders campaign and the following year, 1794, the secretary at war used the opportunity to take the first hesitant steps down the path of reform. The apothecary-general—the position had become hereditary in the Garnier family—was sidelined and the other three general officers, the physician, surgeon, and inspector of hospitals, were brought together in a formal Army Medical Board, with its own London office, and henceforth required to take their decisions collectively.[18] The leadership was still far from ideal. Neither the physician-general, Sir Lucas Pepys (1742–1830), nor the new surgeon-general, John Gunning (d. 1798), had ever served in the army, while the inspector-general of regimental infirmaries, Thomas Keate (1745–1821), surgeon to the Foot Guards and the Chelsea pensioners, was a notorious and well-connected pluralist who held a clutch of civilian appointments including a surgeoncy at St George's Hospital, London.[19] Nonetheless, the new troika, although still only giving two to three hours a day to the service for their £2 per day pay, seem to have operated relatively efficiently, especially after they were allowed to employ three secretaries from 1796. Moreover, the government had the good sense to reduce the board's workload by creating independent medical establishments for Ireland and the Ordnance department, whose remit included the large Woolwich Arsenal, in 1795 and 1797.[20]

In the four years following their appointment, the new board oversaw a dramatic expansion in the size of the army medical service and also began to extend its authority. The general medical officers still had limited powers over the appointment of regimental surgeons and their mates (from 1796 called assistants) and positions continued to be purchased in the new regiments established in the first years of the war.[21] Indeed, when the first expedition to Flanders was launched, the board had no control even over the staff appointments once the troops were abroad, for the king gave the right to fill vacancies to the principal medical officer with the invading army, Dr Hugh Alexander Kennedy (d. 1795).[22] Nonetheless, the board greatly increased its power of patronage by turning the existing infirmary wing at Chelsea (rechristened the York Hospital after George III's

[18] Cantlie, *Army Medical Department*, i. 178–82. The first Garnier to hold the post of apothecary-general was the French-born Isaac Garnier in 1733.

[19] None of the three is in the database. Pepys (Drew, no. 1223) was a leading light in the Royal College of Physicians and physician to George III. Gunning (Drew, no. 1193) was a surgeon at St George's. Keate (Drew, no. 899) supposedly gained £1,200 p.a. from his various offices; and he had a significant private practice, too.

[20] Cantlie, *Army Medical Department*, i. 110–11, 205–8. The independent Irish Medical Board survived till 1833; the Ordnance Service was reintegrated in 1853.   [21] See e.g. p. 37.

[22] Thomas Keate, *Observations on the Fifth Report of the Commissioners of Military Enquiry...* (London, 1808), 13–18. Kennedy (not in the database; see Drew no. 656) was one of the most distinguished doctors in the service at the outbreak of the war: he had been the physician serving with Albermarle at the siege of Havanna in 1762.

second son, the duke of York, commander-in-chief from 1798) into a hospital for serving soldiers and adding new general hospitals at Plymouth (1795), Gosport (1796), and Deal (1797), as well as a number of ad hoc creations on the east coast to deal with the wounded and sick returning from the continent.[23] In addition, the board gained the power to supervise closely the activities of the apothecary-general, who from 1796 was given the task of supplying medicines, bandages, and capital surgical instruments to the regimental surgeons as well as the staff officers, thus bringing all aspects of medical supply under central control.[24]

However, despite the troika's success, when Surgeon-General Gunning died in 1798, the government decided to abolish the board (while retaining its physical identity) and issued new regulations that ordered in future 'the Physician General, Surgeon General, and Inspector of Regimental Hospitals shall each have his distinct Province of business, and of recommendation; and be each made openly and solely responsible for his own acts'.[25] Why the secretary at war took this decision is impossible to say. When later questioned by a Parliamentary Commission of Enquiry on the move, neither Pepys nor Keate could give an answer.[26] The consequence, though, was to create rather than reduce administrative confusion, since the surgeon-general and the inspector of hospitals were given overlapping roles. With regard to appointments a crude division of labour was set up which broadly followed eighteenth-century practice: the physician-general recommended staff physicians, and the surgeon-general staff and regimental surgeons and their assistants (from 1794 no longer called mates), while the inspector of hospitals nominated ancillary hospital personnel—the surgeons' mates, apothecaries (who looked after the medicines), and purveyors (who looked after the stores and equipment)—at the surgeon-general's behest. As a result, the surgeon-general obtained exceptional patronage power, for there were never more than a handful of physicians in service at any one time, while the number of surgeons (both staff and regimental) was many hundreds. However, the inspector of hospitals was more powerful than he looked. Although he could use the lion's share of his patronage power only when asked to do so, he had the right to interfere in the lives of the regimental surgeons whom the surgeon-general had promoted by dint of being 'responsible for all matters relative to the supply of their medicines, and management of their hospitals'. In consequence, he was free to appoint deputies and meddle in the day-to-day lives of the surgeon-general's clients.[27]

---

[23] Cantlie, *Army Medical Department*, i. 191–3; Keate, *Observations*, 46. Deal was originally a navy hospital. Discussions re the creation of Plymouth began in the spring of 1794: see TNA, WO1/896, fos. 36–8: Army Medical Board to secretary at war, 3 May 1794.

[24] *Fifth Report of the Commissioners of Military Enquiry: Army Medical Department* (London, 26 Jan. 1808), 28–9. Capital instruments were the saws, large knives, and tourniquets needed in major operations, such as amputations. Pocket instruments - probes, small knives, etc. - were bought by the surgeons themselves.

[25] TNA, WO26/37, fo. 358: War Office circular, 12 Mar. 1798 (fos. 358–63).

[26] *Fifth Report of the Commissioners of Military Enquiry*, 5.

[27] TNA, WO26/37, fo. 360.

The 1798 regulations also laid down more precise rules for entry to the service and for promotion. To start with, hospital mates, as well as regimental medical officers, in future had to pass the army surgical examination administered by the royal colleges. The document reads as if this were already a requirement, but, if so, it never seems to have been formally introduced.[28] Second, the regulations demanded that entrants passed a further, novel examination if they wished to progress.

[N]one of those entering into the service after the present period, to be deemed eligible to a Regimental Commission, unless they shall have also passed a Medical Examination; if at home, by the Physician General, and assisted by the Surgeon General, and Inspector, or one of them, or, if Abroad, by a Board of Hospital Officers.[29]

A limited attempt, too, was made to establish an integrated career structure and to restrict the rights of nomination by commanding officers. Assistant surgeons were to be taken from among hospital mates and the regimental surgeons from the assistants, 'who are to be preferred according to length or merit of service; and not, on the recommendation of their commanding officer, to succeed regimentally, unless they otherwise have reasonable pretensions for the promotion'. Otherwise, staff and regimental appointments were kept strictly separate, except that apothecaries were to be chosen from mates or assistant surgeons and purveyors from among either the senior staff or regimental officers, 'if any are found among them properly qualified for the duties of that Department'. The traditional distinction between physicians and surgeons was also carefully maintained, although a narrow window of opportunity was opened for the appointment of physicians to the forces from non-conventional backgrounds.

In the case of Physicians, a Medical Degree at Oxford or Cambridge, or a Licence from the College of Physicians in London, although always desirable, not to be deemed indispensable requisites; if the Candidate should otherwise have strong pretensions from Military service, local Knowledge and Experience, or other circumstances of special cogency; or if he should be a Medical Graduate of any university in Great Britain or Ireland, and be found properly qualified in other respects and be found properly qualified, on one or more examinations by the Physician General, assisted by two Army Physicians.[30]

In the following years, the new regulations seem to have been generally honoured, Keate now acting as surgeon-general in place of Gunning and his own post being filled by John Rush (d. 1801), previously surgeon to the second troop of the Horse Grenadier Guards.[31] Until January 1801, it still seems to have been possible for hospital mates to be appointed who had not passed the army examination, but thereafter the requirements were enforced and mates in service who were uncertificated were ordered to regularize their position or face expulsion. One who

---

[28] Hospital mates were not examined before the war: see Hamilton, *Duties of a Regimental Surgeon*, ii. 169–70.   [29] TNA, WO26/37, fo. 361.
[30] Ibid., fos. 361–3.   [31] Not in the database: see Drew, no. 1012.

hastened to do so the following month was George James Guthrie, son of a London surgical goods manufacturer and later one of the most prominent surgeons in the kingdom, who had been appointed by Rush to the York hospital in June 1800 at the tender age of 15.[32] A small attempt too was made to offer further formal training to the lucky few once they had joined the service. In 1805 a decision was taken to offer one or two cadetships a year to entrants willing to commit to the army for a minimum period: in return for signing on for a definite length of time, cadets would be paid to walk the wards of a London hospital for six months to a year after becoming a medical offier. However, as Susan Lawrence has noted, no mention of these cadetships appears in hospital governors' minutes or newspaper advertisements, and they seem to have been filled by patronage. In 1806 for instance one was initially offered to one of the cohort, Alexander Lesassier, thanks to the influence of his uncle James Hamilton, Edinburgh professor of midwifery.[33]

Furthermore, despite the potential for friction, the three general officers seem to have muddled along for the first few years under the new dispensation. But when Rush died in 1801 and the inspector's office was given to Francis Knight (d. 1832), surgeon in the Coldstream Guards, harmony began to break down.[34] Essentially, Keate and Knight had a very different view about the value of general hospitals both at home and abroad. Keate, who owed his livelihood to hospital medicine, was a great supporter of the institution, believing that the staff surgeons who ran them were much more competent than regimental surgeons. He and Gunning, he insisted, had chosen well-educated, active young men, 'who after qualifying themselves to become good operators in the London hospitals, had served as hospital mates'. From his appointment as surgeon-general therefore he continued to champion the institutions that the old board had helped to set up, creating another set of temporary hospitals at Harwich, Yarmouth, and Colchester in 1799 to ensure the sick and wounded returning from the continent in that year were properly housed.[35] Knight, on the other hand, who was given a wider brief as inspector of army hospitals than Rush and had the power to shut redundant establishments, believed general hospitals were a waste of money and in the course of four years (1802–6) closed Gosport, Plymouth, and Deal, leaving only the London York Hospital and Newport Isle of Wight (where Chatham had been relocated in 1801).[36]

[32] T. J. Pettigrew, *Medical Portrait Gallery*, 4 vols., (London, 1838–40), vol. iv, *sub* Guthrie, 2–3. Rush had been overseeing the young Guthrie's education, see Ch. 3.

[33] Lawrence, *Charitable Knowledge*, 140; Rosner, 38–9. Lesassier declined the cadetship and it was given to David Maclagan, also in the cohort.

[34] Not in the database: see Drew, no. 955. Knight had come to the notice of the duke of York because of the well-regulated regimental hospital that he had set up: see McGrigor, 124. For McGrigor's contribution to the army medical service, see pp. 37 ff.

[35] Keate, *Observations*, 18–19, 46–60.

[36] Cantlie, *Army Medical Department*, i. 184, 195. Newport replaced Chatham when the army depot was moved to the Isle of Wight.

To add fuel to the flames, Knight also greatly extended his role as regimental inspector by gaining the authority from September 1803 to demand regimental surgeons produced weekly accounts and monthly lists of the sick, then using his right to appoint assistants (called deputy inspectors from May 1804) to establish an independent team of subordinates who could police the regulation.[37] His final insult was to introduce into his office in 1805 as his personal assistant, Dr James Borland (1774–1836). Borland was a man whom neither Pepys nor Keate could stomach in that he was the close friend of Dr Jackson, the Army Medical Board's constant critic, and even assisted the latter in composing his last diatribes of 1808.[38]

The divisions within the Army Medical Board remained largely out of sight of the public gaze until 1807, when Parliament launched an inquiry into the service. There is no evidence that this was done because there was thought to be anything amiss. It was just one of several investigations launched on the Treasury's initiative at this juncture into different government and army departments.[39] The commissioners, however, took evidence from the leading critics of the Army Medical Board as well as its general officers, and apparently prepared by reading the early works of Jackson. Inevitably, therefore, the tone of its subsequent report, published in January 1808 was critical. Looking to save waste rather than lives, the commissioners came firmly down on Knight's side and queried Keate's penchant for general hospitals.[40] In its conclusions the Commission made three basic recommendations.

First, the Army Medical Board should be once more remodelled so that its members might again control all aspects of the service collectively. Their number should still only be three, but henceforth there should be a chairman and two junior commissioners, and there was no suggestion that one should be a physician. Since the monopoly position of the apothecary-general was strongly questioned for causing unnecessary expenditure, the post of the fourth general officer was by implication to lapse.[41]

Second, the commissioners took up a suggestion pushed by Jackson that an army medical school should be set up, where medical officers could be properly

[37] *Fifth Report*, 29.

[38] Keate to Pepys, 31 Mar. 1810: letter published in *The Times* (14 May 1810), 3, col. E. Borland (not in the database; see Drew, no. 1244) entered the service in 1794 and 1810–16 was principal medical officer in the Mediterranean. He was the author of Jackson's 'Life': see above, n. 14. Pepys especially hated Jackson because he had been promoted to physician to the forces by the duke of York without an Oxbridge MD. Relations between Jackson and Keate got so bad that in 1809 Jackson thrashed the surgeon-general with a cane and received six months' detention: see [Borland], 'Life', pp. lxv–lxvi, lxxv. On Jackson's contacts in the Army High Command, see Ch. 4.

[39] Martin Howard, *Wellington's Doctors: The British Army Medical Services in the Napoleonic Wars* (Staplehurst, 2000), 5.

[40] One fact that caught the commissioners' eye was that the expense of running the board's office had doubled over seven years, from £3,415 to £7,448: *Fifth Report*, 8.

[41] Ibid. 82–4. The apothecary-general took no part in the provision of medicines but lived in the countryside and left his job to deputies. Nonetheless, he garnered a 10 per cent sinecure from a drugs bill which came to £67,340 p.a.: ibid. 39–48.

prepared for their role both as surgeons and administrators, in imitation of a school apparently already established by the Ordnance Department at Woolwich.[42] Although prospective entrants to the service had been able to attend lectures on military surgery at the University of Edinburgh from 1806 thanks to the foundation of the Regius chair there by the new Whig government of Lord Grenville, this was clearly felt to be a too ad hoc arrangement. For all the merits of the first incumbent, its promoter John Thomson (1765–1846), who held the chair until 1822, the course, which did not count towards an Edinburgh degree, only slowly gained an audience: in 1807/8 only fifty prospective entrants to the navy as well as the army enrolled. The commission wanted the establishment of compulsory in-service training under the army's control, presumably along the lines already devised by the Revolutionaries for entrants to the French army medical corps at the Paris hospital of Val-de-Grâce.[43]

Finally, some thought was given to creating an integrated career structure. The proliferation in the hospital inspectorate, both at home and abroad, under Knight had been to the benefit of regimental surgeons, for it was from their ranks, not from the general staff, that the officials had been chosen. According to one of his appointees, James McGrigor, later head of the army medical service, the inspector-general 'deemed it necessary that, for the correct execution of his duties, the inspector ought himself to be acquainted with the duties required of the subordinate officers; should be well acquainted from experience with the habits of officers, with the diseases incidental to them; with the many tricks practised by the soldier in assuming disease or what is termed malingering'.[44] Pepys in his evidence to the commission took umbrage at this policy on the grounds that the physicians (whom he had appointed) were frequently forced to take orders from 'people of inferior education' (i.e. surgeons).[45] It is doubtful that the commissioners fell for this piece of special pleading, but they did understand the need to merge the two sides of the service. They therefore recommended the establishment of a career ladder where promotion would be based on seniority (see Table 1.1). Although the possibility of a regimental surgeon becoming a deputy inspector was still envisaged, it was assumed that in normal circumstances he would first have been on the staff. Implicitly, therefore, staff surgeoncies were no longer to be filled by civilians recruited for a campaign but from regimental surgeons, while the position of physician to the forces was slated to disappear.

[42] Ibid. 82–5. Jackson, *System of Arrangement*, 27–33, 76–80. Bell, too, called for an army medical school in his 1800 *Memorial*, 7–41. Presumably the Ordnance Service's medical school was part of the Woolwich artillery school.
[43] Matthew H. Kaufman, *Surgeons at War: Medical Arrangements for the Treatment of the Sick and Wounded in the British Army during the Late Eighteenth and Nineteenth Centuries* (Westport, Conn., 2001), ch. 3; id., *The Regius Chair of Military Surgery in the University of Edinburgh, 1806–55* (Amsterdam, 2003), 65–8. Thomson, who is not in the database, began giving lectures privately in the winter of 1803–4. He was temporarily attached to the army medical service after Waterloo (see Drew, no. 3961) as a staff surgeon. His chair was established through the good offices of the Whig Earl Spencer, the dedicatee of Bell's earlier pamphlet and then in charge of the Home Department.
[44] McGrigor, 124–6. [45] *Fifth Report*, 5.

Table 1.1. Ranks in the Army Medical Service

1804	Equivalent army rank	1830	1840	Status
Hospital mate[a]	Subaltern			
Regimental assistant surgeon	Subaltern	Regimental assistant surgeon	Regimental assistant surgeon	Lieutenant
		Staff Assistant[b]	Staff assistant surgeon	Lieutenant
Apothecary to the forces[c]				
Regimental Surgeon	Captain[d]	Regimental surgeon	Regimental surgeon	Captain
			Staff surgeon class II[e]	Captain
Staff surgeon		Staff surgeon	Staff surgeon I class	Major
Physician to the forces[f]				
		Assistant inspector of hospitals[g]		
Deputy inspector of hospitals		Deputy inspector-general	Deputy inspector-general of hospitals	Lieutenant colonel
Inspector of hospitals		Inspector-general	Inspector-general of hospitals	Brigadier

[a] From 1813 called hospital assistants.

[b] New rank replaces hospital mate/assistant and ranked above regimental assistant surgeon. Initial entrants to the service were sent to be trained at Fort Pitt, Chatham, where they were called supernumeraries until gazetted to a regiment: see below, p. 43.

[c] Rank abolished in 1830. Serving officers of this rank became an assistant inspector of hospitals (AIH).

[d] Regimental surgeons ranked as captain under the 1796 warrant.

[e] Post could be held while attached to a regiment.

[f] Rank abolished in 1830. Serving officers of this rank became an AIH.

[g] Post initially existed from 1795 to 1804 and then replaced by deputy inspector of hospitals.

Note: Under the 1804 warrant, appointment to senior posts was not determined by length of service. Under the 1830 warrant an assistant surgeon had to serve five years before becoming a regimental surgeon and a regimental surgeon seven years before promotion to the staff. A staff surgeon had to serve a further ten years before he could be appointed an assistant inspector, another two before he could become a deputy inspector, and five more before becoming inspector-general. Service in the cavalry and guards always carried a higher status but there was no pay differential after 1804: see Table 1.3.

Sources: Royal Warrant 1804: RAMC 1406: Instructions from the Army Medical Board of Ireland to Regimental Surgeons . . . (1806), appendix 1. Royal Warrants 1830 and 1840: Cantlie, *Army Medical Department*, ii. 432–3.

The commissioners were convinced that the introduction of a career ladder could not but be beneficial. It 'would operate as an encouragement to enter the Service, and be a new stimulus to exertion and good conduct in it'.[46]

As can be imagined, the publication of the Parliamentary Report nettled Keate in particular, and he quickly composed an apology. So too did the army physician, Edward Nathaniel Bancroft (1772–1842), his physician-colleague at St George's

[46] *Fifth Report*, 86–7. Throughout the report the commissioners were impressed by the system pertaining in the navy, where by an order of January 1805 no one could be a physician to the fleet or a physician to a naval hospital who had not served as a ship's surgeon for five years: see Christopher Lloyd and Jack L. S. Coulter, *Medicine and the Navy 1200–1900*, iii: *1714–1815* (London, 1960), 33. It seems to have been the case that this system already largely operated in practice in the eighteenth century.

and Fellow of the Royal College of Physicians, who defended the practice of appointing civilians to staff positions on the grounds of their greater knowledge of the treatment of disease.[47] Neither need have worried because the report had no initial effect on the structure of the army medical service. Presumably, the army command had their hands too full preparing for the ill-judged attack on Sweden and the beginning of the Peninsular war in June 1808 to bother their heads about implementing its recommendations. Indeed, the difficulties that the service had in dealing with the legion of sick and wounded who arrived at Portsmouth after the disastrous evacuation from Corunna in January 1809, thanks to the closure of the army hospital at Gosport, must have convinced many close to the commander-in-chief that a report which judged Knight's activities such a success was not to be taken too seriously. The army had the humiliation of having to lease space in the massive naval hospital at Haslar, which had been founded in 1746 to serve the combined fleets.[48]

It was only with the Walcheren disaster the following summer that hearts hardened. The fever that attacked the British expeditionary force on the island at the mouth of the Scheldt was peculiarly virulent. By 17 September, 8,200 soldiers were incapacitated and 250 men were dying each week. Moreover, there had been too few medical staff officers sent out with the troops and too few medical supplies. Realizing that the army was beginning to fall apart from disease, Francis Moore, deputy secretary at war, asked the three general officers at the end of September to depart immediately for the Low Countries to sort out the mess. All three, not surprisingly, demurred, Knight and Keate claiming it was the province of the physician-general and Pepys pleading age and saying he was too busy organizing the ad hoc general hospitals set up in East Anglia to deal with the flood of repatriated soldiers. Eventually, deputies were sent in their place, including Borland, presumably representing the inspector-general, but they could do nothing to stem the mortality and only recommended that the whole army be shipped back to England.[49]

The refusal of the heads of the medical service to come to the aid of their country in its hour of need signed their death warrant.[50] The secretary at war, Lord Palmerston, was pushing for reform of the Army Medical Board from as early as April 1809 and in early December an ad hoc military committee, specially convened by the commander-in-chief, finally pronounced on its fate. At the beginning of 1810 the three general officers were dismissed, the apothecary-general bought

---

[47] Keate, *Observations*, esp. 46–60: defence of general hospitals. E. N. Bancroft, *A Letter to the Commissioners of Military Enquiry Continuing Some Animadversions on Some Parts of the Fifth Report...* (London, 1808), 1–25, 98–9: on physicians. He is not in the database: see Drew, no. 1460.

[48] McGrigor, 145–50. Lloyd and Coulter, *Medicine and the Navy*, ch. 6: Hasler could accommodate 1,800 patients, including those suffering from mental illness.

[49] Blanco, *Wellington's Surgeon General*, ch. vi; McGrigor, 159–60.

[50] Kate Elizabeth Crowe claims the Walcheren campaign actually delayed the reform of the Army Medical Board. We are not convinced. See Crowe, 'The Walcheren Expedition and the New Army Medical Board: A Reconsideration', *English Historical Review*, 88 (1973), 770–85. Admittedly, York's temporary replacement as c.-in-c. by Sir David Dundas in 1809 may have helped to bury the report in the long grass before the Walcheren disaster.

out, and a new board established along the lines suggested by the 1808 Report. [51] The government could do little else. A Parliamentary commission was appointed, in the teeth of government opposition, to investigate the Walcheren catastrophe which sat from January to June 1810. Since medical men as well as army brass were summoned before it, it was only a matter of time before the behaviour of the troika became public knowledge. In fact, the public did not have to await the publication of the correspondence between Francis Moore and the three general medical officers in the subsequent Parliamentary report, which began to appear in the spring. Someone passed the letters to *The Times* and the 'Thunderer' placed them before its readers on 21 February. Then the following month Thomas Rowlandson published a coloured print called 'Winding up of the Medical Report of the Walcheren Expedition', in which Pepys and Keate were quite literally put in the pillory (see Illustration 1).[52]

The new regulations for the Army Medical Board, issued on 24 February 1810 established for the first time a professional army medical service.[53] No one could enter the corps who had not been examined by one of the three Royal Colleges of Surgeons and received a regimental surgeon's certificate. Entrants then had to begin their career as a hospital mate before advancing to assistant regimental surgeon. Full regimental surgeons had to have been assistants for at least two years and been in the service for five. Staff surgeons were now to be exclusively drawn from regimental medical officers, preferably surgeons but, if none was available, also from their assistants of seven years standing. Finally, deputy inspectors could be found among regimental surgeons, staff surgeons, or physicians, provided they had served five years in their previous position. Deputy inspectors could eventually hope to become full inspectors, while the whole service was ultimately run by a board of three consisting of a director-general and two principal inspectors, who were expected to take decisions collectively. Army apothecaries and physicians were no longer considered a distinctive part of the service hierarchy, although the offices continued to exist: apothecaries were to be drawn from hospital mates, and physicians from regimental or staff surgeons and from MDs of any British and Irish university or from licentiates of the London Royal College of Physicians.[54] Purveyors formed henceforth a completely different organization and were no longer to be medical men. The director-general was to be in control of all appointments, and wherever possible emphasis was to be placed on seniority. Running the service was now to be a full-time occupation and members of the board were expected to give up civilian positions and private practice.

[51] The chief documents can be found in three collections of papers pertaining to the Army Medical Board in PP, 1810, xiv. 157 *et seq.*

[52] *Times* (21 Feb. 1810), 4, cols. A-D; PP, 1810, vii. 46–9.

[53] PP, 1810, xiv, 'Papers Relating to the Formation of the New Medical Department' (document 36), 20–2 (of this collection): 'Regulations for the Conduct of the Army Medical Board'.

[54] It is unclear whether surgeons could gain the post of army physician without a medical degree or licence. Apothecaries, oddly, had precedence over regimental surgeons, and physicians over deputy inspectors.

Not surprisingly, Keate and Pepys protested their dismissal. The latter claimed that his removal was an attack on the royal prerogative, while Keate demanded he first be tried by court martial. According to the erstwhile physician-general, 'a Board of General Officers determining the medical arrangements of the Army is not more incompetent than a college of physicians to decide on the attack of a fortress'.[55] Their whining got them nowhere, however, and the new board, consisting of Director-General Dr John Weir (d. 1819) and principal inspectors Dr Charles Ker (d. *c*.1837) and Dr William Franklin (d. 1833), began its work. In contrast to many of the earlier heads of the medical service, the new troika were all long-serving army surgeons who had risen to the rank of inspector and seen service abroad. Weir was an inspector of fifteen years' standing. In consequence, if they were not necessarily better at their job than their predecessors, they potentially had the respect of the regimental medical officers. They also seem to have worked well together as a team.[56]

Given the prejudices of the 1808 commission and the fact that the fresh set of appointees had been Knight's lieutenants, if not necessarily his protégés, the new board inevitably placed great emphasis on avoiding waste. The director-general kept a particularly close eye on the demand for medical supplies from the Peninsula. That said, the troika did not share Knight's hostility to general hospitals, and several were reopened and used as training-schools for new medical officers. Indeed, under the new regime, it became customary for entrants to the medical service to serve several weeks or months at the York hospital where they learnt the ropes before moving on to a position of responsibility. In this way, the board ensured that surgeons were 'blooded' before they were assigned a regiment and that the medical officers sent out in ever-growing numbers to the Peninsula would have some idea of what was expected of them, and the conditions under which they might have to live. In his memoirs, the Irishman William Gibney recalled how he had spent six weeks at the York in early 1813 before joining the 15th Hussars as an assistant surgeon. He and the other mates acted under the orders of two or three staff surgeons and took turns at being duty officer. Gibney found this experience, which came round all too frequently, monotonous because he had to spend the whole day at the hospital in order to receive any sick or wounded and the food was appalling. 'Our pound of beef was anything in the shape of meat, and as tough as shoe leather; the potatoes bad and badly boiled; one pound of bread of the brickbat nature; and a pint of porter sufficiently sour.'[57]

---

[55] *Times* (5 Apr. 1810), 3, col. B: Pepys to secretary at war.

[56] None in the database: see Drew, nos. 829, 989, 1126: both Weir and Franklin had begun their army careers as regimental mates. The third member of the board was initially Dr Theodore Gordon, another inspector, who had joined the service as a regimental mate in 1788. But he seems never to have taken up his appointment and definitely retired in July 1810, although he lived until 1843: Drew, no. 1189; TNA, WO25/3897, no. 1: half-pay list, individual returns with additions, *c*.1840. He should not be confused with a surgeon of the same name in the cohort.

[57] Gibney, 88–9.

Not surprisingly in wartime, however, this was as close as the board got to establishing an army medical school, as the 1808 commission had recommended. Nor initially did the board show much ability to interpret its remit imaginatively, so that the talented and committed might feel that their efforts would not go unrewarded. A vitriolic if ungrammatical missive from Wellington to Henry, Lord Bathurst (secretary for war and the colonies) in September 1812 suggests that the director-general was overly keen on sticking to the letter of the law about seniority to the detriment of the sick in the Peninsula.

I beg to draw your Lordship's attention to the practice of the Medical Board in promoting to vacancies in this army, instead of promoting the officers on the spot, who deserve promotion highly for their merits and services, officers are selected in England, the Mediterranean, or elsewhere to be promoted. The consequence is increased delay in their arrival to perform their duties, and all who do arrive are sick in the first instance. It would be but justice to promote those on the spot, who are performing their duty; and we should enjoy the advantages and the seniors of the department at least would have experience in the disorders of the climate, and of the troops serving in this country; to which climate they would have become accustomed.[58]

Thereafter, however, the situation seems to have improved. Six months later, Wellington and his medical staff were taking their own decisions on promotions as vacancies occurred in the war zone and merely sending lists back to London to be rubber stamped by the army command.[59] Indeed, there is evidence that Wellington could get his way at the regimental level at least, even before he sent off his letter of complaint to the secretary at war. John Murray of Turriff, Aberdeenshire (1786–1841) arrived in the Peninsula from serving in Sicily and the Ionian islands in January 1811 as assistant surgeon to the 39th Foot, a position he had gained on 2 March 1809 after spending five long years as a hospital mate. Tellingly, despite his relatively junior ranking, he was raised to surgeon of the 66th on 28 May 1812, a little more than a year after joining the campaign. Writing home to his father on the subject of his elevation, Murray boasted that he was the first of the fifteen medical officers to go out to the Mediterranean with Sir James Craig's army in November 1805 who had made full surgeon, even though ten of the number had been in the service many months longer. And the following year he was promoted again. On 9 September 1813, as the British army prepared to cross the Pyrenees, he was gazetted to the staff, a position which he piously assured his family was a fitting reward for his years of sacrifice and hardship in the call of duty.[60]

---

[58] Cited in Howard, *Wellington's Doctors*, 22.

[59] e.g. WL, RAMC 396: Wellington to the commander-in-chief at the Horse Guards, 17 Feb. 1813, list of medical officers for promotion. An endorsement reveals that Horse Guards stuck to the rules, even if Wellington did not. The list was redirected to the director-general for the Army Medical Board to secure his initial approval.

[60] Ibid., RAMC 830, Murray correspondence, nos. 67 and 83: John Murray to his father and family, 6 July 1812 and 27 Sept. 1813. For an analysis of the factors effecting promotion for Murray and his colleagues in the Peninsula, see Ch. 4. Murray, who is not in the database (see Drew, no. 2923) must be distinguished from the surgeon of the same name who is.

THE McGRIGOR YEARS

At the end of the French wars Director-General Weir retired on the grounds of ill-health and was replaced by Sir James McGrigor on 13 June 1815. Although another army surgeon who had served in the guards—he had been surgeon to the Royal Horse Guards Blue—McGrigor was by far the most campaign-hardened medical officer to sit on the Army Medical Board.[61] For eleven years from 1793, he had been surgeon to the newly formed 88th Foot (the Connaught Rangers), a position he had bought for £150 when the regiment was formed.[62] In their company he had travelled to Flanders, the West Indies, India, and Egypt and seen all manner of epidemic diseases, including bubonic plague. Becoming surgeon to the Blues in 1804, he had only a year enjoying a much more comfortable billet before Knight made him a deputy inspector and he became a full-time administrator in charge of the northern and then the south-western districts of England. Conspicuous for his success in finding lodgings for the wounded of Corunna who landed at Portsmouth, he was sent out to head the medical staff at Walcheren when the original chief, Dr, later Sir, John Webb (1772–1852) fell sick.[63] On his return he continued to act as a deputy inspector but at the end of 1811 was sent to the Peninsula as chief medical officer to Wellington's army in place of Dr James Franck (1768–1843), who had also succumbed to illness.[64] Over the next two years, McGrigor brought relative order and efficiency to a demoralized and poorly run service, and, to Wellington's obvious delight, successfully reduced the number of troops reporting unfit for duty, which had been hitherto spiralling out of control. Sharing Knight's suspicion of large general hospitals as the breeders of disease, he insisted the sick were kept close to the front in regimental hospitals, thereby reducing the possibilities of cross-infection, discouraging malingering, and ensuring that they immediately returned to their units when discharged.[65] McGrigor's reward on returning home in 1814 completely exhausted was a knighthood and a summons to Horse Guards to learn that it was the duke of York's intention that he should fill the position of director-general, in succession

[61] The best account of McGrigor's career during the French wars is his autobiography, originally published in 1861: see McGrigor, *passim*. Further details can be found in Blanco, *Wellington's Surgeon General*, and Howard, *Wellington's Doctors*.

[62] McGrigor, 32; Keate, *Observations*, 22–3. McGrigor's colonel for most of his time in the Connaught Rangers was William Carr Beresford, later general in charge of the Portuguese army in the Peninsula. For his putative influence on McGrigor's career, see Ch. 4.

[63] Not in the database: see Drew, no. 1429. Webb began his career as a regimental mate in 1794, the year after McGrigor, and initially prospered more quickly. He was knighted in 1821.

[64] Not in the database: see Drew, no. 1341. Wellington had inherited Franck from his predecessor, Sir John Moore, previously in charge of the Peninsular army. He had entered the service as a physician in 1794.

[65] It was assumed that the regimental surgeon would know better than a staff officer when a soldier was feigning disease. Soldiers who were sent to one of the general field hospitals by their regimental surgeon were often sent back again: see below, Ch. 4, pp. 176–7.

to Weir. McGrigor was well aware that there were others with a better call on the post—especially the two principal inspectors—but he accepted his good fortune with alacrity. 'My ambition at once determined me to accede to this, although my friends were still apprehensive for my health'.[66] He then took up the reins of his new office and only put them down again thirty-six years later in the spring of 1851.

The McGrigor era saw little development in the way the army medical service was structured. Those that occurred consolidated the rationalization introduced by the 1810 regulations. In 1830 the position of physician to the forces was abolished and thereafter no one could become a staff surgeon who had not served first in the regimental grade. Ten years later, in response to the limited possibilities of promotion in the much-reduced peacetime service, the former post was divided in two and the office of staff surgeon second class was created as an honorary position for long-standing regimental surgeons. No regimental surgeon or staff surgeon II, however, could aspire to become a staff surgeon I until they had served ten years on active service, while the latter became eligible for promotion to the post of deputy inspector general (from 1840 rechristened deputy inspector-general of hospitals) after three years further service at home or two abroad (see Table 1.1). The board itself gradually became McGrigor's personal fiefdom. Ker quickly resigned and when his replacement, Dr William Somerville (1771–1860), demitted in turn (to become physician to the York hospital) in 1819, the second principal inspector's post was not renewed. Franklin, on the other hand, served McGrigor loyally for nearly twenty years, but when he finally retired in 1833, his position was also moth-balled. Thereafter McGrigor reigned supreme over an Army Medical Office based in Berkeley Street, assisted by a secretary and six clerks. Under his aegis the director-generalship became a full-time job. He rose early, answered correspondence at home before going to the office, then spent the whole day there until the evening.[67]

McGrigor, however, did take a number of significant steps towards the further professionalization of the service from the beginning of his tenure. In the first place, he instituted the practice of keeping detailed individual career records by demanding that existing medical officers and new recruits completed a pro-forma curriculum vitae which could then be periodically updated.[68] Second, he had one of the most experienced officers in the service, John Gideon Van Millingen (b. 1782), draw up the first official army surgeon's manual, which was published

[66] McGrigor, 247.

[67] Blanco, *Wellington's Surgeon General*, 166–7. McGrigor praised Franklin as the perfect colleague: McGrigor, 251. Somerville, not in the database, had joined the service as a hospital mate in 1795: see Drew, no. 1499.

[68] TNA, WO25/3923–43 contain the pro-forma CVs of all candidates for commissions from 1825–67 in chronological order. It may only be in 1825 that the practice was initiated. The major part of this study is based on the pro forma completed by all medical officers already in service in 1815, which seems to have been distributed in the late 1810s: see Introd.

and distributed in 1819.[69] Hitherto, his predecessors had gone no further than to
publish regulations for the administration of army hospitals in 1803 and 1813.[70]
Third, and most importantly, he laid down for the first time detailed conditions of
entry. The large majority of recruits during the French wars had been admitted
under the regulations of 1798, which merely demanded candidates passed an
examination in surgery and physic.[71] Although in 1811 and 1813 the Royal
College of Surgeons of London, under pressure from the new Army Medical
Board, had decreed that no one could take the army surgical examination unless
he had attended lectures in anatomy, physiology, and surgery, performed dissections, and spent a year in a hospital, no educational cursus for entrants had
ever been officially prescribed.[72] McGrigor did not alter the requirement for candidates to gain a regimental surgeon's certificate from one of the royal colleges, but
he did specify for the first time in two sets of instructions, issued on 30 September
1816 and 1 July 1826, the personal profile and educational background that
he expected hospital assistants to have.[73]

To begin with, they had to be unmarried and have reached 21 years of age.
Next, they had to produce evidence of having had a regular apprenticeship of at
least three years, preferably with a member of one of the royal colleges of surgery,
and to have spent not less than a year attending a celebrated hospital. Those who
had not had an apprenticeship had to demonstrate that they had spent two years
in a hospital and done a year's practical pharmacy. Finally, they had to prove they
had attended specific medical courses 'at established schools of eminence'. Under
the 1826 regulations, besides clinical lectures on the practice of medicine and
surgery, a hospital mate was to have followed a course in anatomy for eighteen
months, one in practical anatomy for twelve, ones in chemistry, surgery, medical
theory, the practice of medicine and botany for six, and finally a course in materia
medica for three. Moreover, 'it will be considered an additional recommendation
to Gentlemen entering the service, to have attended lectures on forensic Medicine
and Public Establishments for the treatment of Diseases of the Eye and Skin and
of Mental derangements'.[74]

In other words, if McGrigor did not demand that entrants had a medical degree
as such or even held a licence from one of the royal colleges, he did expect them to
have studied in one of the country's medical faculties or the burgeoning London

[69] J. G. Van Millingen, *The Army Medical Officer's Manual upon Active Service* (London, 1819).
Hamilton's work of 1787 (see above, n. 5) had not been official. Van Millingen (not in the database:
see Drew, no. 2145) was the London-born son of a Dutch merchant who entered the service as a
hospital mate in 1800.
[70] *Instructions to Regimental Surgeons for Regulating the Concerns of the Sick and of the Hospital*
(London, 1803); *Regulations for the Management of the General Hospitals in Great Britain* (London, 1813).
[71] See p. 28.   [72] Lawrence, *Charitable Knowledge*, 102–3.
[73] *EMJ*, 3 (1816), 124–5; TNA, WO/30/139, fos. 228–9: 'On the Qualifications of Medical
Officers in the Army', 1826.
[74] The 1816 demands were slightly different as far as the length of the courses was concerned and
included one in midwifery.

hospital schools.[75] Indeed, the director-general made it clear that the ideal candidate would have had not just formal medical training but formal instruction in the arts and sciences. He was to have would have had the same kind of liberal education as any aspiring member of the country's elite.

Gentlemen who have had an University education will be preferred, it is desirable that all should have studied Natural Philosophy, Mathematics and Natural History in all its branches, but a liberal Education, and a competent knowledge of the Greek and Latin languages are indispensably requisite in every Candidate.

McGrigor further emphasized that an entrant's educational attainments would effect his future career. The greater his progress in the science of medicine 'in addition to competent professional knowledge', the more eligible he would be for promotion to assistant, then full regimental surgeon once he had completed five years in the service. 'Selections to fill vacancies will be guided more by reference to such acquirements, than to mere seniority.'

McGrigor thereby publicly committed the board to creating a service based upon a mix of experience and meritocracy. In 1826, he also stressed that the new demands would equally affect existing medical officers, who were 'earnestly recommended to avail themselves of adding to their knowledge by attending universities or schools' and asked to pass to the Office the details of any classes that they subsequently followed, so they could be registered.[76] Serving officers were warned that they 'must be prepared for further examination' before promotion or on returning to the service from half-pay, and prospective staff surgeons told that they needed to have spent at least two years in 'a public hospital of celebrity', including one, if possible, in London.[77]

McGrigor's commitment to seniority and merit helped improve the army medical service's image among the reform-minded both in and outside government circles in the decades after Waterloo. So, too, did his enthusiasm for controlling costs. McGrigor as another Knight protégé was a stickler for good accounting. While a deputy inspector in England he had insisted that regimental surgeons produced weekly returns and hounded those who were negligent. Typical were the letters he sent to a surgeon called Macartney on two occasions in the summer of 1807: on 5 June he excoriated the hapless doctor for not properly classifying the diseases of the patients in his regimental hospital; on 23 August he lambasted him for filing his reports uniformly late.[78] In office, McGrigor thus waged a constant war

---

[75] For the provision of formal medical education in early nineteenth-century Britain and Ireland, see Ch. 3.

[76] Presumably the information would be added to the pro forma on which this study is based and which all those in service in 1815 and all new entrants had had to complete.

[77] TNA, WO/30/139, fo. 229[r]. Prospective candidates for the soon-to-be abolished post of physician to the forces were informed that they had to have a medical degree from a British university or be a fellow of the Royal College of Physicians of London. For the half-pay system, see pp. 51–3.

[78] WL, RAMC 799/3 (microfilm), McGrigor's letter book 1805–9, fos. 140, 158. This is not the Macartney in the database.

on waste and mismanagement, although he never succeeded in gaining full control over the expenditure on medicines until the apothecary-general's patent finally lapsed in 1842.[79] He also shared Knight's dislike of general hospitals, so shut down all the existing staff hospitals in England except the depot infirmary at Newport, Isle of Wight. He even closed the York hospital for serving soldiers (about 1820) on the grounds it was too small to be of use, and established a new training hospital at Fort Pitt at Chatham.[80] McGrigor's long period in office then was inevitably one of scrupulous good housekeeping of which his political masters could not but approve.

But the new director-general was a creative as well as an efficient administrator who in an extended era of peace wanted to build a service which would have a wider brief than simply caring for soldiers. This was done by extending the function of the inspectorate into a data-gathering agency. The director-general, it seems, had not long been a deputy inspector himself before he realized the post had a greater potential.

There can be no doubt but that, both on account of the economical concerns of hospitals as well as the inspection of the practice pursued in them, the institution of these appointments was most beneficial to the service. But it struck me how very easily these appointments might be turned to beneficial account professionally and for the advancement of medical science in general, which, as it appeared had never been thought of.[81]

Having weathered the Waterloo campaign, therefore, the director-general set out to make his dream reality. Taking advantage of the fact that by 1815 there were contingents of the British army stationed all round the globe, McGrigor ordered his deputy inspectors and principal medical officers in their various foreign stations to oversee the preparation of ongoing regimental medical histories which would detail the prevalent diseases and their treatments.[82] Specially designed forms had to be filled in every six months and, along with an annual report, sent back to England, where they were stored at Fort Pitt. Army surgeons bound for foreign climes were expected to peruse them before they left in the hope that they would arrive better prepared.[83] By the mid-1830s there were 160 volumes available for consultation, whose contents, in an age obsessed for the first time with the power of statistics, were soon subject to thorough analysis. This task was undertaken

[79] Cantlie, *Army Medical Department*, i. 449–50. The apothecary-general's office seems to have been abolished in 1810, but the government never succeeded in redeeming Garnier's letters patent and it passed to his assistant, Calvert Clarke, who held it until he died in 1842.

[80] Ibid. 438, 444. General hospitals remained at Dublin and Cork. Initially, McGrigor had got Guthrie to give lectures on military surgery at the York. Guthrie who left the service in 1814 continued to give the lectures free of charge at a different venue for some twenty years: Pettigrew, *Medical Portrait Gallery*, iv, *sub* Guthrie, 7–8.

[81] McGrigor, 124. Unfortunately, McGrigor's memoirs end with his becoming director-general.

[82] Blanco, *Wellington's Surgeon General*, 169–73. Heads of foreign stations were usually deputy inspectors but some were staff surgeons, given the temporary title (never a rank) of principal medical officer.

[83] In peacetime the predominant task of the regimental surgeon was treating physical diseases.

from late 1835 by Henry Marshall, a retired inspector (1775–1851), and Lieutenant (later Major General Sir) Alexander Murray Tulloch (1803–64), an expert actuary, who were entrusted by the government with producing a medical history of British troops in the West Indies, where mortality and morbidity were particularly strong. This was completed in 1837 and was followed in the next twenty years by a clutch of statistical surveys of the health of British troops in virtually every part of the world.[84]

At the same time, the inspectors (and other surgeons at home and abroad) were encouraged to collect and send back interesting anatomical specimens and examples of the local flora and fauna. The specimens were then stored at the Chatham military hospital, in a museum which McGrigor had begun in 1816, along with a library. [85] Grasping that the age of the private collector was in decline and that the future lay with institutional collections, McGrigor created a scientific facility for the Army Medical Department that could stand comparison with the collections of the Royal College of Surgeons in both London and Edinburgh and the Hunterian Museum at Glasgow, endowed by John's brother, William.[86] By 1850 both library and museum had become a unique centre for the study of tropical and military medicine. Created entirely by voluntary donations, the library on McGrigor's retirement boasted 67,000 volumes and the museum 41,000 specimens, including more than 500 examples of human crania. It also contained an important collection of anatomical drawings produced by John Alexander Schetky (1785–1824), an army surgeon seconded to Fort Pitt for the purpose in the early 1820s.[87]

McGrigor's long tenure as director-general has earned him the sobriquet of 'father of the Army Medical Department'.[88] The accolade is just, for there can be no doubt that he dedicated his life to building on the work of Weir and his team and creating a professional medical service. Admittedly, for all his interest in ensuring recruits were properly educated, he never managed to establish an army

[84] They all appeared as parliamentary papers, starting with *The Statistical Report on the Sickness, Mortality and Invaliding among the Troops in the West Indies*: see PP, 1837–38, ix. 1–150. Marshall (not in the database: see Drew, no. 2609) had joined the naval medical service in 1803 before switching to the army as a hospital mate in 1806. After the completion of the West Indian volume, Marshall's role was taken over by Assistant Surgeon Thomas Graham (Drew, no. 4449), who had entered the service in 1836: Cantlie, *Army Medical Department*, i. 442.

[85] Blanco, *Wellington's Surgeon General*, 167–8; McGrigor, 258–9.

[86] In the second half of the 1820s and 1830s, McGrigor received numerous specimens from the Edinburgh collection through the generosity of its curators: see Matthew H. Kaufman, 'Specimens Transferred to the Museum at Fort Pitt Chatham in the 1820s': www.rced.ac.uk/journal/vol. 46. The first conservator, Robert Knox (1791–1862), was a former army surgeon (not in the cohort; Drew, no. 3911) who had joined the service in 1815.

[87] Catalogues of the library and part of the natural-history collection were published in the 1830s: see *A Catalogue of the Library of the Army Medical Department* (London, 1833); Edward Burton, *A Catalogue of the Collection of Mammalia and Birds in the Museum of Fort Pitt Chatham* (London, 1838). Schetky is not in the database: see Drew, no. 2410. A short obituary was published by David Maclagan, no. 106: [David Maclagan], *Biographical Sketch of the Late John Alexander Schetky* (Edinburgh, 1825).

[88] His statue, formerly on the Embankment, now stands at the entrance to Sandhurst.

medical school, presumably due to lack of funds. Towards the end of his reign, an official course in military surgery was opened at Dublin in 1846 to complement the one given at Edinburgh from 1822 by Thomson's successor, Sir George Ballingall (1780–1855), and a third was established at London University in 1853. But the first proper school would only open in 1860 at Fort Pitt—later transferred to Netley.[89] Nonetheless, the limited instruction McGrigor provided for new recruits at the Chatham depot seems to have gone some way in preparing them for their new responsibilities. Although the hospital was shabby and some of the wards damp, the entrants received much needed hands-on experience in military ailments and tropical diseases, for the hospital was the general infirmary for army invalids from around the world, especially India. From the moment they entered the depot, the new medical officers (called supernumeraries because they had not yet been gazetted to a specific post in the service) had to take charge of a ward of some thirty patients. Then, for periods of time varying between two and nine months, they learnt on the job under the eagle eye of the principal medical officer and his two assistants.[90] Moreover, besides giving the young army surgeon much needed practical knowledge, the stay at Fort Pitt gave many a useful induction into the mysteries of life as an army officer. According to William Johnstone Fyffe (1826–91) who entered the service in 1848, many of the entrants were rough diamonds who lacked social polish and 'were entirely innocent at first of the ordinary uses of a silver fork or finger-basin at dinner'. In consequence, 'a period of probation at a military Mess-table was not the least useful part of their education'.[91]

Admittedly, too, the medical service which performed so abysmally in the Crimea in 1854–6 was essentially McGrigor's creation. But the deaths of nearly 30,000 men, 18,000 from disease, cannot be laid at his door. This was the first European war with lethal weaponry that the army had fought for forty years and the serving medical officers lacked practical experience of dealing with the results. Moreover, there was a limit to what could be done to treat the thousands of victims of cholera and dysentery, given the state of medical knowledge, while in the first year of the war the surgeons' efforts were handicapped by the poor condition of the buildings used as hospitals, the independence of the Purveyor's Office and the difficulties of transporting the sick and wounded the 300 miles from Balaklava to Scutari. If hygiene was a major problem especially at the beginning of the conflict,

[89] Kaufman, *Surgeons at War*, chs. 3 and 5; Kaufman, *The Regius Chair*, chs. 3–4. Ballingall had been an army surgeon who joined as a hospital mate in 1806 and served in India (ibid. 111–12). He is not in the cohort (Drew, no. 2629). The first Dublin professor of military medicine was another former army surgeon, Thomas Jolliffe Tufnell (1819–85).

[90] cf. the description in William Munro, *Records of Service and Campaigning in Many Lands*, 2 vols. (London, 1887), i. 17–24. Munro (1822–96; Drew, no. 4793) attended Fort Pitt in 1844. Before leaving all officers had to take a natural history examination, presumably to demonstrate their ability to help build up the hospital's collection of fauna and flora. Munro was head of the army medical service 1874–80.

[91] Kaufman, *Surgeons at War*, 43, n. 105. Fyffe (Drew, no. 4977) was an Irishman from County Tyrone who had studied at Trinity College Dublin.

this was not a reflection of the former director-general's lack of interest in the subject. McGrigor had been appointed to the government's provisional board of health established in June 1831 to deal with the first outbreak of cholera, and if he was not a member of the Central Board of Health set up at the end of the year, he was always interested in ways of keeping soldiers free of disease. Above all, through his promotion of Marshall and Tulloch's investigations into the health of the army overseas, McGrigor played an important part in the relocation and reconstruction of insanitary barracks in the colonies. If soldiers' living conditions still remained atrocious in the British Isles when he left office, this should not be allowed to obscure the fact that new more airy and roomy barracks were already beginning to be built. The chief count against McGrigor in the light of the Crimean fiasco would be that he had failed in his long tenure in office to establish a team of stretcher bearers to collect the wounded from the battlefield in imitation of the 'flying ambulances' created by the French in the Napoleonic wars.[92] His successor, the distinguished naturalist Sir Andrew Smith (1797–1872), had to create a hospital corps from scratch at the outbreak of the conflict and it took most of the war to become established.[93]

NUMBERS, STATUS, AND RECRUITMENT

The army medical service took its first tentative steps towards professionalization in an era of unprecedented expansion in numbers; its consolidation as a profession took place in a period of rapid contraction, followed by many decades of stability. The figures speak for themselves (see Table 1.2). In the twenty years before the French wars 340 surgeons joined the service. Then from January 1793 to December 1815, as the British army grew ever bigger to meet the French threat, the service recruited 2,834 medical officers, seldom less than a hundred a year. After 1815, on the other hand, only a further 1,198 new surgeons were taken on before the outbreak of the Crimean war in 1854. In 1814, when Napoleon abdicated for the first time, there were 1,274 surgeons on the army's books, 354 attached to the staff (the large majority in the Peninsular army) and 920 members of regiments or garrisons. Seven years later, however, the figure had been more than halved and the service had reached a level around which it stabilized.[94]

---

[92] Blanco, *Wellington's Surgeon General*, 179–84; Howard, *Wellington's Doctors*, 38–40 (on collecting the wounded); Strachan, *Wellington's Legacy*, 61; Kaufman, *Surgeons at War*, ch. 4. McGrigor was mortified by the vilification of the Army Medical Board for the conditions in the Crimea. For Guthrie's intervention in the debate, see his letters to *The Times* (17 Feb. 1854), 10, col. A; (6 Oct. 1854), 9, col. F; (17 Oct. 1854), 10, col. B; (18 Oct. 1854), 8, col. C; (11 May 1855), 5, col. E.

[93] Smith joined the service in 1816 as a hospital mate. While in South Africa, 1820–37, he played an important part in mapping the flora and fauna of the colony, thereby embodying perfectly McGrigor's ideal of the medical officer as knowledge gatherer: see *DNB*, *sub nomine*. For his army career, see Drew, no. 3998.

[94] Cantlie, *Army Medical Department*, i. 431. According to TNA, WO25/262 (return of staff officers home and abroad in 1814), there were 322 staff in the Peninsular army, including 47 purveyors and their clerks.

Table 1.2. Size of the Army Medical Service

Year	Total new entrants	No. of staff officers	No. of regimental officers and others[a]	Total numbers[b]	Numbers on half-pay
1783	16				
1789	12		152[c]		154
1793	161				
1794	137				
1795	130				
1796	109				
1797	181				
1798	53				
1799	105				
1800	67		449		
1801	83				
1802	58				
1803	122				
1804	129				
1805	136				
1806	112				
1807	105				
1808	89				
1809	194				
1810	180		800		178[d]
1811	119				139[f]
1812	134				
1813	189	229[e]			
1814	91	354	920	1,274	134[f]
1815	95	237[e]			
1816	21				
1817	1				
1818	7	212			438[f]
1819	16	229			
1820	7				
1821	7	238	327	565	905
1828	25				
1830	5	152			723
1831	1	141	385	516	
1841	71	162	380	542	
1856	12				
1898	17				

[a] Includes garrison surgeons and miscellaneous appointments.

[b] Includes purveyors even though post-1807 not necessarily medical men.

[c] Includes full surgeons, not mates.

[d] 77 regimental medical officers who had been placed on half-pay since 1795, plus 101 staff and hospital officers, some of whom had been on half-pay before the war started.

[e] Does not include hospital assistants.

[f] Staff only.

Source: Drew; *Army List*; Cantlie, *Army Medical Department*, i. 431. The *Army List* does not give information about the size of the staff until 1813 and initially does not give the number of hospital mates. Regimental medical officers are listed by regiment and not given under a separate heading. Medical officers attached to the artillery are not included.

Rapid demobilization began immediately after the initial French surrender when most of Wellington's staff, including McGrigor, were stood down and put on half-pay.[95] This, though, only necessitated fresh recruitment in the autumn of 1815 to plug the gap and contributed to the logistical problems of the Waterloo campaign, where there were too few surgeons to cope with the much higher than expected casualties. This experience imposed caution, and in the following year the planned contraction was more sedate. Initially in 1816, only 63 staff, nearly all serving at home, were slated to lose their posts out of a contingent which now numbered 407, and no reduction in the staff serving with the army in France was considered. Once it became clear, however, that Napoleon was gone for good, the lay-offs proceeded apace and the service seems to have been down to 230 staff officers by the end of the year, with a further 57 losses anticipated. [96] In the event, further staff reductions proved difficult before the 1830s because of Great Britain's growing commitments around the world, and the bulk of the losses in subsequent years came from within the regimental service when the army of occupation finally quit France in 1818 and the strength of the British army was significantly cut. An army which had been reduced to 147,000 regulars by 1823 and 109,000 (the low point) by 1835 obviously required a dramatically slimmed down medical corps.[97]

Quite clearly, the primary task of the Army Medical Board between 1794 and 1815 was to find and keep on finding a large number of surgeons willing to serve. This was no easy undertaking. Not only did the army's medical general officers face competition from the navy, which was also recruiting strongly, but both services were fishing for volunteers in a shallow pool: prima facie, compared with civilian practice, the hazards of a military life made a career in either arm unattractive.[98] Probably about a quarter of army medical officers died in service during the war, some on the battlefield, most from disease.[99] The West Indies was a particularly deadly station for medical practitioners as it was for officers and men. Sir Ralph Abercromby's expedition in 1795–6 wisely took twice as many staff officers as it needed: of the eleven physicians who accompanied him, six died during the brief campaign and only one, Edward Nathaniel Bancroft, was still in the service in 1800.[100] Many who survived did so by chance and were forced to convalesce for a considerable time. McGrigor particularly lived on his luck in the

---

[95] McGrigor, 247. There had been a partial demobilization after the Peace of Amiens in 1802.

[96] BL, Add. MSS 48429, fos. 3–32b: assorted documents relating to army estimates for 1816–17: there seems to have been some hope of reducing the staff at home and abroad to 87.

[97] Strachan, *Wellington; Legacy*, 181–2. There was no suggestion that there might be an increase in the number of surgeons allocated to each regiment.

[98] There were 550 naval surgeons in 1793 and the number had risen to more than 1,400 by 1814: see Lloyd and Coulter, *Medicine in the Navy*, iii. 20–1. In contrast to Revolutionary France, there was never an attempt to conscript military doctors during the wars, suggesting the civilian profession was overstocked and there was no need.

[99] Based on a study of the biographical notices in Drew.

[100] Bancroft, *Letter to the Commissioners*, 55, 90.

Connaught Rangers. On his first posting to Jersey he caught typhus and then had a relapse when he belatedly joined the 88th in Flanders, so that he had to be ignominiously carted back in a wheelbarrow to the ships taking off the troops. He was just as unhealthy when he was with his regiment in the West Indies. Sent to the other side of Grenada by his commanding officer, while continually weakened by dysentery and suffering from dehydration, he only survived through a stroke of good fortune.

The morning was warm and I could proceed but a short distance when I was obliged to lie down for rest. In this way a great part of the day was spent. I became alarmed and made little progress. Observing a house at a little distance off I made for it . . . . I scrambled to a settee and lay down on it in great pain, and extremely exhausted. . . . The person in the room approached and upon his opening a jalousie to discover who I was, I saw a face leaning over me which I thought was familiar to me. A very few minutes afterwards I recognized . . . in the gentleman who had returned with some wine that he was my old friend and fellow student, Mr Pemberton, a West Indian who had come to King's College, Aberdeen, and had subsequently studied medicine there and at Edinburgh.[101]

In consequence, the Army Medical Board could not just sit and wait for medical practitioners to volunteer for service. They had to entice them to the colours and find ways of keeping them there. One way this was done was by giving recruits commissions, whatever their background. At the start of the French wars regimental surgeons were already commissioned officers but regimental and hospital mates only held warrants so were excluded from any social contact with the officer class in the mess. The mate's status, however, improved as the war went on. When regimental mates were rechristened assistants in 1796, they were also given commissions, as were hospital mates from 1804, although the latter were not gazetted till 1809. In the second decade of the war, therefore, anyone entering the army medical service in the junior ranks, whatever his background, was an army officer and entitled to be called a gentleman. Assistants were only subalterns, but from 1796 regimental surgeons had a rank equivalent to captain, while after 1841 staff surgeons II were deemed to be majors.[102]

In an age when civilians from the king down liked to strut in uniform before the admiring glances of the ladies, the officer status of the army surgeon gave the appointment much needed glamour, if nothing else. The uniform was expensive to buy, but it could not but appeal to masculine vanity. According to the adjutant-general's circular of 30 September 1797, run-of-the-mill vets, assistants, and regimental surgeons were to sport a plain red jacket with a red cuff and collar

[101] McGrigor, 36–7, 43–6, 61–4 (quotation, 61). McGrigor had attended medical classes at both Aberdeen and Edinburgh.

[102] Cantlie, *Army Medical Department*, i. 198, 426, 428. Hospital mates could be commissioned for general service or warranted for temporary service from 1804. They became hospital assistants in 1813 and from 1830 staff assistant surgeons (see Table. 1.1). The fact that regimental surgeons were commissioned gave the army the recruiting edge over the navy for most of the war. Naval surgeons were only warrant officers until 1808 and even then never enjoyed the full status of a commissioned officer, while naval assistant surgeons were still not allowed in the wardroom by 1840.

over a white waistcoat and breeches, topped off with a plain cocked hat. Although not allowed to wear epaulettes or lapels, they were to wear the appropriate regimental buttons on their jacket and hat, or buttons bearing the royal coronet above the letter HS (hospital surgeon).[103] Medical officers in the royal regiments were even more splendidly attired. When McGrigor transferred to the Blues, the colonel made him acquire the dress uniform of an officer in the Horse Guards and the much travelled medical officer of the 88th became a court dandy.

[W]hen I presented myself in the ancient costume of that distinguished old corps... I burst into laughter at my own appearance, equipped as I was with a broad buff belt, jack boots that came high up my thigh and stout leather gloves which reached nearly to my elbows, with a large fierce-looking cocked hat and a sword of great length as well as weight.[104]

More importantly, the officer status of the army surgeon brought an entrée to the mess and a promise of useful contacts, especially in the prestigious regiments. Once the pattern of recruitment had settled down after 1798, medical officers paid nothing for their commissions. They entered an officer corps, on the other hand, where regimental commissions were generally purchased and where many of their mess mates were well heeled and well connected. Admittedly, there were pitfalls for the unwary. When not on campaign, life could be too comfortable and the young medical officer too easily seduced into a life of idleness, heavy drinking, and needless expense, as McGrigor learnt to his cost in his early days in the service.

When I entered the army, and for several years afterwards, the custom with all was to drink much wine. A bottle of port, the wine chiefly drunk, was a very common dose for each and when there were guests, particularly when two corps of officers dined together on the arrival of a corps at a station where the other had been established, the dose was doubled, and with a proportion of sherry, claret and champagne besides.[105]

But for the medical officer who could live within his income and keep friends with his fellow officers while avoiding their frivolities, the potential gain was great. By winning the respect of the commanding officer and becoming intimate friends with affluent or blue-blooded junior officers of his own age, the young medical officer could forge useful relationships for the future, especially when he returned to civilian life.[106]

Gradually, too, the Army Medical Board also had the good sense to offer medical practitioners financial inducements to join the service (see Table 1.3). For most of the eighteenth century, the pay of junior medical officers had been adequate but not generous: regimental surgeons received 4s per day and their

103 TNA, WO26/27, fo. 310.   104 McGrigor, 113–14.
105 Ibid. 136–7. Needless to say, McGrigor quickly found ways of avoiding debilitating drinking sessions in the mess. William Dent (d. 1824; not in the database; Drew, no. 3179), assistant surgeon to the 9th Foot, was still drinking a pint of madeira a day in the mess when in the West Indies in 1819: see WL, RAMC 536, Dent's letters home, no. 43: 12 Aug. 1819.
106 Discussed further in, Chs. 4 and 5. Recruitment into the army officer corps was 'democratized' to a certain extent during the wars. Too many officers were needed to allow recruitment to be restricted to the sons of the country gentry. Few, however, were not men of substance.

Table 1.3. Army Surgeons' Pay

Rank	1796	1804	1830	1840
Hospital mate	7/6[a]	6/6 to 7/6[b]		
Staff assistant surgeon				7/6 to 10/-[c]
Regimental assistant surgeon	5/-to 7/6[d]	7/6[e]	7/6	7/6 to 10/-[f]
Regimental surgeon	4/-to 10/-[g] 6/-to 12/-[h] 15/-[i]	11/4 to 14/1[j] to 18/10[k]	11/4 to 18/10	13/-to 22/-[l]
Apothecary to forces		10/-	9/6[m]	
Staff surgeon II class				13/-to 22/-[n]
Staff surgeon	10/-	15/-	14/3 to 18/10	19/-to 24/-[o]
Physician to the forces		20/-	19/-[p]	
Deputy inspector of hospitals		25/-to 30/-[q]	23/8 to 28/6[r]	24/-to 30/-[s]
Inspector of hospitals		40/-	36/-to 40/-[t]	36/-to 40/-[u]

[a] From 1793.

[b] Dependent on whether serving at home or abroad.

[c] Higher rate after 2 years.

[d] Dependent on whether serving at home or abroad.

[e] Assistant surgeons seem to have received 9/-a day when abroad, although this was not laid down in the 1804 warrant: see n. 111 below.

[f] Higher rate after 2 years.

[g] Infantry regiments.

[h] Cavalry regiments.

[i] 3 senior surgeons in the Foot Guards regiments.

[j] Rate after 7 years as regimental surgeon or 10 years' service. All regimental surgeons now paid the same.

[k] Rate after 20 years' service.

[l] Highest rate after 25 years' service

[m] Post now called assistant inspector of hospitals (see Table 1.1).

[n] Highest rate after 25 years' service.

[o] Ditto.

[p] Post now called assistant inspector of hospitals (see Table 1.1).

[q] Rate after 20 years' service.

[r] Post now deputy inspector-general (see Table 1.1).

[s] Post now deputy inspector-general of hospitals (see Table 1.1). Highest rate after 25 years' service.

[t] Post now inspector-general (see Table 1.1).

[u] Post now inspector-general of hospitals (see Table 1.1). Highest rate after 25 years' service.

Note: Army surgeons had to pay for their subsistence out of their salary. They were also subject to certain compulsory stoppages such as clerks' fees. Before the French wars, Hamilton estimated that a surgeon's mate (later regimental assistant surgeon) on 3/6*d* a day would be lucky if he cleared £4 17*s*. 6*d*. in a year (Hamilton, *Duties of a Regimental Surgeon*, ii. 173). From 1804 regimental surgeons in infantry as well as cavalry regiments had to keep a horse at their own expense, although they received a forage allowance. Staff officers were expected to retain a number of horses and consequently had a larger subsidy. According to the *Fifth Report*, appendix 19, regimental surgeons and above on campaign also received a weekly lodgings allowance of 15/- to 21/- per week. In addition, in the Peninsula at least, they also received money for rations (see Murray's letters cited below).

Source: WL, RAMC 1406; Cantlie, *Army Medical Department*, i. 198, 432–3.

mates 2*s*. 6*d*., a sum increased to 3*s*. 6*d*. in 1763. Moreover, as prices were slowly rising from the 1740s, the real value of their pay was falling, and the Irishman, Dr Robert Hamilton (1749–1830), was right to complain in his 1787 account of the duties of an army surgeon that the medical officers were insufficiently rewarded and their pay insufficient to tempt practitioners away from civilian life.[107] Steps were taken to remedy the situation from the beginning of the French wars when the daily pay of hospital mates was raised to 7s. 6d. in an evident attempt to attract recruits, but as nothing was done to improve the pay of regimental medical officers this only exacerbated the problem and left the board bemoaning the fact it could not attract well-qualified candidates. In 1796, however, the pay of regimental medical officers was readjusted. Thereafter they were paid a much more attractive wage. Dependent on the regiment and length of service, surgeons could earn 4–15s. per day, while mates could receive 5s. and 7s. 6d. on active duty. The financial attraction of the service was further enhanced by the royal warrant of 22 May 1804 which laid down a pay scale for both sides of the service for the first time. Basic pay for regimental assistants was confirmed at 7s. 6d. per day, while the surgeons' rates now ranged between 11s. 4d. and 18s. 10d. (after twenty years service). Staff surgeons were given 15s. per day, deputy inspectors 25–30s. and inspectors 40s., but hospital mates were henceforth to be only paid 7s. 6d. when serving abroad. At home, they had to make do with 6s. 6d., a reflection of the fact that theirs was now the normal point of entry into the service.[108]

The 1804 pay scale continued to operate until the end of the war and was only slightly modified in 1831 and 1840.[109] Clearly, medical practitioners who entered the service in the second half of the French wars could anticipate earning a salary of more than £200 per annum if they rose to be a regimental surgeon and twice that amount if they made deputy inspector. This must have been an enticing prospect. Many civilian practitioners could not expect to earn such sums, while a regimental surgeon's income compared favourably with the return from many parish livings in the Church of England.[110] Moreover, the pay scale undervalued the rewards of the service because it neglected the additional material benefits that the medical officer enjoyed when on the move or on campaign or overseas. While in barracks in Britain and Ireland, officers presumably received free board and lodging. Besides their professional expenses—the purchase of books, pocket instruments etc.—their primary outlay came in keeping up appearances: the officer had

[107] Hamilton, *Duties of a Regimental Surgeon*, ii. 200–10. Hamilton (not in the cohort) had been a surgeon in 10th Foot.

[108] Cantlie, *Army Medical Department*, i. 60, 172–3, 198–201; TNA, WO1/896, fo. 88: AMB to Sir George Yonge, 8 Mar. 1794 (on low pay). Secretary at War Yonge had run the army in the absence of a c.-in-c. from 1783 to 1793.

[109] Naval surgeons' basic pay lagged behind in the first part of the war, again giving the army the recruiting edge. But rates were broadly equalized from 1805: Coulter and Lloyd, *Medicine and the Navy*, iii. 33–4. Even before this, many naval surgeons may have earned more than their army counterparts thanks to prize money and the extra pay given to surgeons serving on larger ships: see Janice Wallace, 'A Profile of the Surgeon's Life in the Navy and Assessment of the 1805 Reforms', unpublished paper, 20–4.

[110] According to the report of the Ecclesiastical Revenues Commission of 1833, 47 per cent of Church of England benefices produced an income less than £200 and 34 per cent less than £150: see Eric J. Evans, *The Forging of the Modern State: Early Industrial Britain 1783–1870* (London, 1983), 425 (table).

to buy his own horse, retain a batman, and pay his share of the mess-bills, mostly drink. Abroad, however, they were much more likely to have to look after themselves and this was reflected in their pay and other benefits.

When John Murray became surgeon to the 66th in July 1812, he informed his family that his pay would be 14*s*. per day while he was in the Peninsula, but would go down to the standard rate of 11*s*. (he meant 11*s*. 4*d*.) if he returned home. In addition he received an allowance for maintaining the four horses that he needed to convey himself, his servant, and the regiment's surgical stores. His elevation to staff surgeon the following year brought further advantages. He now had a daily pay of 18*s*., again 3*s*. more than the normal rate, but he was also more generously subsidized. In addition to forage for two horses and three mules, he received free rations for himself and two or three servants, which he estimated was worth 10–12*s*. more.[111] And as he rose higher up the service, the rewards only got better. Based on the staff in Paris in 1815–18 with the occupying army, he claimed to be enjoying an income courtesy of the French taxpayer £300 per annum greater than the one he would receive in England and, though living like a gentleman, able to save £100 a year.[112] Twenty years later, now based in Madras as a deputy inspector (a rank gained in 1830) he was living the life of Riley. He had twenty-five servants—the wage bill he assured his Scottish relatives was low—and an income of £7 per day or £2,500 per annum, as much as a government minister or general.[113] Unfortunately, he died after only a couple of years in India, so never managed to capitalize on his good fortune and build up substantial investments at home.[114]

Evidently, in an era when the army medical service had a properly defined career structure, high-ranking officers on foreign duty could hope to live like a prince. But even from the beginning of the French wars, when such an embarrassment of riches must have been beyond the wildest dreams of the average regimental medical officer, the army had more to offer than a steady wage. Those who entered the service were enticed to stay there for a number of years not just for the immediate reward but by the prospect of eventually being retained on half-pay. In the course of the eighteenth century both the army and navy had developed a sophisticated and successful method of ensuring that their officer corps could be painlessly inflated and contracted according to the rhythms of international

111 See above, n. 60: Murray's letters home. Assistant surgeons received a similar increase in their pay. When William Dent was posted to Gibraltar in 1810, he received 9*s*. per day, plus a clothes allowance. His expenses increased once he joined Wellington's army because he now felt the need for two horses, one to ride and one for carrying his baggage: he wrote home asking for £20 to cover their purchase: WL, RAMC 536, no. 17: letters, 17 Sept. 1810, 17 Feb. 1813.

112 Ibid., RAMC 830, letters, 9 Mar. and 10 Dec. 1816, 7 June 1817. In another letter, Murray admitted keeping up appearances could be expensive. After being created staff surgeon in 1813, he had to lay out 100 guineas to buy new linen and he expected to hire a cook at 20 guineas a year and two servants and a boy at £50: letter 28 Dec. 1813. Surgeons gazetted to cavalry regiments and the guards would also have found that they faced heavy bills.

113 Ibid., letter 23 July 1838, written in part by his new wife (his third!).

114 He died at Kurnaul, Bengal, on 21 Oct. 1841.

Table 1.4. Army Surgeons' Half-Pay

Rank	1804	1830
Hospital mate	2/–	
Regimental assistant surgeon	3/–	4/–
Staff assistant surgeon		4/–
Apothecary to the forces		5/– to 7/6
Regimental surgeon	6/–[a] to 15/–[b]	7/– to 10/–[c] to 15/–[d]
Staff surgeon	6/– to 15/–[e]	7/– to 10/– to 15/–[e]
Physician		10/–
Deputy inspector of hospitals	12/6 to 30/–[f]	12/– to 15/–
Inspector of hospitals	20/–	20/– to 30/–

[a] Value of pension after 20 years' service.
[b] Value of pension after 30 years' service.
[c] Value of pension after 20 years' service.
[d] Value of pension after 30 years' service.
[e] Same length of service benefits as regimental surgeons.
[f] Ditto.

Source: WL, RAMC 1406; Cantlie, *Army Medical Department*, i. 432.

conflict. Officers stood down at the end of the war could be placed on half-pay on the understanding that they could be recalled immediately to the service when they were needed. Commissioned army medical officers were also part of the scheme and could look forward to a useful annuity when they returned to civilian life, provided that they had served a requisite number of years. [115]

As in the case of full pay, the conditions pertaining to half-pay in the first half of the nineteenth century were finalized by the warrant of 1804 (see Table 1.4). To encourage recruits to stay in the medical corps, no one was to receive half-pay unless he had served five years at home or three years abroad. On the other hand, anyone who had served for twenty years could retire on a permanent half-pay pension. Rates varied according to rank from 2*s.* per day for a hospital mate to £1 per day for an inspector of hospitals. A surgeon who had seen a reasonable period of service, therefore, during the French wars could look forward to being cushioned on returning to civilian life by an annuity of £100 at least, easily enough to keep a single man in some comfort. Those at the top were treated as special cases and stood down on particularly beneficial terms. McGrigor in 1814 was asked by Wellington to name his own terms.

'Mac, we are now winding up all arrears with the government; I have asked them how you are to be disposed of and I am told you are to be placed on half pay, but I consider your peculiar services will entitle you to a specific retirement. Before I enter on this subject with Lord Castlereagh [Secretary of State for War], I wish to know your own sentiments.' I replied that the last and only case I knew of was Dr Young, who had been inspector-general with

[115] It was also possible for medical officers to be promoted while on half-pay to increase their allowance, though the criteria for advancement in such cases, beyond peculiar favour, remains mysterious.

Sir Ralph Abercromby, and who got £3 per day as a retiring allowance. He suddenly replied, 'To that they can have no possible objection; the demand is moderate'.[116]

Not surprisingly, some surgeons tried to clock up as much service as possible to maximize the benefit. Writing home in March 1817, John Murray calculated that if he could serve for another eight years and gain one more promotion, he would enjoy half-pay of 15s. per day. At present, though, were he stood down immediately that the army redrew from France, he would only get 7s.[117] Not surprisingly, too, the more feckless among the surgeons placed on half-pay after the French wars found their annual cheque from the War Office indispensable. In the late 1820s and early 1830s, the Army Medical Board, presumably in the hope of removing dead wood and reducing its wage bill, began to demand that some officers who had not served for many years should either give up their right to half-pay in exchange for a one-off capital payment or re-enter the service. A number, now middle-aged, rejoined, doubtless to McGrigor's surprise.[118] Those who had failed to make good in civilian life could not afford to lose their annual dole. One such was the Edinburgh physician, Alexander Lesassier, who had retired on half-pay in 1814 and was offered a sum of £500 to commute. Profligate and making scarcely £70 per annum from his civilian practice, Lessassier was completely dependent on his £120 annual cheque and could not afford to lose it for short-term gain.[119]

In the McGrigor era, the need to attract medical practitioners to the service was obviously nowhere nearly so great, but the director-general was anxious to recruit men of character with a good all round education, as we have seen. He continued therefore to boost the attractions of service, even if he was no longer desperate for recruits. Above all, he tackled one of the drawbacks of the half-pay system: the limited assistance that it provided widows and orphans. Although the widows of medical officers who died in service received a pension, those whose husbands had been placed on half-pay received nothing under the terms of the 1804 warrant unless the dead officer was of the rank of surgeon or above and had served at least twenty years.[120] Similarly neglected were the children of medical officers, serving

[116] McGrigor, 241. The duke and McGrigor were close. See Ch. 4. Dr Thomas Young (not in the cohort; Drew, no. 972) had retired on half-pay in December 1802.
[117] WL, RAMC 830, letter 29 Mar. 1817.
[118] The decision to commute half-pay is shrouded in mystery and seems to have primarily affected younger surgeons who had only entered the service in the latter part of the French Wars and been stood down in the years after Waterloo: see Ch. 4. Very few medical officers with the rank of staff surgeon and above were affected. TNA, WO25/3897 is a list of 121 senior medical officers still on half-pay in 1843, including many who had been placed on half-pay even before the war ended. The move was part of broader campaign to reduce the half-pay bill throughout the army officer corps. In 1831, the army had 9,404 officers drawing some form of half-pay compared with 6,768 officers on full pay. Strachan, *Wellington; Legacy*, 113–17.
[119] Rosner, 196–7. Lesassier, who will be encountered in a number of chapters in this volume, was a shirker and philanderer, scarcely the type of officer whom McGrigor would have wanted to employ. He had asked to re-enter the service on at least one occasion in the 1820s and been rebuffed.
[120] In other words, he had already qualified for permanent half-pay. The widows and children of lower ranks could apply for an allowance from the army compassionate fund.

or otherwise, who lost both of their parents. To remedy the deficiency and demonstrate that the service looked after the families of its personnel, McGrigor established two benevolent funds, one for widows, the other for orphans, in 1816 and 1820. The first was an insurance scheme, whereby serving officers of all ranks were encouraged to pay a small annual premium: when McGrigor retired, the fund was supporting 120 widows. The second was a charity: officers and their wives were solicited for annual or lifetime donations and legacies, and the interest on the invested capital used to help with the education of the sons and daughters of erstwhile colleagues.[121] Some unfortunate families had to draw on both. Assistant Surgeon Oliver Dease was a Dubliner who served as a medical officer from 1809 to 1816. On being stood down, his civilian career looked to be on the point of blossoming when he was elected surgeon of a Dublin hospital. Sadly, he died almost immediately, leaving a widow and five children. Worse, his wife, after drawing a pension of £40 per annum from the widows' fund, died in turn in 1826, forcing Dease's mother to approach the orphans' trustees. They looked kindly on the case and for the next decade provided from £15 to £25 per annum to support the children.[122]

McGrigor also fought to get his surgeons properly honoured within the army.[123] Traditionally, they were treated as civilians, their role on the battlefield went largely unacknowledged, and they enjoyed none of the recognition accorded military officers. The first time their efforts were even mentioned in dispatches was in April 1812 after the battle of Badajoz.[124] Admittedly, the medical officers serving at Waterloo received a medal, but so did all the soldiers who fought there.[125] Admittedly, too, individual medical officers were knighted for their services in the first decades of the nineteenth century, while McGrigor, after much lobbying, was eventually invested as a baronet on 30 September 1831.[126] But these were civil honours, and McGrigor and other former medical officers who had served in the Peninsula wanted members of the service to be treated as combatants. They were also irked by the fact that medical officers' pay lagged behind that for comparable military ranks and that the service was frequently treated as an inferior branch of the army. On one occasion in 1836, for instance, the commanding officer of the Grenadier Guards pointedly ordered his surgeons not to attend a ball at St James's to which the rest of the mess had been invited.[127]

[121] McGrigor, 259–60 (editor's additions).

[122] WL, RAMC 206: Minute Book (1820–41), 55 *et seq.* The Deases were an important Dublin surgical family. Unfortunately, it has been impossible to discover Oliver's relationship to the Richard Dease who was professor at the Dublin Royal College of Surgeons in the early nineteenth century.

[123] Blanco, *Wellington's Surgeon General,* 173–9: solid account of the campaign.

[124] McGrigor, 185, 280.

[125] This was the first military medal issued to all soldiers present: Philip J. Haythornwhite, *Waterloo Men: The Experience of Battle, 16–18 June 1815* (Marlborough, 1999), 115–16.

[126] He demanded the honour from Wellington, much to the duke's surprise, in 1814, then approached Lord Liverpool and the Duke of York in 1826: see Ch. 4, pp. 202–3.

[127] *Times* (28 May, 1836), p. 5, col. C.

Even more galling was the fact that when Victoria ascended the throne in the following year, the medical service did not enjoy the general promotion accorded military officers, much to the disappointment of assistant surgeons, some of whom had served more than twenty years in the junior rank.[128]

In a period when the chance of rapid advance to staff positions was extremely limited, such sleights could not but affect morale and must have seemed a threat to the whole professionalization project. Inevitably, then, when McGrigor and his former colleague, the highly fêted London surgeon, Guthrie, were invited to give evidence to the Royal Commission on Promotion in the Army and Navy, convened in 1840, they made their frustrations clear, emphasizing that unless the service was properly treated, it would begin to fall apart. Guthrie in particular went over the top declaring that the army surgeon was 'the most neglected officer in the service' and pretending, quite wrongly, that he had none of the privileges of his fellow officers. 'I have seen a staff surgeon in charge of many hundred wounded... brush his own shoes, clean his own horse, and then go out to do many of the most delicate operations in surgery.' The service, he concluded, faced meltdown. It needed 'medical officers of good administrative knowledge and best professional ability. Such men can only be obtained by adequate remuneration, rewards and honours.'[129]

The commission, chaired by Wellington, suspected McGrigor and his ally with some justice of special pleading and nothing was done to address their grievances. When the royal warrant of October 1840 was issued on army pay and pensions, the rates for medical officers remained largely unchanged (see Table 1.3). But the demand for military honours did not go away and eventually surfaced in Parliament in 1849. By then, too, the *Lancet* was behind the campaign, its radical editor, Thomas Wakley (1795–1862), pointing out that a number of medical officers had fallen in recent conflicts in the east. 'Where then... is the propriety—nay the decency—of classing such officers as civil staff?'[130] This time the citadel fell, and the military division of the Order of the Bath was finally opened to medical officers of the army, navy, and East India service in 1850. Fittingly, McGrigor with the heads of the other two services was created Knight Commander (thereby gaining a second knighthood), while a clutch of other army medical officers, including Dr John Hume, Wellington's physician, made do with a simple CB. Wakley was euphoric, declaring the reform a victory for medicine. 'We believe this a signal triumph—for triumph it is—to be the greatest step ever made by our profession towards obtaining its just recognition by the State... It is the removal of a profound stigma.'[131] From the mid-nineteenth century, in theory, at any rate,

---

[128] Ibid. (14 July 1838), 3, col. D: letter from an anonymous assistant surgeon. Royal brevets of general promotion even applied to officers on half-pay.

[129] PP, 1840, vol. lx, *Report of the Commission into Naval and Military Promotion*, 202–3 (from Guthrie's evidence given on Tuesday 19 Mar. 1839).

[130] *Lancet*, 1 (1848), 77. The latest study of Wakley and his contribution to medical reform is John Hostettler, *Thomas Wakley: An Improbable Radical* (Chichester, 1993).

[131] *Lancet*, 2 (1850), 240.

service in the army medical corps was as honourable as service in the British army
tout court.

CONCLUSION

In the course of the first half of the nineteenth century, the army medical service
had developed many of the marks of a professional corps.[132] By the end of the
French wars, the traditional and clear-cut division between staff and regimental
medical officers had been swept aside and replaced by an integrated promotional
ladder where all entrants to the service were supposed to begin as hospital mates.
At the same time, the wars had seen the introduction of much more attractive
conditions of employment: a hierarchical pay scale, adjusted for length of service,
higher status, and generous retirement benefits (provided a surgeon lived carefully).
McGrigor after 1815 had taken professionalization further. To begin with, he had
laid down the level of educational attainment expected of medical officers for
the first time. If the only paper qualification demanded of candidates seeking a
commission until 1858 remained the army surgeon's certificate bestowed by the
three royal colleges, the director-general made clear that entrants in future had to
have had a proper medical education subsequent to training in the classical
humanities.[133] In addition, if there was still no army medical school before 1860,
McGrigor placed public emphasis on in-service study and additional qualifications and claimed to favour the better educated in the promotion race. In the
second place, by developing the role of the medical officer as information gatherer,
he attempted to turn the army medical service in peacetime into a privileged
instrument of scientific research. The service was more than the health-care
department of the British army.

The professionalization of the army medical service during this period was
shaped by external pressures, direct and indirect. The changes before 1815 were the
result of the exigencies of war and largely imposed on the service from without. In
the early years, the army command desperately needed to attract medical officers.
Later on, as more and more troops were committed to active service, it wanted an
efficient medical service full of well-trained and energized surgeons who would
ensure the maximum number of troops available for action. The government and
Parliament agreed, though their eyes were always firmly focused on the bottom
line of the balance sheet.

---

[132] For literature on professionalization, see Introduction.

[133] In the 1840s the conditions of entry were stated on the pro-forma CVs that candidates for
commissions were expected to fill in: see above, n. 68. By then, to become a physician (a post which
no longer existed!) or a deputy inspector, it was necessary to be a fellow or licentiate of the Royal
College of Physicians, London, or a graduate of Oxbridge, Edinburgh, Dublin, Glasgow, or Aberdeen.
St Andrews was excluded, doubtless because its degrees had been traditionally delivered on request.
With the introduction of national registration under the 1858 Medical Act, all recruits thereafter
had to hold a certificate from one of the nineteen recognized licensing bodies.

McGrigor, in contrast, was apparently free to work his own professional miracle, but he too was a prisoner of his context to a certain degree. It cannot be a coincidence, to start with, that he prescribed the first detailed educational cursus for candidates in 1816, the year after the passage of the Apothecaries Act. Under the new law, medical practitioners in England had to be henceforth certificated. Surgeon-apothecaries acting as general practitioners, who did not hold a university doctorate or were not a member of one of the royal colleges of physicians or surgeons, had to be a licentiate of the London Society of Apothecaries. Army and naval surgeons were not affected by the legislation, but it is not hard to see that McGrigor would have been anxious to demonstrate to the public that his officers deserved their exemption on the grounds of their exemplary education.[134] More generally, too, McGrigor's period of office coincided with a novel interest in staffing the professions (both old and new) with the classically educated—the Victorians' idea of the gentleman—and controlling entry through certification. Admittedly, in the second case, little was achieved before the second half of the century beyond the establishment of a handful of voluntary associations, and the British professions remained stubbornly unprofessionalized. The army and navy medical services were striking exceptions.[135] Nonetheless, throughout the 1840s and 1850s, the process of professionalization was gathering pace. Although there would be no further legislation determining access to a medical career before 1858, there was continual debate on the subject throughout the McGrigor era.[136] Above all, by the time he died in that year, entry to the civil service and the regular army officer corps had become policed by an examination, in which candidates had to demonstrate their knowledge of the liberal arts. In his enthusiasm for educated officers, who knew their Homer and Virgil, McGrigor was swimming with a fast-gathering tide.[137]

Similarly, McGrigor's development of the army medical service into an instrument of knowledge creation needs to be placed in the context of the contemporary utilitarian mania for reducing the world to statistics, which would be so effectively satirized in Dickens's *Hard Times* (1854). From the end of the French wars government commissions and individuals were continually collecting data about the state of the nation in the name of improvement. McGrigor's drive to document

[134] Loudon, *Medical Care*, chs. 6–7 (for the passage of the Act after many years' lobbying).

[135] During McGrigor's years as director-general, the naval medical service, endowed with a professional structure since 1805, as we saw above, was run by Sir William Burnett (1779–1861), a medical knight with similar ideas.

[136] Loudon, *Medical Care*, 282–301. A 'Select Committee on the Education and Practice of the Medical Profession in the United Kingdom' was held as early as 1834: see PP, 1834, vol. xiii, pt. 2.

[137] Richard Jenkyns, *The Victorians and Ancient Greece* (London, 1980); Laurence Brockliss, 'The Professions and National Identity', in Brockliss and David Eastwood (eds.), *A Union of Multiple Identities: The British Isles, c.1750-c.1850* (Manchester, 1997), ch. 1; Strachan, *Wellington's Legacy*, 126–36; Edward Hughes, 'Sir Charles Trevelyan and Civil Service Reform, 1853–5', *English Historical Review*, 64 (1949), 53–88, 206–34. The belief that a professional should be a gentleman educated in the Latin and Greek humanities was the making of the English public school and encouraged curricular reform throughout the secondary school system.

year on year the health of the British army cannot be divorced from the contemporary drive to improve public health, associated above all with Edwin Chadwick. It was part of the belief that a problem could be successfully dealt with once it was quantified, a shibboleth that exercised its fascination throughout the so-called Age of Reform among progressives, Tories as well as Whigs.[138] McGrigor may well have dreamt of harnessing the inspectorate in this way ten years before he became director-general, but he could only have galvanized his officers around the globe into doing his bidding because his ambition was in tune with the Benthamite spirit of the age. The move also made good political sense. In the long era of peace when the army was run down and the expenditure it continued to incur resented by both public and government, it was an astute strategy to demonstrate that the service was value for money and could contribute to the great nineteenth-century project of 'improvement'. McGrigor's dedication to data gathering would ensure that until the Crimean disaster the army medical service had a high and positive public profile, all the more that individual army surgeons, on the director's encouragement, flooded the burgeoning medical press with their weighty observations on topics of great contemporary concern, such as cholera.[139]

Still, however many marks of professionalization the army medical service might exhibit by the mid-nineteenth century, they tell us little about the reality of life in the service during and after the French wars. This chapter has principally explored the external face of the medical corps. It has provided a linear account of a modern profession brought into being through a series of War Office warrants and public documents. Yet the official creation of a promotional hierarchy and a public commitment to the principles of seniority and meritocracy are no guarantee that the army medical service experienced substantive internal change over the period. On the one hand, the official documentation may have largely given effect to developments that were already in the process of occurring. On the other, more probably, it may simply have enclosed the medical service in a paper professional carapace within which change occurred slowly or not at all. Professionalized structures are not hermetically sealed entities. How they operate in practice, especially in their gestation period, will be inevitably affected by the values of the wider society in which they are imbedded. McGrigor might have been swimming with the Reformist current, but reform never commanded universal support in the first half of the nineteenth century. Britain was still a country of place and patronage in which 'getting on' was associated with knowing the 'right people'. It would be naive to expect the army medical service to have become a beacon of meritocracy over night, particularly while Wellington remained in a position of authority.

[138] M. J. Cullen, *The Statistical Movement in Early Victorian Britain* (Hassocks, 1975); F. B. Smith, *The People's Health, 1830–1910* (London, 1979).

[139] See Ch. 7. For the growth of the medical press in the period, see W. Bartrip, *Mirror of Medicine: A History of the British Medical Journal* (Oxford, 1990), chs. 1–2.

In the following chapters, the reality of this paper professionalization is tested by analysing the lives of the people who manned the service. Our prosopographical cohort, drawn from surgeons who became medical officers in the French wars and were still alive in 1815, forms an ideal point of departure for such a study. Having virtually all entered the army at a time when neither the service nor society had experienced reform—indeed, when reform was associated with revolution and atheism—our surgeons would all have been reared in an Ancien Régime world. Yet those who survived to enjoy the fruits of peace for several decades made a career for themselves in or outside the army in a much more contested political atmosphere. In the course of exploring a variety of aspects of their lives—notably their background and education, the trajectory of their professional career, wealth on death, sons' occupations, and their contribution to the wider republic of letters—it will become clear what the medical officers of the war years expected from the army, how far those expectations came to be primarily realized through their professional abilities, and the extent to which they took out into the civilian world progressive and meritocratic values imbued in the service. It will then become possible to assess whether or not the history of the army medical service in the first half of the period was one of continuity or genuine change and whether or not McGrigor's creation was a precocious modern profession or merely a paper facsimile.

2

Background

GEOGRAPHICAL ORIGIN

According to the census of 1811, 57 per cent of the population of the British Isles lived in England and Wales, 33 per cent in Ireland, and only 10 per cent in Scotland. Recruits into the army medical service, on the other hand, were disproportionately drawn from north of the Tweed. The country of birth of 312 of the 454 army surgeons who comprise the database cohort is recorded on the pro forma that they were required to fill in at the end of the French wars. In addition, the putative origins of a further 114 can be deduced from the information that the pro forma provides about the cohort's apprenticeship.[1] As will be shown in Chapter 3, virtually every member of the cohort was indentured in his home kingdom.[2] In consequence, the nationality of all but 28 of the cohort is known. As Table 2.1 reveals, the Irish contingent in the army medical service was broadly commensurate with the Irish share of the overall population. The English and Welsh, on the other hand, were under-represented by a factor of two, and the Scots were over-represented by a factor of three. Only a handful of recruits came from outside the British Isles, including, bizarrely, the Frenchman, Romaine Amiel from Riez, near Toulon, who became a surgeon's mate in November 1794.[3]

There can be no doubt that Scots were more visible in the medical service than in any other branch of the army. Figures for the geographical origin of the rank and file from 1813 would suggest that recruitment largely followed the distribution of the wider population: half were English, a third Irish, and a sixth Scots. Even the army officer corps, which had attracted a disproportionate number of Scots in the eighteenth century, even before its fourfold rise in size during the French wars, only ever drew a quarter of its needs from north of the border.[4] The Scots came to be particularly prominent on the Army Medical Board, as we saw in the previous chapter. If the service for most of the war was run by Englishmen,

---

[1] For the *pro forma* and the database, see Introd.   [2] See Ch. 3 under 'Appprenticeship'.
[3] Toulon was temporarily occupied by the British during the Terror. Perhaps his family escaped from the town when the British left in December 1793 or perhaps he was an aristocrat on the run. When Toulon was evacuated, the British took 7,500 civilians with them: Roger Knight, *The Pursuit of Victory: The Life and Achievement of Horatio Nelson* (London, 2005), 164–5.
[4] J. E. Cookson, *The British Armed Nation, 1793–1815* (Oxford, 1997), 126–8.

Table 2.1. Country of Origin

	Definite	Putative	Total	%
ABROAD	10	1	11	2.42
Canada	[1]			
France	[1]			
Jersey	[1]			
W. Indies	[7]			
ENGLAND	85	45	130	28.63
IRELAND	95	47	142	31.27
SCOTLAND	117	18	135	29.74
WALES	5	3	8	1.76
Unknown	142		28	6.16
Total	454		454	

Note: Definite: country of birth as given in the pro-forma returns.
Putative: country of apprenticeship. (In the few cases where a surgeon was apprenticed in more than one country, the country of his first apprenticeship has been used.)

Source: Doctors' database: Tables: Doctors; Apprenticeship.

such as Pepys and Keate, based in the London hospitals, the four surgeons appointed to the reformed board set up in 1810 were all Scots. Thereafter it became a Scottish fiefdom, as five years later Weir gave way to McGrigor, who in turn was replaced in the mid-nineteenth century by Dr (later Sir) Andrew Smith.[5]

When the geographical origins of the cohort are broken down further, it is equally clear that the army was disproportionately drawing its surgeons from the three capital cities (see Tables 2.2–2.4). One in five of the medical officers from England and Wales came from London (including Westminster), a slightly smaller proportion of their Irish colleagues from Dublin, and about one out of six Scots from Edinburgh, while the Scottish capital provided the largest contingent from any town (19).[6] In other words, in terms of their share of the intake, the three capital cities were grossly over-represented. London may well have had a population of a million in the period of the French wars, but only one out of nine Englishmen lived there, while fewer than one in thirty of Ireland's people were to be found in Dublin and one in twenty of Scotland's in the Athens of the North. That said, the birth places of the rest (and the large majority) of the army surgeons were relatively evenly spread around the counties of the three kingdoms. With the exception of Wales, where officers only came from the west and north of the principality, one or two recruits came from most counties. Even the far reaches of

[5] See Ch. 1, pp. 35, 37–8, 44 (on the history of the Army Medical Board). To what extent Scots came to be advantaged in the service thanks to their compatriots' control of the board is discussed in Ch. 4. Smith ran the Army Medical Board from 1853 to 1858.

[6] The figure is higher if officers from towns close to Edinburgh, such as Dalkeith, are included. Dalkeith was arguably a suburb but very much under the thumb of the duke of Buccleuch.

Table 2.2. Scotland: County of Birth

County	Total	Town (A)	Town (B)	Town (C)	Rural
Aberdeenshire	12 [2]	5	1		3
Angusshire	7 [1]	1	1	1	3
Argyllshire	2	1			1
Ayrshire	5	2		2	1
Banffshire	3 [1]			1	1
Berwickshire	2				2
Dumfriesshire	5 [3]				2
East Lothian	1			1	
Fife	4 [2]	1			1
Inverness-shire	5 [2]				3
Kirkudbrightshire	1				1
Lanarkshire	9 [2]		6		1
Midlothian	24	19		3	2
Morayshire	1			1	
Nairnshire	2	1			1
Orkney	2	2			
Peeblesshire	1 [1]				
Perthshire	10 [3]	3		4	
Renfrewshire	4 [1]		3		
Roxburghshire	2	2			
Selkirkshire	2 [1]	1			
Stirlingshire	4 [1]	2		1	
Sutherland	1 [1]				
West Lothian	1			1	
Wigtonshire	1			1	
County not given	6 [6]				
TOTAL	117 [27]	40	11	16	23
Percentage	[23.08%]	36.36%	9.4%	13.6%	19.66%

Key:
Town (A): county town (including Edinburgh).
Town (B): industrial town (e.g. Glasgow).
Town (C): small market town or port (e.g. Falkirk or Peterhead).
Rural: village, farm or estate (e.g. Kirkconnel Hall, Ecclefechan, Dumfriesshire).
[3]: no specified location within county.

Source: Doctors' database: Table: Doctors.

the British Isles were represented. Two officers came from Orkney (Patrick Patterson and James Low Warren), four from County Donegal, and three each from Galway, Kerry, and Cornwall, among the latter John Davy, the brother of the scientist and inventor, Sir Humphry.

Significantly, there was no obvious bias towards the industrializing and hence most populous areas of Great Britain. Only nine surgeons originated from the Glasgow-Clyde conurbation, one from Hull (William Henry Young), and one each from Dundee (George Ross Watson), Belfast (William Burtt), Manchester (William Newton), Burton-on-Trent (William Greaves), and Birmingham

Table 2.3. Ireland: County of Birth

County	Total	Town (A)	Town (B)	Town (C)	Rural
Antrim	4	1	1	1	1
Armagh	3 [1]	2			
Carlow	1	1			
Cavan	2	1		1	
Cork	6 [1]	3		2	
Donegal	4 [2]	1		1	
Down	5 [3]	1		1	
Dublin	17	17			
Fermanagh	4 [3]				1
Galway	3 [1]	1		1	
Kerry	3 [1]	1		2	
Kildare	1	1			
Kilkenny	1 [1]				
Limerick	2	2			
Londonderry	7 [3]	1		3	
Longford	2	1		1	
Louth	1			1	
Mayo	3 [1]			2	
Meath	4 [1]			3	
Monaghan	5 [4]			2	
Queen's	1			1	
Roscommon	1	1			
Sligo	2 [2]				
Tyrone	3 [1]	1		1	
Waterford	1 [1]				
Wexford	2 [1]				1
Wicklow	1 [1]				
County not given	6 [6]				
TOTAL	95 [32]	36	1	23	3
Percentage	[33.68%]	37.89%	1.05%	24.21%	3.15%

Key:

Town (A): county or cathedral town (including Dublin).

Town (B): industrial town (Belfast).

Town (C): small market town or port (e.g. Bandon, Co. Cork).

Rural: village, farm, or estate (e.g. Killygowan, Co. Wexford).

[3]: no specified location within county.

Source: As Table 2.2.

(Horatio Nelson Holden).[7] No one at all hailed from Liverpool, Leeds, Bradford, Cardiff, or any other part of the industrializing West Midlands, while only one, John Gray Hibbert, was a native of the pleasure city of Bath, the fastest growing town in the country.[8] The overall impression is that the largest group of army

[7] Admittedly, some of the cohort may have been raised in the large industrial and commercial cities. Christopher Richard Alderson was born in Whitby but raised in Hull.

[8] R. S. Neale, *Bath 1768–1850: A Social History, or, a Valley of Pleasure, yet a Sink of Iniquity* (London, 1981).

Background

Table 2.4. England: County of Birth

County	Total	Town (A)	Town (B)	Town (C)	Rural
Berkshire	2			2	
Buckinghamshire	1 [1]				
Cambridgeshire	2	2			
Cheshire	1				1
Cornwall	2				2
Cumberland	2				2
Devonshire	3			1	2
Dorset	1 [1]				
Durham	1			1	
Essex	3 [1]			2	
Gloucestershire	3 [1]	1		1	
Hampshire	3			2	1
Herefordshire	1			1	
Hertfordshire	1			1	
Kent	4	2		2	
Lancashire	2 [1]		1		
Leicestershire	1	1			
Lincolnshire	2	2			
Middlesex	18 [1]	16		1	
Norfolk	1 [1]				
Northamptonshire	2	1		1	
Northumberland	3	1		2	
Nottinghamshire	2 [1]	1			
Shropshire	2			2	
Somerset	6 [1]	2			3
Staffordshire	1		1		
Suffolk	1			1	
Sussex	2				2
Warwickshire	1		1		
Westmorland	1 [1]				
Wiltshire	2 [1]			1	
Worcestershire	2 [1]				1
Yorkshire	3		1	2	
County not given	3 [3]				
TOTAL	85 [15]	29	4	23	14
Percentage	[17.65%]	34.12%	4.71%	27.05%	16.47%

Key:
Town (A): county or cathedral town (including London).
Town (B): industrial town or major port (e.g. Manchester or Hull).
Town (C): market town or small port (e.g. Ludlow or Whitby).
Rural: village, farm, or estate (e.g. Hartlebury, Worestershire).
[3]: no specified location within county.

Source: As Table 2.2.

surgeons in the United Kingdom came from historic market towns and ports. In Ireland's case, a third of surgeons whose place of origin is known exactly came from local centres of secular and ecclesiastical administration, such as Cork and Limerick, which were the birthplace respectively of three and two of the officers.

In Scotland and England, though, the proportion hailing from important local towns was much smaller. Only thirteen of the sixty Englishmen whose provenance is definitely known were born in a county town—one in Maidstone, Leicester, Northampton, Newcastle, and Nottingham (home of the geologist John Jeremiah Bigsby) and two in Cambridge and Lincoln—and only four in non-county-town cathedral cities (Canterbury, Baths, Wells, and Bristol).[9] More typical among English urban recruits was Pennel Cole, later surgeon to the Worcester infirmary, born in Ludlow, Shropshire, in 1750, or the Beverley GP Charles Brereton who came from Bawtry in Yorkshire, on the Great North Road, south of Doncaster.

An important number of English and Scottish surgeons, moreover, came from the countryside. Thomas Keate, nephew of the surgeon-general, was born in Laverton in Somerset, Samuel Ayrault Piper at nearby Colyton, Devon, and Daniel Owen Davies came from Llangrandog in Cardiganshire. Among the officers from south-west Scotland were Archibald Arnott of Ecclefechan, John Lorimer of Sanquhar (both villages in Dumfriesshire), and Alexander Browne of Langlands in the parish of Twynholm, Kirkudbrightshire. It was to this group, too, that Sir James McGrigor, the future director-general of the army medical service, belonged. Although he spent most of his childhood in Aberdeen, he was born at Cromdale in Strathspey, Inverness-shire.[10] Few Irish recruits, in contrast, seem to have hailed from the countryside, though the number may have been greater than recorded. Given the unlikelihood of the clerks in Berkeley Street having even a passing acquaintance with the topography of rural Ireland, several may have preferred to enter as their place of birth the nearest town. Certainly, this is what William Gibney seems to have done. Gibney officially was born in Navan, County Meath, while in reality his home was Dormston (or Dormiston) Castle some miles away.[11] Indeed, there may be large-scale under-recording of rural origins among recruits from all three kingdoms in that it can be mooted that the officers who only recorded the county in which they were born were similarly raised in villages. If this is so, then those raised in the countryside may actually have been the largest group and perhaps even the majority. Among surgeons whose country of birth is definitely known, at least 50 of the 117 Scots probably had a rural background, 35 of the 95 Irish, and 29 of the 85 English.[12]

[9] As Bristol, Newcastle, and Nottingham could equally be classed as major ports and/or industrial towns, seven rather than four English recruits came from substantial centres of trade and manufacturing.

[10] McGrigor, editor's introduction. Although McGrigor cited his place of birth correctly in his army return, he does not mention in his autobiography that he came from Strathspey, perhaps not wishing his readers to know that the director-general of the Army Medical Service hailed from a region historically full of papists and Jacobites.

[11] Gibney, 1–2. The transcription of the 1851 census gives his place of birth as Ardreasan, Ireland. As the original text is hard to read, this may be a misreading of Ardriston (House), Co. Carlow: www.ancestry.com: 1851 census (Jan. 2006).

[12] Figures obtained by adding the number known to have been born in the countryside to the number who provided no specific location.

SOCIAL BACKGROUND

It is much more difficult to gather information about the social origins of army surgeons than their place of birth, since the pro forma provides no details about their family circumstances. It has been necessary, in consequence, to construct their family background from a variety of disparate sources. The Mormon International Genealogical Index (Family Search) has been invaluable in identifying parents and siblings, but seldom provides occupational data.[13] This has chiefly come from biographical dictionaries and databases, obituaries, family letters, and trade directories, sources which can vary significantly in their reliability. Obituaries, for instance, tend to inflate the background of their subject. When the most technically innovative surgeon in the cohort, George James Guthrie, died in 1856, he was described in *The Times* as the son of Mr Andrew Guthrie, a chiropedist. In fact, Andrew dealt in surgical goods and the nearest he got to dealing with injured feet was to sell surgeons the plasters that they used.[14] Wherever possible, therefore, any information about parents and siblings has been double-checked. Despite these constraints, however, it has been possible to uncover the social origins of nearly a quarter of the cohort (and over a half of those whose father's name has been found), in some cases tracing their families back through several generations (see Table 2.5).

Among this quarter identified, the most prominent group were the offspring of medical families. A fifth of the grandfathers whose occupation is known were medical practitioners, a third of the fathers, and nearly half the uncles. The bare statistics, though, almost certainly exaggerate the percentage of army surgeons who came from medical families. The task of discovering whether or not an army surgeon had a family member practising in the town or district in which he was raised was relatively easy thanks to the existence of a detailed database of medical practitioners in eighteenth-century Britain and Ireland compiled by the Wallises.[15] It was simply a case of checking the surgeons' names against the list. Where a match was found and the surname was not problematically common (such as Brown or Smith), then it was a legitimate assumption that a relative had been discovered, even when there was no independent validating evidence.[16] It is possible to say

[13] When the study began the IGI was not on-line and had to be consulted on microfiche in the Guildhall Library. It is possible, then, that a second complete trawl through the source would be even more productive.

[14] *The Times* (2 May 1856), 5, col. D. This mistake found its way into Guthrie's *DNB* entry. The correct occupation of his father is given in Pettigrew: see below, n. 57.

[15] Peter J. and Ruth Wallis, *Eighteenth-Century Medics: Subscriptions, Licences, Apprenticeships* (Newcastle, 1985). This database sprang from a social study of book subscription lists. It is exceptionally full but difficult to use even in its printed version. The database was created before the modern era of relational database packages.

[16] Corroborating evidence exists in the many cases where surgeons' recorded that they were apprenticed to relatives. See Ch. 3, pp. 114–15. Further corroborative evidence comes from wills and biographical notices and memoirs.

Table 2.5. Social and Occupational Background

Occupation	Father	Uncle	Grandfather	Great-grandfather
Agriculture	15	1	6	
Landowner	5[a]		2	
Tenant	8[b]		3	
Other	2[c]		1[d]	
Professions	54	25	13	2
Administration	1			
Armed Forces	2[e]			
Church	12	7	5	
Education[f]	3	1[g]		
Law	4	2	2	1
(Barristers)			(1)	
(Solicitors)	(4)	(2)	(1)	(1)
Medicine	32	15	6	1
(Apothecaries)	(3)		(2)	
(Physicians)	(4)[h]	(8)[i]	(1)	(1)[j]
(Practitioners)[k]	(4)		(3)	
(Surgeons)	(19)[l]	(7)[m]		
(Surgs. & Apoth.)	(2)			
Trade & Business	25	6	7	1
Artisans	5		6[n]	1
Clerks	1			
Manufacturers[o]	2			
Merchants	12	3	1	
Mixed[p]	3			
Shopkeepers	2	1		
Independent[q]	7	1	3	
TOTAL	101	33	29	3
ALL NAMES	181	48	43	7
(Percentage)	(55.80%)	(68.75%)	(67.44%)	(42.86%)
HIGHER EDUCATION	13	14	3	1
Abroad	1			
Inns of Court		1		
Oxbridge	6	6	1	
Scotland	6	7	2	1

[a] Includes copyholders.

[b] A number may have been landowners.

[c] 2 factors or estate managers.

[d] Gardener.

[e] A third is included among the clergymen.

[f] Does not include three professors of medicine.

[g] Professor of oriental languages.

[h] 2 army.

[i] 1 in army; 1 professor of medicine.

[j] Professor of medicine.

[k] Unspecified.

[l] 1 in army, 1 in navy.

[m] 1 in navy.

[n] Includes 1 innkeeper.

[o] Substantial.

[p] Artisans, shopkeepers, and merchants.

[q] Family members classed simply as gentleman. Many may have had a career that the source does not record.

Source: Doctors' Database: Table: Relationships 1.

with some confidence, therefore, that the 32 fathers, 15 uncles, and 6 grandfathers who were medical practitioners comprise the major part of the cohort's family connections with the medical profession prior to their generation. In consequence, probably less than 10 per cent of army surgeons had a medical background. The vast majority of entrants, it can be assumed, were newcomers to the trade. Virtually all of them, moreover, were newcomers to the military medical service, for only six of the fifty-three medical relatives discovered had served in the forces, four in the army and two in the navy. This number, too, includes one of the cohort, John Hennen Snr, who died of yellow fever at Gibraltar in 1828 with the rank of deputy inspector. His son, John Hennen Jnr, is one of the handful of post-war entrants in the sample whose service record was mysteriously intruded into the collection of pro formas which form the basis of this study.[17]

Some of the surgeons who did come from medical families had relatives in the commanding heights of the profession. Half the medical uncles had degrees and one rose to social pre-eminence: the Irishman John Gibney, uncle to William, who took his MD at Edinburgh in 1790 and became a respected Brighton physician and intimate of the prince regent and was eventually knighted.[18] Moreover, two of the uncles were Edinburgh professors—James Gregory (1753–1821), uncle of George, who held the chair of theoretical medicine from 1766 to 1790 and the chair of medical practice from 1790 until his death in 1821, and James Hamilton (died 1839), professor of midwifery from 1800, uncle of Alexander Lesassier.[19] Graduate physicians were less in evidence among the thirty-eight medical grandfathers and fathers—a mere five in all, only two of whom had degrees from Edinburgh, John Ligertwood (MD 1777), father of John, and John Hennen Snr (MD 1819).[20] But they equally included two leading members of the profession in their day, George Gregory's grandfather, John (1724–74), who also held a chair at Edinburgh,[21] and John Alderson (1757–1829), father of Christopher, who was physician at the Hull Infirmary.

Alderson Snr was a typical reform-minded surgeon of the turn of the nineteenth century. He was the third son of a Nonconformist minister from Yarmouth, who after training with his elder brother in Norwich obtained a surgeoncy in the Norfolk militia. When the militia was stationed in Yorkshire in 1780, he resigned his commission and decided to set himself up in the county, marrying Ann Scott of Beverley, then moving to Whitby where Christopher was born in 1788. Prior to this he had studied at Edinburgh for a year, then taken a

---

[17] See Introd. John Hennen Jnr published a posthumous tribute to his father: see 'Life of the Author by His Son Dr John Hennen', in John Hennen Snr, *Principles of Military Surgery* (London, 1829), esp. pp. xv–xvi (on the son's joining the service).   [18] Gibney, Ch. 1.
[19] Gregory and Hamilton quarrelled violently and came to blows. Both have notices in the *DNB*. For Gregory's popularity as a teacher, see Ch. 3.   [20] The degrees of the rest cannot be traced.
[21] The Gregorys were a professorial dynasty going back to the mid-seventeenth century who held chairs at Aberdeen, Oxford, and Edinburgh. Many have individual notices in the *DNB*. George, besides his medical works, wrote an influential but highly sexist book on the education of girls: see *A Father's Legacy to his Daughter*, 1st edn. (1774).

medical degree at Marischal College, Aberdeen. In 1789 he moved to the fast-expanding city of Hull, where he took up the post of physician at the recently founded Infirmary in 1792.[22] He held the post for the rest of his life, living first in Savile Street and then from 1810 at 4, Charlotte Street, in the smart, newly built west end of town. Besides his work as an infirmary physician and private practitioner, he was a tireless devotee of 'improvement'. He was co-founder and proprietor of a refuge for the insane, president at one time or other of the Hull Subscription Library, the Hull Philosophical Society, and the Hull Mechanics' Institute, as well as organizer of the local geological society and founder of the local botanical garden at Anlaby. He was also the chairman of the commission appointed by Parliament to provide essential public services for the new dormitory town of Sculcoates to the north of the city. In other words, he was a local grandee, who was made freeman of Hull in 1813, despite a Nonconformist background, and by his death in 1828 had accumulated a considerable amount of urban and rural property, leaving a taxable estate of £14,000. Moreover, he was not the only member of his family in his generation to become a prominent medical practi-tioner. His eldest brother, James (1742–1825) was a Norwich practitioner of note, whose novelist daughter, Amelia (1769–1853), would marry the fashionable painter, John Opie.[23]

Alderson, however, was an exceptional figure. The majority of the medical relatives of our army surgeons were simple surgeons or apothecaries with a predominantly rural practice. Typical were James Hennen, father of John Snr, who was based at Castlebar, County Mayo, Alexander Anderson, father of Andrew, who lived at Shaw and practised in the Selkirk region, and John Brereton, father of Charles, who was based at Bawtry. Although we know little about their lives, it can be assumed that they dwelt in relatively straitened circumstances, like the surgeon relation of Alexander Anderson, one Thomas Anderson of Broomhill, who practised in Edinburgh, and got himself into financial difficulties in 1817.[24] Arguably, most army surgeons from medical families did not boast promising pedigrees. Only one non-graduate medical practitioner came near to matching Alderson's local importance. This was the surgeon, John Bigsby (1760–1844), father of John Jeremiah, who was the third son of another Nottingham surgeon, James, and the nephew of an Ipswich physician, Thomas, who had studied at Caius College, Cambridge.[25] Although James only left £80 in goods when he died in 1783,

22 *DNB, sub nomine.*

23 The most detailed account of John Alderson's life is J. A. R. Bickford and M. E. Bickford, *The Medical Profession in Hull, 1400–1900* (Hull, 1983), 3–5. His many extra-curricular activities are listed in W. Parsons (ed.), *The Directory, Guide and Annals of Kingston-upon-Hull and the Parish of Sculcoates* (Leeds, 1826), pp. xxxiv, xl, lix, lx–xi. There is an Alderson Family History Society and we are indebted to the assistance of its records officer, Mrs Susan Sharp, in researching the family.

24 Alexander Anderson owned a small property at Shaw: NAS, Selkirkshire sasines, 1814, no. 317.

25 Thomas Bigsby was born in Stowmarket, Suffolk, where, according to his wife's will, he was eventually buried. Presumably, James was a younger brother and had moved to Nottingham to set up in practice.

he had been wealthy enough to send his two elder sons to Oxbridge.[26] John himself was one of the leading medical men in Nottinghamshire society at the turn of the nineteenth century and surgeon to the Nottingham Hospital. He seems to have retired about 1820 and spent the rest of his life at West Retford Hall in the north of the county.[27]

Army surgeons with backgrounds in the other professions were much thinner on the ground. To begin with, only three of the cohort had a grandfather, uncle, or father who apparently had had a commission, even though membership of the army and navy officer corps in the eighteenth century is one of the easier careers to trace.[28] John Boutflower (1736–1818), father of Charles, was a humble naval lieutenant in his twenties and thirties, then abandoned the service for the Church. Although only the son of a ship's carpenter, called Marmaduke, he was descended from a landed family in Northumberland and his initial career was possibly determined by the fact that his father's second cousin was Admiral Sir Chaloner Ogle (d. 1750).[29] Alexander George Home's father (Christian name unknown) was also a lieutenant in the navy who had eventually settled on the West Indian island of Dominica. He, too, came from a landed family, in Scotland, but one whose fortunes had been blighted by Jacobite connections.[30] On the other hand, Samuel Ayrault Piper's father, John (d. 1801), was in the army and retired with the rank of army captain. Either Piper senior made money in the army or he had inherited a sizeable fortune, for his residence, Colyton House, in the village of Colyton, Devon, which he owned, was a fine dwelling with garden and stables. When he died, he left £12,000 in legacies.[31]

The legal profession hardly fared better. Admittedly, identifying lawyers before the mid-nineteenth century is difficult, but the fact that here again so few—only nine in total—have been discovered among the cohort's relatives is surely indicative.[32] Moreover, three of the nine come from the same family.

---

[26] The inventory, taken on 8 Feb. 1783, is in the Nottinghamshire RO, as is his short will, dated 6 Apr. 1782, where he leaves everything to his wife, Sarah. One of the two sons also went to Charterhouse.

[27] John Bigsby is continually encountered in *The Diary of Abigail Gawthern of Nottingham, 1751–1810*, ed. Adrian Henstock (Thoroton Society of Nottinghamshire: Nottingham, 1980). Venn, i. 261, *sub* Charles Bigsby (one of his sons), wrongly describes John as a fellow of the Royal College of Physicians, London. Presumably he owned West Retford Hall.

[28] Especially thanks to *The Commissioned Officers of the Royal Navy 1660–1815*, 3 vols. (n.p., 1954). Bound, typed list: alphabetical. Copies are available on open shelf at the Bodleian Library and TNA.

[29] Douglas Samuel Boutflower, *The Complete Story of a Family of the Middle Class Connected with the North of England (1303–1930)* (Newcastle, 1930), esp. 72–9. One of Guthrie's ancestors, possibly his great-grandfather had served in William of Orange's army which invaded Ireland, but he was not necessarily an officer.   [30] *Burke's Landed Gentry* (London, 1886), *sub* Hume of Ninewells.

[31] John Piper's will exists but no evaluation of his estate: TNA, Prob 11/1360, qs. 359–62. In his will he specified that Samuel was not to be put in the army or navy.

[32] English and Irish barristers can be traced through the biographical registers of the Inns of Court but solicitors are impossible to identify easily in the eighteenth and early nineteenth centuries. From 1836 English solicitors had to take a written exam organized by the fledgling Law Society. Before this they were supposed to be examined orally by a judge and their name placed on the high court roll. A successful career in the law at this juncture depended heavily on patronage and political favours.

Henry William Markham hailed from a Northampton legal dynasty of some local prominence. His father, John (1750–1803), grandfather, Henry William (1725–76), and great grandfather, William (1670–1763) all practised in the town. John Markham owned property in Northampton, but his residence for most of his adult life, Little Holmby House, St Giles Street, belonged to his uncle, Charles Markham (1722–1802), rector of the near-by village of Langton. John only inherited the house, shortly before his own death in 1803, along with two pews in the neighbouring church.[33]

All but one of the nine lawyer relatives were solicitors. Only J. O. Bruce, grandfather of Samuel Barwick Bruce, who was a judge in Barbados at the beginning of the eighteenth century, may have been a barrister and had had a university education. As he was born in Clackmannanshire, he had presumably qualified for the Scottish bar before being appointed to the West Indies.[34] One of the legal uncles, Robert Alderson (1752–1833), was another elder brother of the Hull physician, John, suggesting once more that the Aldersons were a particularly upwardly mobile family. Robert kept an office in Norwich and eventually became the town's recorder, while his own son, Edward Hall (1787–1857), would study at Charterhouse and Caius and become a baron of the exchequer in 1834. The only solicitor father practising in a capital city was Henry Harrison, whose son, William, joined the army medical service in 1798. Henry probably attended TCD, then served from at least 1790 to 1806 as solicitor in the Dublin courts of King's Bench and Exchequer.[35]

Clergymen, too, if clearly more visible—twenty-three have been found—cannot have been very numerous among the relatives of army surgeons. Like officers in the armed services, ordained ministers of the established Churches can be identified relatively simply through the Fasti of the Church of Scotland and the biographical registers of Oxford, Cambridge, and Trinity College Dublin.[36] As only twenty-one of the 272 fathers, grandfathers, and uncles whose names are known belonged to this category—sixteen were ministers of the Church of England, four of the Church of Scotland, and one the Church of Ireland—few in the sample can have had connections with the parsonage or the manse. Admittedly, Nonconformist ministers are as difficult to track as lawyers, but here again the fact that only four have come to light in the course of research would suggest they would be rare birds in an army surgeon's family tree. In fact, apart

[33] Charles was the elder brother and had no children. A number of wills of the Markham family exist but no valuations: TNA, Prob 11/884, qs. 224–6 (his great grandfather); Prob 11 /1216, qs. 35–9 (his great uncle); Prob 11/1401, fo. 143 (his father).

[34] It has so far proved impossible to trace him in university archives, probably because the class-lists do not survive for this early date.

[35] Burtchaell, 374, gives a Henry Harrison, son of William, armiger, born Limerick, who matriculated at the university in 1773.

[36] All ministers of the Church of England and Ireland had to have an MA from one of the three Anglican universities. Much more information will be available about C. of E. ministers once the ongoing compilation of the *Fasti* of the C. of E. is complete: see **www.theclergydatabase.org.uk** (July 2005).

from Christopher Alderson, whose grandfather and an uncle had been dissenting ministers,[37] only one other surgeon in the sample—Stewart Crawford—had free-church relatives. Both Crawford's father, William, and grandfather were Irish presbyterians, the former (d. 1800) taking his MA at Glasgow in 1763, then serving the congregation at Strabane from 1766 to 1798 before moving to Holywood, County Down, for the two years before his death.[38]

Given the number of Irish and Scots in the service, the almost complete absence of Church of Ireland ministers and the paucity of Scottish presbyterians among the surgeons' close relations is particularly striking. Only one of the four Scots, moreover, was of any consequence. This was Gavin Gibb (d. 1831), father of James Richardson, who served as minister of Fintry (1787–91), Strathblane (1791–1807), and St Andrew's Glasgow (1809–31), a particularly rich parish. Gibb was a man of learning and substance. A Glasgow graduate who took his MA in 1783 and became a DD in 1804, he was elected moderator of the Church of Scotland for 1817 and was professor of oriental languages at the University of Glasgow from 1809 until his death.

The Church of England ministers were equally a mixed bag. Only one, William Keate (1739–95), father of Robert, was the scion of an Anglican clerical dynasty and could boast not just a father but a grandfather, both also called William, who were parish clergy. The first William seems to have been minister at Seaton in Devon, while the second was an Oxford man who held the very lucrative living of St Cuthbert's, Wells. Father William, on the other hand, was educated at Eton and Cambridge, and went on to be a Fellow of King's College (1762–8), master of Stamford Grammar School, minister of Laverton in Somerset (1768–95), and canon of Wells (1773–95). He was clearly a man of substance and importance in the Church and probably had an income in excess of £1,000 per annum.[39] The one other Anglican minister of any significance was William Gregory (1759–1803), father of George and brother of John, the Edinburgh professor of medicine. Born in Aberdeen, he entered Balliol College, Oxford, and gained his MA in 1783 before becoming rector of St Andrew's, Canterbury, master of the local Eastbridge hospital, and one of the six preachers of Canterbury cathedral. His annual earnings possibly came to £400. By comparison all the other Anglican ministers were small fry, for the most part in charge of rural parishes and doubtless forced to get by on an income of £200 or less.[40] Only Jeremiah Bigsby (1748–97),

[37] Christopher's uncle, Robert Alderson, initially served as minister to the Octagon Presbyterian Chapel in Norwich, but on the advice of his brother-in-law entered Lincoln's Inn in 1791 (he does not seem to have been called to the bar). He is recorded in Table 2.5 as a lawyer. Later in life he conformed and there is a memorial to him and his second wife in Norwich cathedral.

[38] William Crawford received his DD from Glasgow in 1784.

[39] Keate Snr preached the sermon at the Wells assize in August 1775. He wrote a number of pamphlets against dissenters and ending establishment: e.g. *A Free Examination of Dr Price's and Dr Priestley's Sermons* (1790).

[40] Estimates based on the valuations in [Richard Gilbert], *The Clerical Guide or Ecclesiastical Directory, Containing a Complete Register of the Dignitaries and Benefices of the Church of England . . .* (London, 1836). The valuations were based on information collected by the ecclesiastical commissioners in the

uncle of John Jeremiah and rector of St Peter's, Nottingham, 1783–97, a church in the town centre, was likely to have drawn a decent substance from his living: in the 1830s his benefice was thought to return £336 per annum net.[41] Two of the number, furthermore, were curiosities in that they had entered the Church late in life and had already had another career.

The first was John Boutflower, encountered above, who abandoned the navy for the Church in 1777, five years before his son Charles was born. In that year he entered St John's, Cambridge under an arrangement whereby mature students could read for a BD by keeping one term in three for ten years, while, in the interim, taking orders and beginning their ministry. Having helped out at Chingford and Waltham Cross, he was eventually given the parish of Seamer in East Yorkshire, some time after 1782, the year Charles was born in Enfield. There he became a noted supporter of the evangelical cause. This was a modest, though not impoverished living worth £243 per annum, and Boutflower, like many other clergymen, could only sustain his large family by taking in pupils. It was in this way that he was able to pay for the surgical apprenticeship of one of Charles's elder brothers, John Johnson (1768–1854), who later practised in Manchester. John Jnr was sent to Francis Weaver Watkins of Wellingborough. In return Watkins's son, William, went to Seamer to learn Latin, Greek, and French.[42]

The second was Charles Este (1752–1829), father of Michael Lambton, who similarly became a ten-year man at St John's in December 1776. Charles was born in St Martin in the Fields, London, to an apothecary and, like a number of his relatives, attended Westminster School. Although his uncle, another Charles, was a graduate of Christ Church, Oxford, who became bishop of Ossory, Waterford, and Lismore, his immediate family did not have enough money to send him to university and he chose to begin life as an actor at the age of 17. Next, presumably under parental pressure, he trained to be an apothecary in his father's shop but in his mid-twenties he saw the light and decided to take advantage of the St John's provision and enter the ministry. Unlike Boutflower, however, he lacked scholarly assiduity and took his name off the books in 1782. This, though, did not harm his career in the Church, for, patronized by the bishop of London, he became one of the king's reading chaplains at Whitehall and an afternoon preacher at the Percy Chapel in the well-heeled parish of St Pancras. He also found plenty of time to indulge his literary ambitions, writing for a number of newspapers and magazines, including the *Morning Post* and publishing several books, notably an account of

early 1830s. Presumably, the return in the late eighteenth century would have been somewhat lower. For St Cuthbert's Wells, Laverton, a Wells canonry, St Andrew's, Canterbury and a Canterbury's preacher's stipend: see ibid., Table II, n.p., *sub* Canterbury and Wells, and Table III, 44, 116, 212.

[41] Ibid., Table III, 152. John Jeremiah was educated at Lincoln, Oxford, and initially held a parish in Suffolk. He is buried in the vault at St Peter's. John Jeremiah had a second uncle in the Church: Thomas (1756–1821), who was educated at Jesus, Cambridge, and was vicar of Burton Joyce, Notts., 1782–1821.

[42] Boutflower, *Story of a Family*, 82, 87; [Gilbert], *Clerical Guide*, 175. The advowson of Seamer was owned during Boutflower's tenure by Joseph Dennison of Jeffries Sq., St Mary Axe, London.

his travels in Europe with son Michael in 1793. When Charles died in 1829 he was a rich man, leaving at least £17,000.[43]

Even humble teachers and professors—a growing proportion of the professional population across the eighteenth century with the expanding provision in education, both institutional and freelance[44]—were seldom to be found among the surgeons' fathers, uncles, and grandfathers. Only seven of the 157 relatives whose occupation is known earned their bread from teaching, all Scots. Three spent part or all of their career in a municipal academy, one initially ran a private school, and five eventually held a chair in a Scottish university. Apart from the three professors of medicine already mentioned, the most celebrated of the group was John Anderson (1726–96), uncle of Alexander Dunlop, who taught natural philosophy at Glasgow from 1757 to 1796. Commonly known as Jolly Jack Phosphorus and a notorious Whig, Jacobin, and hardline Calvinist, Anderson's posthumous gift to the city where he had worked and thrived was the Andersonian Institute (now the University of Strathclyde). The most varied career, however, was that followed by William Wallace (1768–1843), father of William. William the elder began his adult life as an apprentice bookbinder, then after spending some time as a bookseller became professor of mathematics at the Perth Academy (1794–1803), one of the leading schools of the Scottish Enlightenment. From there he moved to teach the subject at the new Army Military College at Great Marlow, Buckinghamshire (1803–19), which was where his son was born, and finally, through the patronage of the Edinburgh mathematician and geologist, John Playfair, he returned to the Scottish capital to take up a chair at the University, which he occupied until 1838.[45]

Furthermore, one final professional group, government officials, were almost completely unrepresented although it must be admitted that they form a category particularly difficult to investigate. Despite the rapid growth in the number of excisemen and postal workers across the eighteenth century—by 1800 there were more government employees than clergymen in England—only one of the 157 relatives has been found on the government's administrative payroll. This was Hugh Buchan, father of James, who seems to have been a tax collector in Edinburgh.[46]

[43] Charles Este, *A Journey in the Year 1793 through Flanders, Brabant and Germany to Switzerland* (London, 1795). The best account of his varied life is the obituary which appeared in the *Gentleman's Magazine*, 1 (1829), 643–4. But for his early years, see his autobiographical pamphlet, *My Own Life* (London 1787), 7–13. Charles in his will (TNA, Prob 11/1138) bequeathed legacies worth £17,000. But he gave nothing to Michael Lambton: see Ch. 6, pp. 269–70.

[44] Nicholas A. Hans, *New Trends in Education in the Eighteenth Century* (London, 1951). For the growing number of freelance science lecturers, see Jan Golinski, *Science as Public Culture: Chemistry and Enlightenment in Britain 1760–1820* (Cambridge, 1999).

[45] William Wallace was another one of the sample who joined the service after 1815. The Army Military College was founded in 1802 to prepare boys for the army officer corps. It later transferred to Sandhurst. Another father of a cohort member, John Riach, father of John, taught English language at the Perth Academy.

[46] According to the dedication of his son's Edinburgh medical thesis sustained in 1792, Hugh was a 'quaestor'. It seems probable that more of the cohort must have had fathers who were government officials and we have failed to trace them. We know of one naval surgeon during the wars, William Beatty, who came from a dynasty of excise gaugers: see Laurence Brockliss, John Cardwell, and Michael Moss, *Nelson's Surgeon: William Beatty, Naval Medicine and Trafalgar* (Oxford, 2005), Ch. 2, sect. 1.

Given the relative visibility of members of the professions at the turn of the nineteenth century, it is unlikely therefore that more than 15 per cent of army surgeons had fathers with liberal careers. Perhaps a further 5 per cent had close elder relatives in the professions, but only a handful of the cohort, such as Thomas Keate, Henry William Markham, and William Gregory, hailed from families which had been embedded in professional life for several generations.[47] Where the large majority seem to have originated was among the reasonably comfortable but less educated middling sort who were the chief creators of Britain and Ireland's wealth outside the industrializing heartland, their fathers probably enjoying annual incomes of £200–300.[48]

Those born in the countryside (perhaps as many as 50 per cent in Scotland and Ireland) seem to have had fathers who were a mix of estate managers, tenant farmers, and small landowners. John Grant, the father of John, was a factor on the huge Gordon estates in Strathspey; while Andrew Murray, the father of another John (mentioned in the previous chapter and not in the cohort) was a tenant farmer on the outskirts of Turriff in Aberdeenshire. Andrew occupied a mixed arable and pasture farm belonging to Lord Fife and many of John's letters home comment on the state of the harvest and the problems of keeping up the tenancy in the agricultural depression after the war.[49] On the other hand, the father of Archibald Arnott, George (1721–1801), owned an estate at Ecclefechan in Dumfriesshire. By origin a member of a landed Fife family down on its luck, he had had the good fortune to marry Janet Knox (1735–96), heiress to Kirkconnel Hall.[50] Another landowner was William Williams (c.1720–75), father of James, who lived at Perry House in the parish of Hartlebury, Worcestershire. According to his will, he owned property in Hartlebury and a number of neighbouring parishes, in particular Emley Lovett and Elmbridge. In his case, the land came not from his wife, Mary Randle (c.1738–1811), whom he married at Ombersley, Worcestershire, in 1755, but from his father, another William, a successful brick manufacturer, who had built Perry House in 1741, and invested in real estate.[51]

It is not usually clear whether the landowners were gentleman farmers or rentiers, although this must largely have depended on how much land was owned. Robert Davy (c.1746–94), father of John, drifted between the two. The Davys were an established landed family in the parish of Ludgvan, a few miles from

[47] Conclusion based on the assumption that the majority of fathers with professional careers has been identified (52 out of 454 = 11.45 per cent) and the fact that not many of the cohort with professional grandfathers and uncles did not also have a father in a liberal career.

[48] L. Davidoff and C. Hall, *Family Fortunes: Men and Women of the English Middle Classes, 1780–1850*, rev. edn. (London, 2002). See the parts of the study devoted to the middle classes in Essex and Suffolk; and esp. Table 1, which distinguishes the upper from the lower middle classes, judged to be two-thirds of the group.

[49] WL, RAMC 830, 9 Mar. 1816: John suggests his father and Fife's other tenants should seek a decrease in rent.

[50] James Arnott, *The House of Arnott* (Edinburgh, 1918), 110–18 (history of the estate).

[51] We are indebted to the researches of Mrs G. M. Lawley for the major part of our information about the Williams of Hartlebury. It is possible that the family also eventually inherited property in Ombersley through Mary Randle.

Penzance, where they had lived for 200 years, sometimes being called yeomen, sometimes gentlemen. Robert's own father, Edmund was 'a respectable builder' but he himself had expected to inherit the estates of his uncle, another Robert (d. 1774), who was worth £600–700 per annum, a really handsome sum which placed him in the upper ranks of the middling sort. However, the inheritance never materialized and Robert was left dependent on the income from a much smaller farm in the parish, known as Varfell, which only brought in £150 a year. Marrying the younger daughter of a Penzance merchant, Grace Millett (c.1756–1826) in 1776, Robert first set up house in the town, where his elder, more famous son Humphry was born, and rented out his farm. But when Humphry was 9 (in 1787) the family moved to Varfell, where a modest but modern farm-house had been built, and for the rest of his short life, Robert Davy was a gentle-man farmer, albeit with limited means.[52]

In other cases, it is impossible to determine whether fathers were landowners or tenants. According to his own testimony, William Gibney of County Meath was born into an Irish landed family of Norman origin, distantly related to the duke of Wellington's. 'So far back as the year 1600 we were possessors of the property at Clongill in the county of Meath; my great-grandfather marrying, in 1690, Margaret Wesley, or Wellesley, a sister of Gerard Wesley, afterwards Lord Mornington.' By the late eighteenth century, though, they were in relatively reduced circumstances, like the Arnotts. Michael, William's father, possessed Dormston or Dormiston Castle, but it seems likely that the property was not large enough to support his family and that he was also compelled to lease land. Significantly, when William's younger brother matriculated at Trinity College Dublin in 1817, he gave his father's occupa-tion as 'agricola' not 'armiger'.[53] The background of William Dent (another surgeon not in the cohort) remains equally difficult to fathom. Hailing from Mickleton-in-Teesdale on the Yorkshire–Durham border, he belonged to a farming family which had been settled in the area since at least the 1520s. But if his farming brother, Kitt (1792–1874), certainly owned land, it is impossible to tell from his letters what his father's status was, or whether the cousin whose mill burnt down in 1812 owned the property.[54]

Members of the sample born in towns or cities seem to have been predominantly the sons of men who owned their own businesses or workshops. Of the twenty-five fathers known to have been involved in some way with commerce and manufacturing, only Robert Maclagan, father of David, a teller in the important

---

[52] The *DNB* describes Robert Davy as a wood-carver. This was not his occupation but a hobby, taken up instead of a career in the days he expected to become a substantial landholder: see John Davy, *Memoris of the Life of Sir Humphry Davy*, 2 vols. (London, 1836), i. 5. This is the best source for information about John's background.

[53] Gibney, 1–4; Burtchaell, 324. Of course many landowning families leased land and/or received leases as part of a marriage settlement. In Gibney's case, though, this may have been out of necessity rather than the speculative pursuit of profit.

[54] WL, RAMC 536, esp. letters 8 Sept. 1812 and 29 Oct. 1820 (originals and typed transcription). See also W. Dent, *A Young Surgeon in Wellington's Army*, ed. L. W. Woodford (Old Woking, 1976), 1, and inside end cover (family tree): this is a printed transcription of the letters.

Edinburgh bank of Ramsay, Bonar and Co. (now part of the Royal Bank of Scotland), was an employee. A few of these businessmen may have been little more than artisan craftsman—John Arthur, for instance, father of John Jnr, was apparently a Dublin shoemaker. One too, the Quaker George Brown of North Shields, father of Joseph, apparently got into financial difficulties.[55] But several were substantial members of their local community. John Robb's father, John Snr, was a significant merchant and banker in Ayr trading with India, rich enough to buy an estate, while John Kinnis, father of John Jnr, was a prominent table-linen manufacturer in Dunfermline, and John Davies Greaves (1750–84), son of William, a substantial brewer in Burton-on-Trent. Guthrie's father, Andrew, who, we noted earlier, made and sold surgical goods in London, seems to have been a singularly successful businessman, although he sadly ended up squandering the fortune that he had carefully accumulated, as his son was also to do.[56]

[Guthrie's] father assisted and afterwards succeeded his maternal uncle, a surgeon in the navy, who retiring from service after the peace of Aix la Chapelle [1748], established himself in business for the sale of the *Emplastrum Lythargyri* of a better description than had hitherto been made, after a process he had become acquainted with during his service abroad. Succeeding to this business after the death of his uncle, he realized by it, and by the sale of most other surgical materials during the early part of the war, combined with habits of great industry and economy, a considerable sum of money, so as to be enabled to secure unto his daughter on her marriage ten thousand pounds, which are now enjoyed by her children. Unfortunately for his son [the army surgeon], he alienated himself from his family late in life, entered into other pursuits and speculations, and on Mr Guthrie's return from the Peninsular war, he found he had little or nothing to expect except from his own exertions.[57]

Some of the fathers, too, who have been identified as artisans were much bigger fish than the appellation implies. When the younger brother of Edward Walsh, Robert, entered Trinity College Dublin in 1789 he described his father as a *faber lignarius* or carpenter. According to Walsh's obituary in the *Dublin University Magazine*, however, he came from a substantial Waterford family, whose members were frequently to be found among the 'chief magistrates'. Since, moreover, Edward's father, John, had the means to send the future army surgeon to school in England, it is unlikely he was a humble chippy. It is much more probable that he was one of the elite corps of Irish carpenter-architects who planned and built the great houses of the Ascendancy.[58] Much the same can be said of the Dublin carpenter James McGauley (*c*.1723–83), father of James Macauley. James senior was also a builder, a timber merchant, grazier, and real estate dealer. At the end of

---

[55] TWA, Acc. No. 1132: Joseph Brown to his sister 10 May 1808. The letter describes Joseph's horror on learning of his father's 'errors and misfortunes'. The archives contain a photocopy of the original and a typed transcript. Quakers usually belonged to the upper echelons of the middling sort, so the family may have been originally prosperous.   [56] See p. 267.

[57] Thomas J. Pettigrew, *Medical Portrait Gallery*, 4 vols. (London, 1838–42), iv. 2.

[58] Burtchaell, 855. *Dublin University Magazine*, 3 (1834), 63.

his life, he was the owner-occupier of Stormanstown House, Drumcondra, an elegant early seventeenth-century mansion outside Dublin, surrounded by ornamental gardens and 21 acres of good pasture.[59]

Too great a division, however, should not be made between town and country. Not only, as we have seen, did several of the fathers in trade purchase small estates, but a number had rural backgrounds. Robert Shekleton's father, Joseph, was a Dundalk merchant, but he had been rasied as a landed gentleman's younger son. James McGrigor's father, Colquhoun McGrigor, was a successful Aberdeen merchant, but he too had been brought up in the countryside. Colquhoun belonged to a branch of the MacGregors of Roro, a proscribed clan which had been settled in Strathspey in the early seventeenth century and it was there that he had spent his formative years. Colquhoun was originally an innkeeper, small-time merchant, and, like his forebears, a tacksman or tenant of the duke of Gordon.[60] It was only in 1775, when James was four and the proscription on using the clan name finally withdrawn, that Colquhoun took his family to Aberdeen and established himself as a general merchant, specializing in hosiery, in Gallowgate.[61]

Whatever the limitations of the data, it is evident that army surgeons in the early nineteenth century came from a wide variety of middling social backgrounds. Even if the proportion of fathers, uncles, and grandfathers with a professional career is not so grossly over-represented among the limited number of identified relatives as we suspect, it seems incontestable that the army medical service drew only a minority of its surgeons from professional families and almost certainly less than 10 per cent from medical backgrounds.[62] Understandably, given the limited educational requirements for entering the professions at this date, even a smaller proportion would have had fathers or forebears who had been to university, perhaps 3 per cent at the most.[63] The majority of surgeons, it can be concluded, came from trade and agriculture and belonged to families which in earlier generations had invested little in formal education of any kind.

[59] Robert Burke Savage, *Catherine McAuley: The First Sister of Mercy* (Dublin, 1949), 5–9. James Macaulay Anglicized his name: see below for a fuller account of his background.

[60] The MacGregors (or MacGrigors) were a notoriously lawless clan in the sixteenth century and in 1603 the whole clan was outlawed. Until the mid-eighteenth century anyone using the surname risked death. Most MacGregors called themselves Whyte but James's grandfather used the name Gordon.

[61] McGrigor, 11–13, 14 (editor's introduction). McGrigor, 27, simply says his father was an Aberdeen merchant.

[62] On the assumption that we have identified most of the medical fathers (32 out of 454).

[63] Only 7 per cent of the 181 identified fathers attended university. The true percentage must be much lower, given that the failure to discover the name of a surgeon's father almost certainly indicates a relatively humble occupation. Admittedly, we cannot claim to have found all of the identified fathers who received a higher education. There are reasonably accurate published matriculation registers for Oxbridge, Glasgow, and TCD but only graduate registers for Aberdeen, Edinburgh, and St Andrews. This is significant given the growing importance of Edinburgh University in the second half of the eighteenth century, and a detailed study of the unpublished class lists in the university archives might reveal further names. It is unlikely, though, that the general conclusion will be invalidated.

Nor is it likely, though this is more speculative, that the majority from a non-professional background hailed from wealthy families. Although many of our sample must have had farmer or businessmen fathers who were comfortably off, none belonged to the great mercantile and industrial families of late Hanoverian Britain and Ireland. Like most of the surgeons from professional families, it can be assumed that the majority from other middling backgrounds came from homes which enjoyed a modest sufficiency rather than great wealth. John Kinnis Snr may have been a big wheel in Dunfermline and been elected Provost, but he was only worth £979 when he died in 1834, scarcely a fortune (although the sum did not include the value of his factory).[64]

It is worth noting that several of the better-placed members of the cohort, whatever their background, actually grew up in an environment where the family fortune had taken a tumble. James McGauley's steady rise to gentility counted for little when he died three months after his son's birth, causing his widow, Elinor Conway (*c*.1756–98), to sell Stormanstown house and move into lodgings in Dublin.[65] And this was only the most extreme of a string of such cases: David Maclagan's father also died just after (or perhaps even before) he was born, William Gibney's when he was 'but a youth' (leading to the loss of Dormston Castle) and George Gregory's in 1803 when George was 13, while Theodore Gordon had lost both parents by the age of 5.[66] It must always be borne in mind that a man's social origins can flatter to deceive. The death of John Davy's father in particular cast the family into penury, because he left behind him debts amounting to £1,300. The day was saved only by the determination and adaptability of his 34-year-old widow. Grace Davy abandoned Varfell, took the family back to Penzance, and opened a milliner's business with a French émigrée. Within five years she had cleared the debt and was able to dissolve the partnership when she unexpectedly inherited another small estate that increased her income to £300 per annum.[67]

SIBLINGS

Discovering how many brothers a surgeon had is as difficult in most cases as identifying his father's occupation, but thanks above all to the on-line International Genealogical Index, it has been possible to establish the family position of about a fifth of the group. As can be seen from Table 2.6, less than a third were the first-born (including four only sons), while slightly more than a third were the third son or below. Admittedly, given the mix of sources, the data is likely to be once more skewed towards surgeons from professional families, but this does not completely undermine the significance of the statistics. At the very least, the information in

---

[64] NAS, SC20/50/8, fos. 347–51: his will.   [65] Savage, *Catherine McAuley*, 19–20.
[66] A tablet commemorates Gregory's father in the south walk of the cloister of Canterbury Cathedral.   [67] Davy, *Life*, i. 7–8.

Table 2.6. Army Surgeons' Ranking among Siblings

	Ranking	Unknown	1	2	3	4	5	6	7	8	Total
No. of sons											
1			4								4
2		10	11	6							27
3		4	5	5	7						21
4		3	2	4	3	5					17
5			1	2	2	3	2				10
6			1	2			1				4
7			1			1			1		3
8									2		2
	Total	17	25	19	12	9	3		3		88

Note: Vertical axis represents number of sons born to surgeons' father.

Source: Doctors' Database: Table: Sons.

the table indicates that the large majority of army surgeons were not at the top of the pecking order, while many, especially the three seventh sons, must have had to have been satisfied with the scraps from the family table, when careers were handed out. However advantaged a surgeon's background prima facie, therefore, in reality his prospects may have been greatly weakened, if he came from a large family and was not an elder son.

Some flesh can be put on this assertion when family ranking is matched with father's occupation (see Table 2.7). Although the information is limited, it seems clear that surgeons from rural backgrounds were usually not the first-born. It is significant that the only member of the cohort known to have been a landowner or farmer's eldest son was the orphan, William Gibney, and he, of course, no longer had any land to inherit. Alexander Thomson, whose father was factor to the Murrays of Broughton and Cally and bought a small estate at Torhousemuir in Wigtownshire in 1799, was the second son. The estate passed to his elder brother, Charles William, who sold it in 1823 and took out a tenancy on Machermore castle, Newton Stewart, Wigtownshire, where Alexander was to die thirty years later.[68] Another second son was John Murray of Turriff (not in the cohort), whose elder brother Alexander, born in 1784 farmed at Backhouse near Peterhouse and wrote letters suggesting a limited education. In this case, though, the farm did not pass to the eldest son but the youngest, William, born in 1792, who worked for his father and eventually took over the tenancy.[69] Other surgeons from the countryside, on the other hand, were much further down the ranking. Archibald Arnott of Ecclefechan was the fifth and youngest son, and James Williams of

---

[68] P. H. MacKerlie *History of the Lands and Their Owners in Galloway with Historical Sketches of the District*, 5 vols., (Edinburgh, 1870–9), ii. 334.

[69] WL, RAMC 830, *passim*, esp. 7 June 1817: John to William. William is about to take over the lease and John suggests the three brothers should buy a house for their parents in Turriff.

Table 2.7. Sibling Ranking According to Father's Occupation

Father's occupation	Sibling ranking								
	1	2	3	4	5	6	7	8	TOTAL
Agriculture	1	4	1	1	1		1		9
Professions									
Armed Forces		1							1
Church	2	2	2	3					9
Education	2								2
Law			1						1
Medicine	6	4	3						13
Trade	6	2	3	1			2		14
TOTAL	17	13	10	5	1		3		49
Only, Younger or Youngest Son	3	3	4	2					12

Source: Doctor's Database: Relationships 1; Sons.

Hartlebury the seventh of eight, suggesting that neither family, however wealthy they might be, placed much value on a medical career.[70] In the Williams family, the lion's share of the land went to the eldest son, John, who died in 1825 leaving 660 acres and an estate valued at £5,000.[71] Archibald's eldest brother, William, however, died at 18 and another was lost at sea, and it was the fourth in line, John, who eventually inherited and farmed the estate of some 100 acres in 1801, when Archibald's father died.[72] Nothing better attests to the relative indigency of the Davys of Ludgvan after Robert Davy's death than the fact that the first-born, Humphry was immediately apprenticed to a local Penzance surgeon by his mother's guardian, John Tonkin.[73]

Surgeons whose fathers were in trade and the professions, in contrast, were much more likely to be first or second in line. The largest number by far were the offspring of medical practitioners who presumably commonly expected their eldest son to embrace some sort of medical career. But sons of clergymen, such as the first-born William Richardson Gibb, could also be highly ranked, as could the sons of tradesmen. Colquhoun McGrigor for one did not keep the future

[70] As James's brother, Samuel, died in 1783 aged 9, he was effectively youngest of six surviving sons.

[71] According to William Williams's will (TNA, Prob 11/1006, qs. 220–1), his wife Mary had a life interest in the Hartlebury estate while John inherited most of the other property when he was 21. Some rents were reserved to pay for bringing up his other children. William's second son, William (1765–1824), also inherited a great deal of landed property, through the will of his uncle, George Williams (d. 1782), also of Hartlebury, who had no children: Prob 11/1092, qs. 311–14. For John's will and valuation: see Prob 11/1706, qs. 473–5; TNA, IR 26/1070, fo. 970.

[72] Possibly the third brother, George, had also died by then. John Arnott (*c*.1769–1830) was a lieutenant in the Dumfriesshire Volunteers: see Arnott, *House of Arnott*, 118–20. The size of the estate is revealed in the 1851 census. Given the high child mortality of the period, it was frequently the case that the eldest son did not live to see his inheritance.

[73] Both of Grace Millett's parents had died within a week of one another in 1757. Tonkin was also a surgeon.

director-general manacled to the shop counter.[74] James was his first son, and it was his second, Robert, who became a merchant. John Kinnis of Dunfermline, in contrast, was more cautious and only trained his second son for medicine. The elder Kinnis, William, inherited the linen manufacture and made the fortune which had eluded his father, leaving £42,935 in 1851.[75]

In the case of medics' sons, there is little sign that there was any correlation between their ranking and their father's wealth and standing. Both John Jeremiah Bigsby and Christopher Alderson were the eldest sons of prominent practitioners. Among other professional and commercial groups, however, the evidence is more ambiguous. Even if the number is too small to be conclusive, it is surely not a coincidence that four of the six from commercial and professional backgrounds ranked fourth or below came from comfortably-off families. Two—Robb and Alexander Dunlop Anderson[76]—were sons of affluent Scottish merchants, while Charles Boutflower and Robert Keate were sons of clergymen. Keate is a particularly good example of a surgeon from a well-to-do family whose career-path must have been largely determined by his ranking. His father, William, it will be recalled, was a canon of Wells cathedral and he came from a clerical dynasty. Had Robert been born higher in the order, he would never have entered medicine, let alone the army medical service. His eldest brother, William Burland (1770–1816/17) went to Cambridge and became rector of Laverton in succession to his father. His second brother, John (1773–1852), also went to Cambridge, took orders, then went into teaching. He became the infamous headmaster of Eton 'flogger' Keate, and his daughter, Emma, would marry a bishop of Chichester.[77] His third brother, Thomas Morris (b. 1775), again studied at Cambridge, then became a lawyer and entered the service of the East India Company as a judge. Robert, however, was the fourth and youngest son, for whom medicine or trade inevitably beckoned. In his case, medicine was the obvious choice. When young Robert reached his mid-teens—the age at which a decision would have to be made—his uncle Thomas, his father's younger brother and his natural patron, was well ensconced as surgeon at St George's and general inspector of army hospitals.[78]

The relatively stellar lives of Keate's elder brothers also reminds us that it is essential to look at the careers of a surgeon's male siblings not just his family position, if we are to gauge accurately his family's circumstances and the strategies

[74] William Greaves was also the first-born of a tradesman father. John Davies Greaves (1750–84) was a Burton brewer, but he died when William was 13 and ordered in his will that the business be sold. The decision to place William in medicine would have been taken by John's two brothers, wife, and brother-in-law. The brother-in-law, William Newton, was a Derby surgeon. TNA, Prob 11/1124, qs. 174–6.
[75] NAS, SC70/4/23, fos. 240–74: will and valuation. John Kinnis Snr also placed his third son in medicine. Medicine and the textile trade had a natural affinity: a successful dyer, like a medical practitioner, needed a knowledge of chemistry.
[76] Anderson's father, Andrew, was a Greenock merchant, who had married into the Glasgow medical and academic family of Dunlop.
[77] Keate flogged 80 boys on the same day on 30 June 1832 but remained surprisingly popular. He was probably worth about £30,000 on his death: see the bequests in his will: TNA, Prob 11/2151, qs. 175–7.   [78] In which guise, Robert Keate appears frequently in Ch. 1 above.

deployed in placing sons. This again is difficult to do given the nature of the sources, but enough information has come to light to allow some conclusions to be made. The clear impression from the data gathered in Table 2.8 is that the large majority of siblings entered the professions (62 out of 81 careers identified). This is unlikely given the background of our cohort and the fact that the careers of only a third of the brothers' identified has been traced—there must have been far more than 25 per cent of siblings (elder or younger) who inherited land or leases or went

Table 2.8. Brothers' Occupation

Brothers' occupation	
Agriculture	4
Professions	62
Administration	3
Armed Forces	11
Church	13
Law	6
Solicitors	(5)
Barristers	(1)
Medicine	29
Apothecaries	(1)
Physicians	(6)
Practitioners[a]	(4)
Surgeons[b]	(18)
Trade & Business	9
Bankers	(2)
Manufacturers[c]	(2)
Merchants	(5)
Independent[d]	6
TOTAL	81
Number of individual families	(57)
Number of names known	257
Number of individual families	(120)
Percentage identified	(31.57)
Higher education	21
Oxbridge	9
TCD	3
Scotland	9
Number of individual families	18

Note: A number of the 257 brothers discovered would have died before they began a career. Four are definitely known to have died in infancy or childhood and one died in his teens. Seven are possibly wrongly attributed.

[a] Unspecified.
[b] Includes four army, navy and East India Company surgeons.
[c] Substantial.
[d] Simply identified as gentlemen. They may have had an unidentified career.

Source: Doctors' Database: Table: Relationships 1.

into their father's or another trade. It simply once more reflects the bias of the sources towards professional and better-off families.

More reliable, if still not to be accepted uncritically, is the information relating to higher education, which suggests about 8 per cent of male siblings attended a university (and less than 4 per cent expensive Oxford and Cambridge, which cost about £200 per annum).[79] The percentage is revealing. We will see in the next chapter that a large proportion of the cohort had attended a medical faculty, even if they had not taken a medical degree prior to entering the service.[80] Arguably, then, few army surgeons belonged to families who had either the desire or the wealth to put more than one son through higher education. Noticeably only one of the eighteen members of the cohort whose families definitely did so hailed from the countryside: the rest were split equally in their origins between trade and the professions. Clearly, Robert Keate came from an exceptional background. Many of the surgeons' brothers may have had some sort of education, but the army doctors, it can be suggested, were far better educated than most of their siblings.[81]

The limited information garnered, however, does reveal several valuable details about the career strategies of our sample's better-placed families (see Table 2.9). In the first place, a small number of the most ambitious and affluent were taking advantage of the recruitment needs of the French wars to place the odd son in the officer-corps proper. At the very least, one of the surgeons had a brother in the navy, one in the Royal Artillery, three in the Royal Engineers and six in the army proper, the last including James Riach, a Perth teacher's son, whose younger brother, William Alexander (1793–1843), rose to be a major in the 79th Foot, and Director-General McGrigor whose younger brother, Charles (third in line, d. 1841), eventually held the rank of lieutenant colonel.[82] One surgeon, Samuel Ayrault Piper, himself the son of an army officer, even had two siblings in the services. His elder brother, John, rose to be lieutenant colonel of the King's Own, while his younger, Robert Sloper (1790–1873) became a general in the Royal Engineers. Others, moreover, had close peer-group relatives in the officer corps of the armed services, notably the clergyman's son, Michael Lambton Este, whose cousin, Charles William Este, reached the rank of major general and was lieutenant-governor of Carlisle Castle when he died in 1812, worth at least £13,000.[83]

---

[79] See what was said above, n. 63, about the incompleteness of the university records.

[80] See Ch. 3 under 'Lectures and Classes'.

[81] It should be said that this was still an impressive commitment to higher education when possibly only about 0.5 per cent of English 18 year olds attended Oxford and Cambridge, and from 1 to 1.4 per cent of Scottish teenagers went to Scottish universities: see Robert Anderson, *Universities and Elites in Britain since 1800* (London, 1992).

[82] Searching for brothers in the *Army List* and *Navy List* is a time-consuming and difficult task and a number may have been missed. One army surgeon not in the cohort, Sir James Fellowes (1771–1857), who joined the service at the start of the French wars as a hospital mate, had two brothers in the navy; one, Sir Thomas (1778–1853) eventually became a rear admiral. Their father, William, was an army surgeon with aristocratic connections: see 'Tales of Family Fortunes: Fellowes-Gordon formerly of Knockespoch' at **www.burkes-peerage.net/sites/common/sitepages/page13i-dec.asp** (July 2005).

[83] He left most of his money to his illegitimate children: TNA, Prob 11/1531, qs. 107–8 (proved 9 Mar. 1812). We have no idea what was the occupation of his father and Michael Lambton Este's uncle.

Table 2.9. Family Career Strategy (i): Families with Three Sons or More

Mix of sons' careers	Number of families
All medicine	3 (3)
Medicine/armed forces	1
Medicine/church	2 (1)
Medicine/law	2 (1)
Medicine/trade	1 (1)
Medicine/armed forces/law	1 (1)
Medicine/armed forces/trade	1
Medicine/church/administration	1
Medicine/church/independent	1
Medicine/church/law	1
Medicine/law/trade	1 (1)
Medicine/armed forces/church/administration	1
TOTAL	16 (8)

( ): Families with more than one son in medicine.

Source: Doctors' Database: Table: Relationships 1.

On the other hand, the small number identified suggests this was a strategy adopted by few families. The initial outlay in making a son a military officer was probably a cheaper option than training him to be a medical practitioner. Although commissions had commonly to be bought in the army, the navy was free from venality, while neither service required any prior specialist education of its officers and accepted them in their mid-teens. In consequence, it might have been expected that many army surgeons would have had brothers in the lowest ranks of the armed services, especially in the navy.[84] That this does not seem to be the case emphasizes again that most of the sample came from moderate middling-sort backgrounds and had fathers unable to give their sons in their early years the breeding and deportment a military officer needed to survive in the mess or the wardroom, and who generally lacked the necessary patronage contacts. This would also explain why the brothers who did go into the armed services proper tended to be the cohort's younger siblings (see Table 2.10). Thus Peter Rutledge Montagu Browne (1795–1864), who became a captain in the prestigious 9th Foot, was a whole generation younger than his army surgeon brother, Andrew, who had entered the service as a surgeon's mate in the year he was born. Presumably in the interim, their medical practitioner father, based in County Mayo, had come good and made enough wealth to make the investment realistic.[85] This would be

[84] See Ch. 3 for the cost of becoming a surgeon. During the war an ensigncy in the army could be obtained for a couple of hundred pounds, to which sum had to be added the cost of uniforms, accoutrements, and perhaps a horse. More prestigious ranks and positions in the posher regiments, of course, cost much more.

[85] Peter Browne made a good marriage with the heiress, Mary Jane Smythe, and settled at Janeville, St John's Point, Ardglass in County Down. He was a major in the Downshire militia, a JP, and deputy lord lieutenant for the county. Unfortunately, we do not even know the Christian

Table 2.10. Family Strategies (ii): Career Orientation
and Sibling Ranking of Cohort's Brothers

Occupation	Elder brother	Younger brother
Agriculture	1	
Professions		
Administration	1	2
Armed Forces	1	6
Church	5	2
Medicine	9	6
Independent	1	
Trade	2	2
TOTAL	20	18

Source: Doctors' Database, Table: Relationships 1.

perfectly plausible: from the outbreak of the long war until its close was a period of rising prosperity that would have benefited virtually all sections of the middle class, regardless of their source of income.

Second, it is clear that the best-placed families, just like the Keates, tried to distribute their sons among the professions, whichever number son was earmarked for medicine. John Alderson, physician to the Hull Infirmary, had four sons who reached manhood.[86] The eldest, Christopher, trained as a surgeon and entered the army medical service; the second, John (1789–1829), practised as a Hull solicitor, presumably having been apprenticed to a local firm; while the third, Ralph Carr (1793–1849) rose to the rank of lieutenant colonel in the Royal Engineers, which would have required him to attend the Woolwich Academy for a number of years at considerable cost to his father. The fourth, Sir James (1794–1882), admittedly became an Oxford MD and court physician who left an estate valued at £17,000, but medicine was not his intended career. John had initially determined him for a trade and placed him as a clerk to a wine merchant based in Portugal shortly before the outbreak of the Peninsular war, when he then joined the army commissariat. It was only on his return to England that his career path was changed, perhaps on his own insistence and at his own cost. In 1818, he was allowed to go up to Pembroke, Cambridge, and four years later he took his BA as sixth wrangler and was elected a Fellow. He then began his medical training at the ripe old age of 28 with the aim of becoming Fellow of the Royal College of Physicians, a position he obtained in 1830 after taking his MD at Oxford.[87]

name of his father, simply that Andrew was his apprentice. Details of Peter's life are given in the various biographical notices of his more famous son, Major General Andrew Smythe Montagu Browne (1836–1916).

[86] A fifth son died shortly after he was born. John also had six daughters, only one of whom survived to adulthood.

[87] Given John Alderson's religious opinions, it seems unlikely that he would have happily sent his son to Cambridge: see pp. 69, 92. Perhaps James had made enough money in Portugal to finance his own studies and make his own career choice.

The Bunnys of Newbury showed a similar profile. The army surgeon, John Mort Bunny, was the second of four sons. His father, Joseph (1740–1810) was an affluent surgeon born in Andover, who at some date in the second half of the eighteenth century set up his plate in the Berkshire town. When he died, his estate was worth £7,500.[88] His eldest, Joseph Blandy (1767–1834), took over the family practice and became very wealthy in turn: his estate was valued at £12,000.[89] The third and fourth sons were also able to stay at home. Edward Brice (b. 1785) became a banker in the local firm of Toomer, Bunny and Slocock, and equally prospered. In the Berkshire Directory for 1854, he was listed as living outside the town at Speen Hill and was a JP and deputy lieutenant for the county. The youngest, Jeremiah (b. 1789), was a solicitor in Northbrook Street.

Even families down on their luck with the right kind of pedigree tried to ring the professional changes. George Gregory was the second son of a branch of one of Scotland and England's great late seventeenth- and eighteenth-century academic families, whose clergyman father, William, as was earlier noted, died in 1803 when George was 13, leaving his widow £2,000 to bring up his four boys.[90] In their case, though, the future was far from bleak. After several years of study at the King's School, Canterbury, they were all found respectable careers, presumably with the help of their uncle, James, the Edinburgh professor of medicine. The eldest, James (1789–1859), appropriately for a clergyman's son, entered the Church, although the family could only afford to send him to Trinity College Dublin, not Oxford where his father had studied. George became an army surgeon, while the third brother, William (1794–1853), was sent to Woolwich and entered the Royal Engineers, rising to the rank of captain. Finally, the fourth, John (1795–1853) became a secretary in the foreign service and ended his days in 1853 as governor-general of Barbados worth £10,000.[91]

Third, and finally, some of the cohort's poorer professional families denied access by circumstance to the most prestigious careers operated a single-profession strategy and placed all their eggs in the medical basket. This was true of Charles Boutflower's father, John, who had five sons from two marriages and who placed all but one in medicine. The eldest, John Johnson (1768–1854) eventually practised as a surgeon in Manchester; the second, Henry (1769–1806), entered the medical service of the East India Company; the fourth was Charles; while the fifth, Andrew (1784–1817), took his MD in Edinburgh in 1812 and set up as a physician in Hull, the nearest big city to the rural parish in which he had been raised.[92] Only the

---

[88] TNA, IR 26/157 (*sub* March 1810, month probate granted, alphabetically listed).

[89] TNA, IR1826, fo. 409.

[90] Valuation of his estate: TNA, IR 26/73 (*sub* March 1803, month probate granted, alphabetically listed). Will: Prob 11/1388, qs. 256–7 (31 Mar. 1803).

[91] TNA, IR 26/1965, fo. 648; TNA, Prob 11/2179, q. 223 Captain William in contrast left only a modest fortune of £800 when he died in the same year: IR 26/1965, fo. 729; Prob 11/2180, quire mark obscured.

[92] Boutflower, *Story of a Family*, 84; *Nomina eorum qui gradum medicinae doctoris in academia Jacobi sexti Scotorum regis, quae Edinburgi est, adepti sunt* (Edinburgh, 1846), 153.

third son, Samuel (1777–1824), was given different marching orders and he was placed in the East India service proper. Even their sister, Mary-Anne (1780–1827) married a medical man, the York and Ripon physician, Frances Whaley, who graduated at Edinburgh in 1812 (d. 1825). Given that John was a clergyman, the bias seems odd at first sight until it is remembered that John was a ten-year St John's man and probably lacked the means to send any of his children to Oxbridge without outside help.[93]

A similar preference was shown, more understandably, by Andrew Anderson's father, Thomas (1745–1810), who practised surgery in Selkirk and the Border country. Thomas had none of the Gregorys' pedigree. Although he made enough money to buy the small property of Broomhill outside the town in 1793, he was the son of an innkeeper of nearby Earlston called Alexander (d. 1798), and had practised in his home village until 1785.[94] Thomas, too, had five sons, four of whom were placed in medicine, while one of his daughters, Alice or Allison (1772–1840), was married to the celebrated surgeon-explorer, Mungo Park (1771–1806), who practised in Peebles. Thomas's eldest son, Alexander (1770–1805), who had presumably been intended to inherit the family practice, perished with Park in Africa; his second son, John (1777–1809) became a surgeon in the Royal Navy;[95] Andrew joined the army; while Thomas (1786–1850) eventually took over from his father about 1808, becoming in time town baillie and provost. Only Andrew's twin, George (1784–1846) had a different, unknown career.[96]

Of course, most families from which the cohort sprang can have had no intention of placing all their sons in a profession, of if they harboured such an aspiration it must have remained a pipe-dream. For many, tenant farmers and small business men, it must have been satisfaction enough if one sibling could be hoisted into educated society. There must have been many army surgeons, like John Murray, whose brothers were literate but not cultured farmers.[97] Moreover, even where non-professional families did place more than one son in the professions, they usually kept one sibling at home running the farm or tending the shop. One of John Kinnis's two brothers became a doctor but the other worked in the

---

[93] John's second wife, Susannah Peach, whom he married in 1776, did provide a dowry of £2,000, but the income almost certainly could not have been used to educate the two sons of the first bed: Boutflower, *Story of a Family*, 85, 87. Henry Johnson was apprenticed to John Sherwen of Enfield, Middlesex, in 1783, the village in which Charles had been born six years before and where John had been based before moving to Seamer: see TNA, IR/1/62–3, fo. 28: apprenticeship records.

[94] The sasine records reveal Thomas was buying property in Earlston in 1782, which he sold in 1793. He bought property adjoining Broomhill in 1806 but he seems to have been the victim of a bank failure and all the land was sold in 1817 by the trustees of his creditors. He inherited the inn which he sold in 1803.

[95] He is in Brockliss and Moss's naval surgeons database: see above, p. 20.

[96] 'The "Doctors Anderson" of Selkirk', *Border Magazine*, 2: (Jan.-Dec. 1897), 155–9, 174–6; Kenneth Lupton, *Mungo Park: The African Traveller* (Oxford, 1975), 8, 226; 'List of pre-1855 gravestones, Selkirk Churchyard' (information courtesy of Scottish Borders Archive and Local History Centre). Another Scottish army surgeon whose two brothers were medics was William Paton.

[97] For instance, Crawford Dick's brother farmed the family's tenant farm on the Kilkerran estate in Ayrshire.

family business in Dunfermline manufacturing table linen, just as one of McGrigor's two siblings entered the hosiery trade.

On the other hand, the price of placing the whole of the next generation in the professions could be that the family home was deserted, if there was no cosy local billet into which they could be tucked. John Riach's younger brother, we have seen, became an army major. Another, John Pringle, trained as a medic and entered the East India Company's service, dying at sea in 1860. For some years he was attached to the embassy in Persia and in 1836 became doctor to the Shah.[98] Evidently, Riach Snr thought respectability adequate compensation for the permanent lack of filial company. Many others would not have set their sights so high, nor thought the gain worth the candle. The Greaves were a landowning family with many branches that had long lived on the Staffordshire and Derbyshire border. One of William's paternal uncles, George (1747–1828), was a clergyman and the other, Robert Charles (1749- 1823), the land-agent and man of business of Sir Robert Burdett. His father, however, the Burton Brewer, the youngest of the three brothers, had very limited ambitions for his family and clearly did not want them to stray far from the family hearth. Dying young in 1784, he left instructions in his will how his young boys were to be prepared for a career. There were no specific instructions. His executors were merely empowered to release monies from his estate in trust 'as they shall think proper for the placing out of any child or children apprentice or apprentices to such trades or businesses as they shall think most advisable'.[99] In this and other cases, it would be interesting to know whether the children had any choice as to where they were placed. What is not surprising is that besides William only one of John Davies Greaves's five other sons has left any occupational trace.[100]

RELIGION

One other variable remains to be explored before we will have plumbed the background of our cohort as fully as possible: their religious affiliation. Discovering the religious allegiance of Britons before the mid-nineteenth century is even more difficult than uncovering their occupations, but enough information has been gleaned from the International Genealogical Index and other sources to give some indication of the confession in which the English and Irish surgeons were raised. Not surprisingly, as Table 2.11 reveals, the large majority were Protestant and had been brought up in the established Churches, although an important minority were Nonconformists of one kind or another. Unfortunately, very little is known

[98] *Perth Courier*, 17 May (1736), 3, col. 2.

[99] TNA, Prob 11/173, q. 176; **www.gravesfa.org/gen228.htm** (Sept. 2005); Georgiana Galbraith (ed.), *The Journal of the Rev. William Bagshaw Stevens* (Oxford, 1965), *passim*.

[100] This was John (1776–1823), who was also a Burton brewer: see *Victoria County History: Staffordshire*, vol. ix, pp. 66, 68.

Table 2.11. Confessional Allegiance Prior
to Entering Army

Confession	Number
Catholic	14
Church of England	25
Church of Scotland	2
Episcopalian (Scotland)	2
Independent (England)	3
Presbyterian (England)	4
Quaker (England)	1
Unidentified Protestant[a]	24
TOTAL	75
Percentage of cohort identified	16.51

[a] Protestants attending medical lectures at TCD, chiefly Irish: see nn. 101, 110 below.

Source: Doctors' Database: Table: Religion.

for certain about the religious allegiance of the Scottish contingent, but it seems reasonable to assume that they were little different.

Roman Catholic recruits were understandably almost exclusively Irish. Thanks chiefly to the information relating to religious persuasion given in the class lists of the medical faculty of Trinity College Dublin, we know the broad religious preference of thirty-seven of the ninety-five surgeons definitely born in the kingdom. Of these, thirteen were Catholics, more than a third. On the assumption that Protestants were more likely to train at Trinity than Catholics, especially Catholics from outside Leinster, then the true proportion was probably even higher.[101] Given George III's notorious reluctance to employ papist officers in the armed forces during the French wars, the Catholic presence among the Irish contingent is remarkably high, even if the number of Catholic regular officers was unofficially growing. It can only be assumed that the confessional purity of medical officers was thought to be of as little account as the religious allegiance of the army rank and file.[102]

[101] 29 of the sample appear in the TCD records, 10 of whom were Catholics, 19 Protestants: not all of the faculty registrands were born in Ireland: TCD, MS 758. The Trinity faculty of medicine only began to develop after 1790 and was deliberately non-confessional: see Ch. 3. Several other Irish surgeons were almost certainly Catholics, notably Eugene McSwiney of Cork City, whose will reveals that he owned property in Macroom, County Cork, where the McSwineys were a Catholic family, according to the 1766 census.

[102] Irish Catholics could be recruited as soldiers from the time of the War of American Independence and Catholic officers could serve with the army in Ireland from 1793. But no Catholic could officially be an officer in the British army in Britain during the wars. Attempts to lift the restriction were stymied by the king. Catholic officers did serve outside Ireland in the period but never officially. The number is unknown but they cannot have formed a large proportion of the officer corps. See J. R. Western, 'Note', *English Historical Review*, 70 (1955), 428–32; T. Bartlett, 'A Weapon of War Yet Untried: Irish Catholics and the Armed Forces of the Crown, 1760–1830', in T. G. Fraser and K. Jeffrey (eds.), *Men, Women and War* (Dublin, 1993). We have encountered no reference to religious affiliation in the official papers of the Army Medical Board.

Indeed, given the indeterminacy of religious allegiance in Ireland at the turn of the nineteenth century, some of the students who declared themselves to be Protestant may have been brought up as Catholics and were so-called prudential converts. One of the Trinity registrands—James William Macauley—certainly had a Catholic background: he was baptized at St Michael's Roman Catholic Church, Rosemary Lane, Dublin. James only became a Protestant (presumably a member of the Church of Ireland) because of family misfortune. Not only did his father die when he was three months old, but his mother passed away when he was 15 and he and his two sisters moved in with a maternal relative, William Armstrong. Armstrong was a director of Apothecary's Hall, Dublin, 1794–1819, and a devout Protestant, and seems to have had no difficulty in persuading James and his elder sister, Mary (b. 1780) to change their allegiance. Only his second sister, Catherine (b. 1781), remained true to Rome. She never married but moved in with William Callaghan, a retired druggist who belonged to the Church of Ireland, and his wife, a Quaker, and went on to found the Sisters of Mercy, paradoxically with money left her by her employer.[103]

Some Irish Catholics, too, may have providentially changed their faith when they entered the army. Gabriel Rice Redmond came from a Wexford gentry family, the Redmonds of Killygowan House (various spellings), who had held the adjacent townland (118 acres) about a mile from Oulart since the mid-seventeenth century. All the major facts about his life point to him being a Protestant. His background, his marriage—he married a lady from Dumfriesshire, Philadelphia Barbara Johnstone (1784–1848), in Minorca in 1801 according to the rites of the Church of England, and three of their six children were baptized in the Church of Ireland (St Peter's and Camden Street, Dublin)—and his burial with the rest of his family in Meelnagh or Millinagh churchyard, Co. Wexford. But the complexity of his pedigree suggest a residual, perhaps dominant, recusant loyalty. The army records reveal that Redmond was the son of John of Newtown (1737–1819) and Catherine Cooke (1745–1798).[104] According to the information on the tombstones, however, John's husband was Anne (Cooke?, 1743–1821). Catherine Cooke was married to his brother who had a name ominous to Protestant ears, Thomas Ignatius (1742–82). It seems possible then that Gabriel Rice tried to hide the fact that his father was a Catholic by claiming descent from his uncle, the owner of Killygowan House from 1780 on the death of his grandfather, Matthew (b. 1710), but who was in fact only his guardian. There again, his mother may have been a Protestant, whomever she married, since she was descended from Sir Richard Cooke, the Irish chancellor of the exchequer in the early seventeenth century. Thereby, Redmond, too, it should be noted, was distantly related to the duke

---

[103] Savage, *Catherine McAuley*, esp. 23–32, 64–70, 418–19. Sister Mary married a Protestant apothecary, William McAuley (or Macauley), of Presbyterian stock, in St Mark's (Church of Ireland), Dublin, in 1804. On her deathbed in 1827, she was reconciled to Rome.

[104] TNA, WO 42/39/053: birth certificate. One of a number of certificates presented to the War Office by his widow in seeking a pension.

of Wellington, for Cooke had married the daughter of Christopher Peyton, Irish auditor-general, while another Peyton daughter had married into the Colleys.[105]

Catholics, equally understandably, were not very visible among surgeons from England and Scotland. But there was at least one—Joseph Constantine Carpue. Carpue came from a family of London Catholics and was baptized at the chapel in Lincoln Inn Fields. Destined for the Church and sent to the English College at Douai to train, he eventually rebelled and tried his hand as a printer-publisher—his uncle was Thomas Lewis of Great Russell Street—and thought about becoming a lawyer and an actor before taking to medicine.[106] Yet, if there were few British Catholics, there were numerous Protestant Nonconformists. The religious background of thirty-three of the eighty-five surgeons definitely born in England and Wales has been uncovered, and eight or a quarter belonged to Protestant dissenting families. Joseph Brown of North Shields was the son of a Quaker; John Hanmer Sprague had been baptized at the Independent chapel in Bishop's Hull, near Taunton, on 18 May 1786; while John Mort Bunney belonged to a Newbury Presbyterian family. Christopher Alderson of Hull was also brought up as a Presbyterian. His grandfather (d. 1760) had been a dissenting minister at Lowestoft and his father, John, the Hull surgeon, steadfastly maintained the family tradition, as did initially his brothers in Norwich. Christopher, John's eldest son was baptized in the Presbyterian church at Whitby, while the names of his many other children appear in the register of the Bowl Alley Lane, Presbyterian or Unitarian chapel, in Hull, where the family worshipped. John never deviated from his religious allegiance, although he did purchase himself a family vault in the new churchyard attached to St Mary's Sculcoates, a village a mile to the north of the city undergoing development.[107] He put his sons through the Revd George Lee's Unitarian school in Hull and pointedly refused to take his turn in holding civic officers because he was a dissenter.[108]

It seems likely too that many of the Scottish surgeons were Episcopalians or other Nonconformists, especially among the large contingent from the north-east. McGrigor is a particularly likely candidate, given his father was originally a tenant

[105] Colley was the duke's middle name. Presumably, John became his guardian when Gabriel Rice was 14. John had his own son, John Cooke (1770–98), but he was murdered by the Irish rebels, thus making Gabriel Rice his heir. We are indebted to Miss Bride Roe of New Ross, Co. Wexford, and Mr Nicholas Furlong, Drinagh, Co. Wexford, for helping us unravel Redmond's genealogy. The article on Redmond in the *Journal of the Army Medical Corps*, 17 (1911), 542–6, says he was brought up in a Catholic milieu. His middle name 'Rice' further suggests a Catholic link; he is almost contemporaneous with Edmund Ignatius Rice of Waterford, founder of the Christian Brothers.

[106] *Proceedings of the Royal Society*, 66 (1846), 638: obit. Lewis, *c*.1750–1802, was probably a Catholic: his own father, William, had been at school with Alexander Pope: see Ian Maxted, *The London Book Trades, 1775–1800: A Preliminary Check List of Members* (Folkestone, 1977), 138.

[107] East Riding RO, PE46/4, burial Sculcoates 1792–1812, 1: leave given to Dr Alderson (as a dissenter) to construct two family vaults 27 feet by 9 feet at the north-west wall. Christopher was buried there on 11 Feb. 1829.

[108] Hull RO, BRL 2157: confirmation of Alderson's disqualification from serving as chamberlain, 30 Sept. 1814. Lee would later edit the *Rockingham* and was one of the chief promoters of the Hull Mechanics Institute.

of the duke of Gordon. So far, though, it has only been possible to identify two Episcopalians: the Edinburgh-born David Maclagan, presumably brought up by his mother's family, the Smeitons, and Alexander Lesassier, whose Hamilton relations did not belong to the kirk.[109] It has been equally difficult to differentiate Irish dissenters from members of the Church of Ireland.[110] But they too may have formed a respectable proportion of the total. So far, though, only two have been uncovered, both Presbyterians, the father of one of whom, Stewart Crawford, it will be recalled, was the long-serving minister at Strabane.

Arguably, then, at least a quarter of the cohort and perhaps as many as a third did not belong to the established Church in their respective countries. The recruits to the army medical service reflected the growing religious hetereogeneity of the British and Irish middle classes at the turn of the nineteenth century as much as their occupational diversity. In consequence, initially at any rate, many surgeons must have been as fish out of water in the officer's mess. Although the officer corps of the regular army in the French wars was no longer exclusively filled with the sons of gentry, it was scarcely an institution of the middling sort. Nor was it filled with dissenters. The religious background of many medical officers must have been an uncomfortable reminder to the English Tories in the mess in particular that nonconformity was beginning to challenge the religious establishment from within.[111] It would be interesting to know if the dissenters during the French wars found allies among the growing number of evangelicals in the officer corps, and to what extent the army suffered from the same divisions as beset the Church of England as a whole with the rise of Tractarianism in the 1820s and 1830s.

ENTERING THE SERVICE

The average army surgeon in the French wars came from the Celtic fringe, had a non-medical background, and was usually a younger son, in some cases a long way down the pecking-order. He was also sometimes a nonconformist. Only a few, moreover, came from families which had invested heavily in the professions in previous generations. These, too, families such as the Bigsbys, Keates, Estes, and Markhams, were predominantly English, even though the English were grossly under-represented within the service. Among the Irish recruits, only Stewart Crawford belonged to a professional dynasty, albeit a dissenting one, while the only Scot to have a grandfather and father in a profession was Alexander Lesassier,

[109] Norman L. Walker, *David Maclagan* (London, 1884), 32: this is a biography of one of Maclagan's sons; Rosner, 4.

[110] The TCD faculty of medicine matriculation register unhelpfully only distinguishes between Catholics and Protestants.

[111] Admittedly, the threat was theoretical rather than real. There is evidence that surgeons adopted the confessional clothes of their regimental messmates. All Carpue's children, for instance, were baptized into the Church of England, at St Anne's Soho.

who belonged to a family of medical practitioners on both sides. And he spent most of his early life in England.[112] Even George Gregory, who came from a distinguished line of Scottish episcopalian university professors, had been born in Canterbury. His father William had been reared in Edinburgh but had decided to pursue a career in the Anglican Church and join the elder branch of the family which had long been settled south of the border.[113] The large majority of surgeons, therefore, came from families who were either placing one or more sons in the professions for the first time, such as the McGrigors, or consolidating a first-generation professional status. Many, probably most, army surgeons, whether raised in the town or countryside, were professional parvenus leading or co-leading their families on a novel occupational journey.

To an important degree the cohort's background must have mirrored the wider medical profession's. Although there is no comparable prosopographical study of another group of early nineteenth-century medical practitioners, it would be surprising if the profession did not chiefly recruit from the middling sort, including the minor landowning families in Ireland and Scotland especially. Contemporaries certainly believed that it was a career eschewed by the peerage and the more affluent gentry. According to the army surgeon, Borland, aristocratic children, even younger sons, were put off by the rigorous moral demands of the profession.[114] Given, too, the contemporary assumption, endorsed by historians, that the profession was expanding rapidly in the first half of the nineteenth century in response to the growing popular demand for health care, it is highly unlikely that the majority of recruits were the sons of medical practitioners.[115] Many, too, must have come from Nonconformist backgrounds, given the anecdotal evidence. A number of famous practitioners in the period 1750–1850 were Nonconformists, notably the Quaker physicians, John Coakley Lettsom (1744–1815) and Thomas Hodgkin (1798–1866), after whom the glandular disorder is named. Doubtless, many were also younger sons, though this will be impossible to know until further comparative research has been done.

On the other hand, it is unlikely that the English were so under-represented in the British medical profession *tout court* in the first half of the nineteenth

[112] Lesassier's surgeon father was cold-shouldered by his Edinburgh grandfather, the man midwife, Alexander Hamilton (1739–1802), and forced to set up practice in Manchester: see Rosner, 4–12.

[113] The first member of the family to settle in England was the mathematician, David Gregory (1661–1708), who became Oxford's Savilian professor of astronomy in 1691. The founder of the family had been a Church of Scotland minister ejected from his living by the Covenanters: hence their Episcopalian allegiance.

[114] For this, read 'lack of social status'. See (Borland], 'The Life of Robert Jackson MD.', in Robert Jackson, *A View of the Formation, Discipline and Economy of Armies*, 3rd edn. (London, 1845), pp. xvii–xviii. Lisa Rosner, *Medical Education in the Age of Improvement: Edinburgh Students and Apprentices 1760–1826* (Edinburgh, 1991), 27–30, claims Edinburgh-trained physicians were 'genteel but not aristocratic' in the main. Her opinion, which she accepts is impressionistic, is based on information concerning 300 Edinburgh graduates in the years 1760–1805 whose father's occupation could be traced.

[115] Unfortunately, before the 1851 census, there are no precise figures: see P. J. Corfield, *Power and the Professions in Britain 1700–1850* (London, 1995), 157–9.

century.[116] Although it would be dangerous to assume that doctors practising in England in 1851—the first census year in which occupation was carefully recorded—were necessarily born there, the fact that they make up 80 per cent of the overall total surely indicates that a large majority of practitioners in the British Isles were English.[117] The fact, too, that the English habitually made up 50 per cent of the medical students attending Edinburgh, the one truly all-British medical school, in the first decade of the nineteenth century again suggests that the wider medical profession was not bursting at the seams with Scots and Irish during the French wars.[118] It would also be surprising to find that the general body of medical practitioners divided so neatly into two contrasting groups: recruits from the three capital cities and those from small towns and the countryside. Presumably, the geographical background of medical practitioners en masse mirrored much more closely the national and local distribution of the population.[119]

If the army medical service was distinctive in these respects, it would go a long way to explain why the cohort had joined up in the first place. The large majority of recruits entered the service in their late teens and early twenties immediately or almost upon completing their training (see Table 2.12). Only the few in the early stages of the war who moved straight into a staff position came from established civilian careers.[120] Indeed, even some of the officers who were directly appointed to senior staff positions (in the years before 1810 when this was still possible) were often wet behind the ears. Recruits were always supposed to be 21 years old before they could be accepted, but several were much younger than this.[121] George James Guthrie was a mere 15 when he became a mate at the York Hospital in 1800 and was an assistant regimental surgeon a year later; Alexander Lesassier, who joined in 1806 was only 18; while Robert Keate who had been appointed a hospital mate at 17 in 1794, celebrated his coming of age by being made a staff surgeon.[122]

Most tyro practitioners would never have thought of making such a daring move. It was a commonplace for the young doctor, once he had completed his

---

[116] Since the British Medical Association contained members from all three kingdoms until 1922, the term 'British' here can be legitimately used to include Irish practitioners.

[117] Corfield, *Power and the Professions*, 158 (Table 6.2 gives detailed figures for medical practitioners in the three kingdoms).   [118] *Nomina eorum qui gradum medicinae doctoris adelphi sunt.*

[119] The dominant position of the Celtic fringe in the army medical service continued until the late Victorian era, except the Irish provided an increasingly disproportionate number of recruits. In the 1860s and 1870s they formed 52.3 per cent of the intake, while the English still only commanded 27.2 per cent and the Scots a mere 9.2 per cent. In consequence, the Royal Army Medical Corps was known as the Irish Royal Army Medical Corps: see Nelson D. Lankford, 'The Victorian Medical Profession and Military Practice: Army Doctors and National Origins', *Bulletin of the History of Medicine*, 54 (1980), 511–28.

[120] See Table 4.1. Some staff surgeons continued to be appointed late in life, even after 1810. The Edinburgh professor of surgery, John Thomson, it will be recalled, was given an acting staff surgeoncy after the Battle of Waterloo and sent out to help organize the treatment of the wounded: see Ch. 1, n. 43.

[121] McGrigor only standardized the accepted position in 1816: see Ch. 1.

[122] Rosner, 6–7, 14, 37–8. Apparently the examiners did not always bother to ask candidates their age.

Table 2.12. Age of Entry to the Service

Age at entry	Number of surgeons
14	1
15	1
16	4
17	6
18	18
19	30
20	43
21	46
22	48
23	40
24	32
25	21
26	14
27	8
28	12
29	2
30	5
30–49	11
Unknown	113

Note: The date of birth of 112 of the 454 surgeons in the cohort is not known. The youngest recruit was the Irishman Robert Sheckleton (no. 57) and the oldest, Richard Henry Heurtley (no. 259), who was 49 when he became a hospital mate in 1813 and had been apprenticed to a surgeon of the same surname in Sheffield.

Source: Doctors' Database: Tables: Doctors; First (Dated) Army Appointment.

education, to return home. A medical practice large enough to keep body and soul together could only be launched through contacts, and, apart from the lucky few who had patrons elsewhere, only the intrepid would risk setting themselves up where they were unknown. Readers of George Eliot's *Middlemarch* will recall the essential role played by the banker Bulstrode in getting the outsider, Tertius Lydgate, accepted.[123] The better part of valour was to return to the family hearth and start out by becoming a locum to an ageing practitioner with a marriageable daughter.[124] For most young doctors military medical service can have had little attraction. Although as the war progressed, the pay and conditions improved, as the government attempted to entice recruits into both the army and navy, service always remained dangerous and arduous.[125]

[123] The novel was published in 1871–2 but set in Coventry in the early 1830s.
[124] Irvine Loudon, *Medical Care and the General Practitioner, 1750–1850* (Oxford, 1986), 29.
[125] See Ch. 1.

That our surgeons did not go home but chose to join the army becomes more understandable given their provenance. Too many came from unpromising parts of the United Kingdom. The chances of making a decent living in a small town or a village, especially in Ireland or even Scotland, where there were few affluent clients, must have seemed slim, however supportive one's family. Without the help of relatives who were medical practitioners, it would have been all but impossible to find a niche in a restricted market. Indeed, where the potential custom was very small, the presence of a medical relative may even have seemed a drawback, especially for those with a modicum of drive and ambition. The inducements of the service must have weighed particularly strongly when the alternative was curing a peasant's colic in County Kerry or lancing the boils of a burgher of Bawtry.[126]

Similarly pessimistic thoughts probably also lay behind the decision to volunteer of many of the army surgeons born in the three capital cities. At first sight, it might be thought that a young medical practitioner from London, Edinburgh, or Dublin, who knew the turf, would have had no difficulty in elbowing his way into the vibrant medical marketplace of his native city, whatever his contacts. This, though, may have been true of the metropolis and would help to explain why the number of medical officers who came from London was actually smaller than the numbers from the two other capitals, a tenth and a fifth of its size. Edinburgh and Dublin, on the other hand, Edinburgh in particular, were much more provincial and stuffy cities where contacts and pedigree continued to count and where the royal colleges still remained powerful institutions. It was hard to build up a practice in Edinburgh, if your face did not fit, as Alexander Lesassier would find when he was retired from the army after the Peninsular campaign.[127] In all three cities, moreover, it was probably the case that supply was outweighing demand, however buoyant, as more and more experienced outsiders flooded into the marketplace looking for lucrative pickings. Also, the growing importance of Edinburgh, Dublin, and London as centres of medical education during the French wars, when continental schools were closed to students from the British Isles, may well have encouraged more of their sons to train for the profession than the home market could bear.[128] As a result, many young metropolitan practitioners may have found the army medical service as comfortable a billet as their country cousins.

In some cases, too, the choice would only have been strengthened by a surgeon's religious allegiance. In England, many young doctors from unpromising backgrounds might have first risked setting up in 'foreign' territory rather than taking the king's shilling regardless of their religious persuasion. If the county and cathedral towns were dominated by the Anglican establishment and were unlikely to offer rich rewards, they could have always set up their plate in the booming commercial and industrial cities, including London, where nonconformity was well established. The fact, all the same, that a significant proportion of the small

[126] Loudun, *Medical Care*, 112–13, on the slim pickings in Scotland.
[127] Rosner, Chs. 9–11.   [128] For further information about this development, see Ch. 3.

English contingent did not belong to the established Church would suggest that the supply of Nonconformist medical practitioners was outrunning the demand. Too many Nonconformist fathers saw their sons as the next Lettsom. In Ireland and Scotland, on the other hand, there were far fewer openings for ambitious Nonconformists. In Ireland, Catholics can have had few opportunities to build up a lucrative practice outside Dublin, given the power of the Protestant (both Church of Ireland and Presbyterian) elites in the towns. In Scotland, the medical establishment was stolidly Church of Scotland and Tory. Scottish Episcopalians, too, might also find the English dislike of the migrant Scot stymied their chances if they tried to move south of the Tweed. Entering the army, then, must have seemed to many nonconformist Irish and Scots the obvious way of escaping from the material consequences of their confessional allegiance.

Of course, over time the 'pull' factor may have begun to play as great a part as the 'push' in attracting young medical practitioners from sleepy backwaters and over-medicalized capital cities into the army medical service. At the beginning of the French wars, not only did the army reward its medical officers poorly but no one could have known how long the conflict was going to last. Once war became the normal state of affairs and service became more attractive, however, many young men with limited prospects as civilian medical practitioners may have undertaken medical training in the knowledge that they could join the army or navy and make a decent career. This was certainly suggested by Thomas Speer in 1823: 'While the war raged, our Fleets and Armies required a constant and continued fund of Medical aid; and from the system on which the establishments of both were conducted, particularly that of the latter, talents and industry were sure to meet with their merits.' As a result, parents had been prompted to put their sons through a medical education: 'crowds flocked to the schools, went through their ordeal and entered the field.'[129] Presumably, then, after the war had lasted twenty years, many recruits must have started training on the eve of Wellington's rapid advance in the Peninsula on the assumption that the war would go on for ever and been initially disappointed when the military medical services were quickly run down in 1814 and again after Waterloo.[130] If so, the number of recruits coming from unpromising backgrounds may well have risen across the war as more and more young men chose a medical career as an escape route from the bounded horizons and limited opportunities of small-town and rural life.

This is not to say, of course, that every recruit to the army medical corps during the French wars came from a disadvantaged background or that a lack of prospects was the only factor encouraging surgeons to join up. Some definitely came from

---

[129] T. C. Speer, *Thoughts on the Present Character and Constitution of the Medical Profession* (Cambridge, 1823), 37–8. Speer, 39, then went on to complain that, whilst that demand had dried up, the same kinds of numbers were still flocking to receive a medical education, but with no employment for them on completion.

[130] In fact, many surgeons forced out of the service after the war went on to illustrious civilian careers: see Ch. 5.

wealthy families and were even elder sons. There was no obvious pecuniary reason why the Hull hospital physician, John Alderson, should have placed his first-born in the army. Admittedly, the Aldersons were dissenters, but there is no evidence that this had a detrimental effect on their social status in the city: John had been made a freeman in spite of his Nonconformity.[131] Other recruits, if relatively poorly off in their youth, were already well positioned when they decided to enter the service. Thus, John Davy of Penzance may have had the misfortune to lose his father early in life and been brought up by his widowed mother on limited means, but when he joined the army medical corps a few months before Waterloo there was again no economic reason for his choice. His elder brother, Humphry, was already a leading light of the Royal Institution, an FRS and a knight, while John himself, who had been his brother's laboratory assistant, had published a number of scientific articles under his own name. He could easily have set up in London.[132]

Alderson, Davy, and many others, advantaged and disadvantaged, presumably entered the service in part from a sense of duty. Whatever misgivings there might have been about the conflict among the middling sort in its early stages, the fight with France eventually came to be seen as a grim necessity. Once Napoleon was firmly in the saddle and the representative institutions of France and her satellite states effectively emasculated from 1804, the war became one around which conservative and reformer, Tory and Whig, established churchman, evangelical, or dissenter, all could rally. In the end, it became a great patriotic war, a struggle against tyranny. Many young surgeons must have joined up out of patriotism, regardless of their parents' or relatives' wishes.

William Dent for one certainly entered the service 'to do his bit', encouraged by the surgeon at St Thomas's, Sir Astley Cooper (1768–1841), with whom he was studying in London during the disastrous Corunna campaign.[133] In February 1809, Dent informed his mother that Knight, inspector-general of hospitals, had asked Cooper to send 'all the students that possibly can leave town, for to go to different districts to attend and dress the Sick and wounded soldiers that have arrived from Spain'. Cooper had encouraged everyone to go for a month or six weeks, partly as a humanitarian duty. Dent informed his mother that he was to leave for the garrison town of Colchester the following day, apologizing for not having had time to ask her permission: 'I beg your pardon for not asking your leave before I went, but as it is on such urgent business I hope you will be led to

---

[131] He became a freeman in 1813.

[132] Humphry was knighted in 1812; he had even been honoured by the French Institut for his discoveries by being made a corresponding member in December 1813. Through his brother, John was also part of the circle of Lakeland poets; Humphry, an enthusiastic versifier, had proof-read the 1798 *Lyrical Ballads*. The Institut was set up by the French Revolutionaries in 1795 to replace the Académie des Sciences founded by Louis XIV. Its members included the cream of Europe's experimental philosophers: see Maurice Crosland, *Science under Control: The French Academy of Sciences 1795–1814* (Cambridge, 1992), esp. Ch. 2.

[133] See Ch. 3 for the army surgeons' training in the London hospitals.

excuse me, and that my conduct will meet with the approbation of yourself and all my friends.'[134] The trainee surgeon enjoyed the experience and ended up serving in the military hospital at Colchester for about six months. It clearly influenced his decision to enter the service after he had taken his diploma at the Royal College of Surgeons. He knew that his mother wanted him to return home, but argued that his youth would prevent him from being able quickly to establish a civilian practice. He thus took the army exam and was duly posted to Portsmouth as a hospital mate, only telling his mother after the event. In a letter of 25th May 1810, in which he asked for another £10 for clothing, he merely expressed his belief that the news could not have come as a surprise to her.[135]

Patriotism alone, however, was probably seldom a sufficient motive.[136] As Dent's case makes clear, there was also a professional incentive in joining up. As he wrote to his mother in a letter of 5 March, the army provided much needed hands-on experience in dissecting. When a soldier died in the Colchester hospital, the body was turned over to the surgeons. In London, on the other hand, it was impossible to gain a body to anatomize for under three guineas.[137] More broadly, once safely ensconced in the army, he emphasized in a later letter that the service would not only give the young medic experience but be a good finishing school. 'I think the Army an excellent school for a young man, who has the desire to excell in either his profession or to become acquainted with the manners of the world.'[138]

John Murray of Turriff waxed even more lyrical about the professional benefits of army service. Writing home from Messina on 17 August 1809, he claimed that the workload in the local military hospital was heavy but the cases always interesting and instructive.

On every occasion in a large army but particularly on actual service the surgeons and medical men have the finest field for information open to them[;] in the space of a single month, they perhaps see more and get more experience (if they pay attention) than a man in private practice may during his whole life time[;] and I really think that after a young man has finished his first studies at the classics, the best school for getting experience is at the General Hospital of a large army, where disease is to be seen in every form, and where nothing is wanting that may be thought requisite for the cure.[139]

Doubtless an Alderson or a Davy would have concurred.

Davy, furthermore, might well have been specifically enticed into the army medical corps with the possibilities that it opened up for the pursuit of his interest

[134] WL, RAMC 536, no. 4, William Dent to his mother from London, 17 Feb. 1809.

[135] Ibid., no. 14, William Dent to his mother from London, 21 May 1810.

[136] Cf. the various motives for joining the Volunteers in Cookson, *The British Armed Nation*, esp. introd.

[137] WL, RAMC 536, no. 5. The lack of subjects for dissection in the country's medical schools encouraged body-snatching and eventually led to the 1832 Anatomy Act: Ruth Richardson, *Death, Dissection and the Destitute* (London, 1987).

[138] Ibid., no. 15, William Dent to his mother from Portsmouth, 24 June 1810.

[139] WL, RAMC 830, Murray to his father, 17 Aug. 1809. By the 'classics' he may mean the classical medical texts rather than works of classical literature.

in natural history.[140] Others may have been lured into the service in part simply by the prospect of seeing the world. The army after all offered young men from the lower middling sort the unprecedented opportunity to go on an extended Grand Tour. When John Murray of Turriff was based in the Mediterranean early in his career he took advantage of any chance to go sight-seeing. He ascended both Etna and Vesuvius and gained permission to go to the Lipari islands with four companions, where he ascended, with difficulty, another volcano, saw the local antiquities, and collected various local minerals to keep as souvenirs.[141]

At least one of our cohort, moreover, was on the run and joined up to escape a legal imbroglio. Stephen Panting came from a respectable family. His grandfather seems to have been a tenant farmer in Gloucestershire, but his father (b. 1733) was somehow sent to Balliol and became perpetual curate to the urban parish of Wellington, Shropshire, and sometime vicar of the neighbouring parishes of Wrockwardine and Wornbridge. His elder or twin brother, Lawrence (d. 1844), was in turn sent to St John's Cambridge where he was a fellow in the 1790s, while a younger brother, Thomas, became a solicitor. Stephen himself, born in 1767, seems to have worked in Lichfield after finishing his apprenticeship, where he acted as the locum for Garrick's ageing brother, Peter. Taking advantage of Peter's advancing years, he and Thomas seem to have defrauded the old man of £525. Garrick's sister took the pair to court, and Stephen took to his heels and covered his shame by taking the king's shilling in 1796.[142]

This said, though, the economic motive should not be pushed too far to one side in understanding how the majority of surgeons ended up in the service during the wars. As we shall see at the end of the following chapter, a number of recruits were directed to the army by their families, *faute de mieux*, even when they were the beneficiaries of patronage. Some, too, who entered of their own free will, did so because they had failed to make a go of civilian life. After McGrigor had finished his training, Dr George French, his old master and professor in Aberdeen, encouraged him to seek his fortune in London.[143] Although this move had his family's blessing, it turned out to be a poor decision. Despite an armful of recommendations, McGrigor was unable to set up in practice and ended up becoming an assistant to a surgeon in Islington, then a village to the north of the city. As he reported to his uncle, David Grant, the position was scarcely ideal: '[The surgeon]

140 Davy published an important account of Ceylon in 1821. See Ch. 1, for McGrigor's enthusiasm for using the service for gathering data about the flora and fauna of foreign stations.

141 WL, RAMC 830, Murray to his brother, 24 Sept. 1809. The contemporary interest in volcanoes was huge, epitomized by the enthusiasm of Sir William Hamilton, the long-serving British ambassador to Naples: see David Constantine, *Fields of Fire: A Life of Sir William Hamilton* (London, 2001), *passim*.

142 Merrial Docksey, *The Trial between Mrs Docksey (Sister of the Late David Garrick) Plaintiff and Stephen Panting of the City of Lichfield, Apothecary* (1796). According to Foster, 1063, Panting's grandfather was registered as being a plebeian when his father matriculated at Oxford. Both Stephen and Lawrence were baptized on 17 June 1767 at Wellington.

143 Professor of chemistry at Marischal College, 1793–1833 (when he died).

is an old gentleman and the first man in this place ... but what with ye gout ... he lets a good deal of his practice evolve on me. The salary with bed, board, and lodging which he allows me is reckoned equal to be £70 per annum—not much here.'[144] The ambitious young Scot looked around for other openings and decided to take advantage of the fact that new regiments were being formed in the early years of the war. He negotiated the purchase of a surgeoncy with the army agents, Cox and Greenwood. Probably the first thing that his family knew of this decision was when he wrote to his father, asking him to send a bill to cover the cost.

In conclusion, then, most of the cohort primarily volunteered for army service because they were relatively disadvantaged compared with other entrants to medical marketplace. Pushed or pulled, our practitioners preferred becoming a medical officer with its good pay and chance of mixing with better-off regular officers to immediately entering civilian practice where the prospects were limited, wherever they set up.[145] One army surgeon not in the cohort with a particularly unfortunate background could have done little else. This was James Miranda Barry (?1794–1865), the nephew of the querulous painter, James Barry (1741–1806).[146] Barry was Irish, a Catholic, poor and illegitimate: his mother was Mary Ann Bulkley née Barry and his father, probably, the Latin American exile, General Francisco de Miranda.[147] To add to these disadvantages, James was also a woman, a fact only discovered when she died. The deception was the invention of his mother, who seems to have decided to solve her pecuniary difficulties—her husband had gone bankrupt—by turning her daughter into a professional gentleman. Having moved to London to seek help from her brother the artist but to no avail, Mary Ann seems to have convinced David Steuart Erskine, earl of Buchan, that James, conveniently presented as five years younger than he was, was a child prodigy. Buchan therefore financed the child through medical school, sending him to Edinburgh when he was supposedly only 10 years old and forcing a reluctant Senate to grant him a degree two years later. Spring 1813 found James walking the wards in London, but a few months later he was in the army, was gazetted as a hospital assistant, then posted to Plymouth, where Joseph Skey, at that date physician to the forces, complained about his youthful appearance. Presumably, the army was the best place for a slightly built female medical practitioner with a high voice to hide: James, purportedly still under 14 years old,

[144] McGrigor, 18–19, 22–3, 30–2. McGrigor's time in Islington is fully discussed in the editor's introduction and not in the autobiography itself, where he merely notes that he went to London, in part because his mother did not want him to go abroad.

[145] Lankford (see n. 119 above) reached much the same conclusion in his study of the national origins of army medical officers in the second half of the nineteenth century. By the late Victorian era, however, there were many more outlets for disadvantaged medics—as poor-law doctors and doctors employed by friendly societies and workingmen's clubs. There was also much greater opportunity to relocate in the empire. The choices of practice open to medics is discussed in M. Jeanne Peterson, *The Medical Profession in Mid-Victorian London* (Berkeley and Los Angeles, 1978), Ch. 3.

[146] Barry became a member of the Royal Academy but was eventually expelled.

[147] For this colourful character see David Sinclair, *Sir Gregor MacGregor and the Land that Never Was* (London, 2003).

could hardly bring home the bacon as a civilian practitioner, while the services were full of boy officers in their mid-teens. Presumably, too, Buchan encouraged the Army Medical Board to accept the young imposter, whatever their qualms about breaking the rule that entrants should be a minimum age of 21.[148]

Barry's case is instructive in more ways than one. However disadvantaged by her sex and origins, she was clearly well educated. So, too, as we will see in the following chapter, was virtually every entrant to the army medical service during the French wars. Although there was no attempt to lay down a detailed educational programme that candidates were expected to have followed before McGrigor's pronouncement of 1816, army medical officers in the 1790s and 1800s were as well if not better qualified than doctors immediately entering civilian practice.[149] It was their background not their ignorance that made them chary of entering the medical marketplace. The army might have had difficulty finding recruits, especially in the first part of the war, but it did not have to accept the dregs of the profession, although some contemporaries wrongly implied this was so.[150]

---

[148] June Rose, *The Perfect Gentleman: The Remarkable Life of Dr James Miranda Barry, the Woman who Served as an Officer in the British Army from 1813 to 1859* (London, 1977), esp. 18–30. This is the best of many historical and fictional accounts of Barry's life. Our interpretation of Mary Ann's behaviour is our own. Rose, ignoring Barry's age on her gravestone in Kensal Green cemetery, treats James as a prodigy. For his service record, see Drew, no. 3632.

[149] For McGrigor's promotion of educational standards, see Ch. 1.   [150] See Ch. 3.

3

Education

MEDICAL EDUCATION IN EARLY NINETEENTH-CENTURY BRITAIN

One of the most crucial aspects of a nascent medical practitioner's early education was instruction in the classics. It was a long-established precept, from R. Campbell in *The London Tradesman* in 1747, through Robert Hamilton's *Duties of a Regimental Surgeon Considered* of 1787, to the pseudonymous Aesculapius's *Hospital Pupil's Guide*, published in 1818, that doctors should know Latin and Greek.[1] During the Royal Commission on the Scottish Universities in 1826, as Michael Moss and Derek Dow have outlined, much discussion took place as to the degree of classical knowledge required by candidates for the MD. Some promoted the idea that all medical students should have previously taken an MA and recommended an improved grounding in classics and languages. However, others feared that such stipulations would drive away students, cause a decline in numbers, and thereby make the institution less attractive to the best medical professors.[2] Nevertheless, most believed some classical education necessary to enable a full understanding of medical history and terminology.

Having completed schooling, a student would then usually be indentured to a medical practitioner for a number of years. Recent scholars have shown that apprenticeship remained crucial as a staple of medical education despite, from the mid-eighteenth century, both increasing attacks on the system and, perhaps more importantly, competition presented by the new London teaching hospitals, the fast-growing Edinburgh medical faculty, and, for the affluent, the medical Grand Tour. However, it became the accepted wisdom that an apprenticeship should precede formal medical instruction.[3] This was already evident by 1747, in

---

[1] R. Campbell, *The London Tradesman* (London, 1747), 50–1; R. Hamilton, *The Duties of a Regimental Surgeon Considered*, 2 vols. (London, 1787), ii. 288–9; Aesculapius, *The Hospital Pupil's Guide, being Oracular Communications Addressed to Students of the Medical Profession* (London, 1818), 20–6.

[2] Derek Dow and Michael Moss, 'The Medical Curriculum at Glasgow in the Early Nineteenth Century', *History of Universities*, 7 (1988), 231–2.

[3] See, for example, J. Lane, 'The Role of Apprenticeship in Eighteenth-Century Medical Education', in W. F. Bynum and R. Porter, *William Hunter and the Eighteenth-Century Medical World* (Cambridge, 1985), ch. 3; Susan C. Lawrence, *Charitable Knowledge: Hospital Pupils and Practitioners in Eighteenth-Century London* (Cambridge, 1996), 96, 112; and Irvine Loudon, *Medical Care and the General Practitioner, 1750–1850* (Oxford, 1986), 35.

Campbell's recommendation of a course of training consisting of five years under the tuition of a master before a year at Edinburgh, attending classes in anatomy and materia medica, and one in Paris, walking the wards at the hospitals and studying midwifery.[4]

The expansion of formal medical education, reflecting broader trends of improved educational facilities and increasing professionalization in the Enlightenment period, was enhanced when continental hospitals and universities became closed to prospective British students during the Napoleonic wars. Institutions and individuals took advantage of the new market opportunities and the number of medical lectures on offer increased substantially. By the end of the wars not only the University of Edinburgh but also the University of Glasgow and Trinity College Dublin were running courses in a wide range of subjects open to all those who wished to study.[5] Over the same period, a comprehensive programme of instruction came to be established at the Dublin College of Surgeons, and other courses of lectures were put on under the auspices of the London and Edinburgh colleges.[6] In addition, increasing numbers of doctors unaffiliated to the universities and colleges began to build on earlier initiatives and provide private lectures, especially those attached to the leading London teaching hospitals.[7] Some of these were given on the grounds of the institutions, but doctors at St George's, the Middlesex, and the Westminster held classes off the premises until the 1830s. Many doctors, too, had their private lecture theatres, modelled on the Great Windmill Street academy, set up by the famous man-midwife, William Hunter (1718–83), brother of the anatomist and army surgeon, John.[8]

[4] Campbell, *London Tradesman*, 52. In the eighteenth century, Paris was the centre of European surgery: see esp. Toby Gelfand, *Professionalizing Modern Medicine: Paris Surgeons and Medical Science and Institutions in the Eighteenth Century* (Westport, Conn., 1980).

[5] For Edinburgh University, see Sir A. Grant, *The Story of the University of Edinburgh, during its First Three Hundred Years*, 2 vols. (London, 1884); Lisa Rosner, *Medical Education in the Age of Improvement: Edinburgh Students and Apprentices, 1760–1826* (Edinburgh, 1991); C. J. Lawrence, 'The Edinburgh Medical School and the End of the "Old Thing" 1790–1830', *History of Universities*, 7 (1988), 259–86. For Glasgow University, see J. Coutts, *A History of the University of Glasgow, from its Foundation in 1451 to 1909* (Glasgow, 1909); Dow and Moss, 'Medical Curriculum at Glasgow', *passim*. For Trinity College Dublin, see R. B. McDowell and D. A. Webb, *Trinity College Dublin, 1592–1952: An Academic History* (Cambridge, 1982).

[6] For the College of Surgeons in Dublin, see Sir C. Cameron, *History of the Royal College of Surgeons in Ireland, and of the Irish Schools of Medicine* (Dublin, 1886); J. D. H. Widdess, *The Royal College of Surgeons in Ireland and its Medical School, 1784–1966* (Dublin, 1966). For the College of Surgeons in London, see C. Wall, *The History of the Surgeons' Company, 1745–1800* (London, 1937); Z. Cope, *The Royal College of Surgeons of England: A History* (London, 1959).

[7] See Lawrence, *Charitable Knowledge, passim*; Susan C. Lawrence, 'Entrepreneurs and Private Enterprise: The Development of Medical Lecturing in London, 1775–1800', *Bulletin of the History of Medicine*, 63 (1988), 171–92.

[8] Lawrence, 'Entrepreneurs and Private Enterprise', 182–3; Lawrence, *Charitable Knowledge*, 191–3. For these hospitals, see J. Blomfield, *St George's, 1733–1933* (London, 1933); G. C. Peachey, *The History of St George's Hospital* (London, 1910–14); H. S. Saunders, *The Middlesex Hospital, 1745–1948* (London, 1949); Sir W. J. E. Wilson, *The History of the Middlesex Hospital during the First Century of its Existence* (London, 1845); J. G. Humble and P. Hansell, *Westminster Hospital, 1716–1966* (London, 1966); J. Langdon-Davies, *Westminster Hospital: Two Centuries of Voluntary*

One of the key aspects of the new formal, medical education, and one of the most notable developments of the second half of the eighteenth century was the practice of walking the wards. Susan Lawrence has calculated that at least 5,921 students signed up to gain experience in London hospitals between 1763 and 1805, and Lisa Rosner has shown that, of the 7,784 men who matriculated at Edinburgh between those dates, 4,966 registered to walk the wards at the Royal Infirmary.[9] Students could gain the practical experience available in such establishments in a number of capacities. The first to learn on the wards were those apprenticed to hospital surgeons, but these increasingly became supplemented by pupils who desired further experience having already served an apprenticeship.[10] Walking pupils attended rounds, visited patients, watched operations and dissections, and, unlike apprentices, were affiliated to and charged by the hospital as a whole rather than an individual surgeon.[11]

The prosopographical data available in the service returns in the National Archives make it possible to conduct a thorough investigation into the way in which a group of medical students conducted themselves through and negotiated this myriad of educational opportunities. Much of the secondary literature has relied on anecdotal material, whilst thorough statistical examination has been restricted to research into particular institutions, namely Rosner's work on Edinburgh University and Lawrence's study of London hospitals. However, the information gathered on the training of army medical practitioners makes it possible to track the educational profile of individuals in detail and to collate key information on apprenticeships, hospital experience, and lecture courses together with the attainment of degrees, diplomas, and other qualifications. Crucially, this allows investigation of the dominant contemporary viewpoint that, until the end of the Napoleonic wars, those medical practitioners who opted for service in the armed forces were poorly trained.

This judgement was particularly promoted by the Edinburgh surgeon, John Bell (1763–1820). In his *Memorial Concerning the Present State of Military and Naval Surgery* of 1800, presented to the first lord of the Admiralty, the second

Service, 1719–1948 (London, 1952). For the teaching hospitals, see V. C. Medvei and J. L. Thornton (eds.), *The Royal Hospital of St Bartholomew, 1123–1973* (London, 1974); F. G. Parsons, *The History of St Thomas's Hospital*, 3 vols. (London, 1932–6); E. M. McInnes, *St Thomas's Hospital* (London, 1963); H. C. Cameron, *Mr Guy's Hospital, 1726–1948* (London, 1954); S. Wilks and G. T. Bettany, *A Biographical History of Guy's Hospital* (London, 1892); A. E. Clark-Kennedy, *The London: A Study in the Voluntary Hospital System*, 2 vols. (London, 1962–3); W. Morris, *A History of the London Hospital* (London, 1926); G. Risse, *Hospital Life in Enlightenment Scotland: Care and Teaching at the Royal Infirmary of Edinburgh* (Cambridge, 1986).

[9] Lawrence, *Charitable Knowledge*, 108, citing L. Rosner, 'Students and Apprentices: Medical Education at Edinburgh University, 1760–1810', Ph.D. dissertation (John Hopkins University, 1986), 394. For the Royal Infirmary in Edinburgh, see A. Logan Turner, *Story of a Great Hospital: The Royal Infirmary of Edinburgh, 1729–1929* (Edinburgh, 1937).

[10] M. E. Fissell, *Patients, Power and the Poor in Eighteenth-Century Bristol* (Cambridge, 1991), 26–8; Lawrence, *Charitable Knowledge*, 110–34.

[11] Fissell, *Patients, Power and the Poor*, 128; Lawrence, *Charitable Knowledge*, 124–5.

Earl Spencer, Bell argued that it was only the doctor whose lack of educational opportunities had prevented him from securing a lucrative civilian practice who was opting for this unattractive career path: 'he . . . enters at once into the service from hard necessity and the difficulty of pursuing his studies; he enters, my Lord, into the public service, not from enthusiasm for that service, but in despair.'[12] According to many accounts, all this changed once Sir James McGrigor took control of the Army Medical Board in 1815. For example, the antiquarian and surgeon, T. J. Pettigrew (1791–1865) in his biography of McGrigor in his *Medical Portrait Gallery* of 1840 praised the director-general for having had 'the great satisfaction of having introduced to the army a body of medical officers, of much higher attainments than it ever before possessed'. Apparently, McGrigor had demanded qualifications that surpassed even those required by the Royal Colleges of Surgeons and Physicians.[13] Moreover, this narrative was greatly bolstered by the director-general himself, who claimed in his autobiography to have aimed to give the nation's brave soldiers the medical care they deserved. As a result, at the time of writing, he could declare that 'in the ranks of the medical officers of the army men are to be found upon a level at least with those in the colleges of physicians and surgeons of London, Edinburgh and Dublin'.[14]

Bell's jeremiad, however, must be placed in its context. Along with a number of other surgeons, including that thorn in the army medical department's flesh, Robert Jackson, he was anxious that the state establish a specific army medical school that would 'breed men worthy of being employed'.[15] The obvious way to shock the state into action was to claim that the soldiers were being looked after by a bunch of incompetents. The tactic worked with the 1808 Parliamentary Commission of Enquiry who called for just such a school. On the other hand, the fact that the state took no notice of their lobbying, beyond the foundation of the chair of military surgery at Edinburgh in 1806 and the decision, the year before, to subsidize the continuing hospital training of a certain number of recruits to the service, provided they promised to serve a stipulated amount of time in the army, would suggest that the government thought the argument exaggerated.[16]

Certainly, entrants to the army medical corps in the period under scrutiny had no educational provision beyond what was on offer for those destined for civilian medical careers. However, *pace* Bell, the findings of this study reveal that, far from having limited access to or taking limited advantage of the existing educational opportunities, army surgeons were remarkably well educated. Admittedly, the

[12] J. Bell, *Memorial Concerning the Present State of Military and Naval Surgery* (Edinburgh, 1800), 16. Sir Neil Cantlie, *A History of the Army Medical Department*, 2 vols. (Edinburgh, 1974), *passim*, esp. vol. i, p.180, reinforces this view.
[13] T. J. Pettigrew, *Medical Portrait Gallery: Biographical Memoirs of the Most Celebrated Physicians, Surgeons etc. Who Have Contributed to the Advancement of Medical Science*, 4 vols. (London, 1840), iv. 9.
[14] McGrigor, 81.
[15] Bell, *Memorial*, 6–7. Robert Jackson, *A System of Arrangement and Discipline for the Medical Department of Armies* (London, 1805), 76. [16] See Ch. 1.

drop in demand for army surgeons with the end of the Napoleonic wars did enable McGrigor and the board to tighten up their appointments policy. Admittedly, too, those who sat for the exam at the Army Medical Board before 1815 did not have to be the most rigorously educated or most thoroughly qualified. Sheer demand meant that the examiners' requirements were fairly relaxed.[17] Nonetheless, the cohort had undertaken a respectable amount of training before entering the army. Many had those qualifications later to be demanded by McGrigor, and it would seem that his regulations rather supported and promoted current practice than instituted an entirely new regime. Most of the cohort undertook apprenticeships, walked the wards, attended courses at universities such as Edinburgh and listened to private lectures, investing a considerable amount of time and money in their education.

SCHOOLING

It is only possible to ascertain the locations where thirteen of the cohort were schooled and details of specific institutions for eleven. The schooling of at least two of the cohort, Robert Keate and McGrigor, supports Irvine Loudon's claim that the typical medical practitioner was the grammar school boy.[18] Keate was sent to King Edward's School in Bath by his father, then rector of Laverton and canon of Wells, whilst McGrigor attended Robert Gordon's School in Aberdeen. A further two of the cohort attended elite Anglican establishments. Like his brothers, George Gregory attended the King's School, Canterbury, entering in 1797 and becoming a King's scholar in 1799. He was sent by his father who was both Master of Eastbridge Hospital in the city and one of the six preachers of the cathedral. George Paulet Morris attended Westminster School from 1770 onward, where his father, Michael, a physician at Westminster Hospital, had also been educated in the 1730s.[19] Alexander Lesassier, on the other hand, attended the non-denominational Manchester Free School, while Joseph Constantine Carpue, a descendant of a Spanish Catholic family, was educated at the Catholic English College in Douai, and Joseph Brown and Christopher Alderson at Unitarian schools.[20] The Irishman, Edward Walsh, was also sent abroad to be educated, for he attended an unnamed boarding school in England, where his father thought he would a receive a better classical education than in Waterford.[21] The schooling of another handful of the cohort can also be guessed at. It can be assumed that John Riach attended the Perth Academy and William Wallace the

[17] See Ch. 1.   [18] Loudon, *Medical Care*, 34.
[19] G. F. Russell Barker and A. H. Stenning, *The Record of Old Westminsters*, 2 vols. (London, 1928), ii. 667.
[20] V.G. Plarr, *Plarr's Lives of the Fellows of the Royal College of Surgeons of England*, 2 vols. (London, 1930), i. 196.
[21] *Dublin University Magazine*, 3 (1834), 63: 'Memoir of the Late Edward Walsh MD'.

military school at Great Marlow, where their fathers were masters. It can also be surmised that Charles Boutflower was educated by his father at home in Seamer in Yorkshire. As there is evidence that John Boutflower took in pupils and schooled them in Latin, Greek, and French, it seems logical to assume that he would have also overseen the education of his own sons.[22]

Despite the limited evidence, however, it can be assumed that the large majority of army surgeons would have had a good classical education. Even before McGrigor in 1816 made a knowledge of Latin and Greek a prerequisite for entry, there are signs that the board expected recruits to have studied the classical humanities. Thomas Backhouse for one was refused the position of surgeon's mate in 1811 for not having attended regular classical lectures and was initially forced to accept the role of dispenser instead.[23] Some doctors also emphasized their classical learning on their service returns. Thomas Rolston included a letter to McGrigor with his form, dated 28 May 1818, in which he proudly noted that he had studied both Latin and Greek before becoming a medical practitioner, enabling him to consult ancient texts on the subject. He even stated that he was in the process of reading Hippocrates and was comparing him with contemporary writings.[24]

Furthermore, many doctors showed their proficiency in the classics in their later publications, where they quoted frequently from the ancients in the original.[25] In addition, the fact that 102 of the cohort obtained a degree from Edinburgh University, as will be discussed later in the chapter, shows that a considerable proportion must have become highly adept in the Classics. This institution not only required graduates to undertake written and oral exams in Latin, but also to write and publicly defend a thesis in the language.[26] William Gibney, who obtained his MD from Edinburgh in 1813, had received a good classical training as a child, his mother and uncle having decided after the death of his father that his education should be 'thorough and liberal'. According to his memoirs, he attended an excellent school which his mother could scarcely afford and turned down the opportunity to join "a large mercantile house" in order to stay there and devote 'more time than hitherto to study, and acquiring a fair acquaintance with Latin, Greek, French, Euclid and Algebra; in fact, in all those things which at that time were considered in the term "a liberal education". This, together with his own reading, apparently set him up for the thesis and exams required for his MD. Although the prospect of facing 'six learned Professors' in the oral exam was still daunting, 'I found the replying in Latin not a very difficult task. I spoke fairly, fluently, grammatically, and correctly, and more than once inwardly felt grateful for the good grounding I had obtained at school.' Once he had passed, Thomas Charles Hope (1766–1844), professor of chemistry, congratulated him on a

[22] D. S. Boutflower, *The Complete Story of a Family of the Middle Class Connected with the North of England (1303–1930)* (Newcastle, 1930), 87. [23] TNA, WO25/3904, fo. 22.
[24] TNA, WO25/3904, fo. 144. [25] See Ch. 7.
[26] Grant, *University of Edinburgh*, i. 329–32.

good examination and on his diligence as a student of the University, 'especially commending my knowledge of the classics'.[27]

A small number of the cohort even took an arts degree at university. Nineteen obtained a masters from a Scottish institution, mostly from Aberdeen. McGrigor qualified for his MA at Marischal College in 1788, sixteen years before being awarded his MD by the same institution. Theodore Gordon obtained a masters degree from Edinburgh and then went on to undertake a medical education at Aberdeen whilst John Mair, later to be awarded an MD from Edinburgh, qualified for his MA at King's College, Aberdeen, in 1815. Benjamin Haywood Browne was the only surgeon in the cohort who did not obtain his MA from a Scottish University, qualifying instead at Merton College, Oxford, in 1795, where he had been awarded a BA three years previously. Another six of the cohort also qualified for a Bachelor of Arts at Trinity College Dublin before going on to further study.[28]

APPRENTICESHIP

Like most of those intended for the medical profession, the large majority of the cohort went on to become apprentices once their schooling was complete.[29] Apprenticeship details for 381 men are known, 83.9 per cent of the total number studied. Thus, although the Army Medical Board did not make apprenticeship obligatory, it does seem to have been accepted as a standard element of training for the army medical practitioner.[30] Certainly, those who had not been apprentices felt obliged to explain themselves. Michael Fogerty cited a 'near relative' in County Tipperary in the section of his return concerned with details of apprenticeship, but stated that he had not been indentured. However, he assured the board that 'Dr. Fogerty' had taught him anatomy and surgery and given him access to a dispensary before he had gone on to continue his studies in Dublin.[31] Alexander Broadfoot similarly admitted that he had not served an apprenticeship but claimed that he had studied his profession as an autodidact. He recorded that he had read anatomical and other medical books as well as studying the human skeleton and practical pharmacy.[32]

The data collected supports the view of most historians that the normal age for starting an apprenticeship was between 14 and 16 (Figure 3.1).[33] Of those doctors

[27] Gibney, 4–6, 75–80.

[28] In Scottish universities the MA was the first degree, at Oxbridge and Dublin the BA.

[29] At least one continued his schooling while apprenticed. Charles Clarke, who seems to have come from somewhere in Munster, revealed on his pro forma that he continued to be privately tutored in classics while indentured in Waterford: TNA, WO25/3904, fo. 37.

[30] As seen in Ch. 1, after 1815 the Army Medical Board demanded hospital practice for at least one year if the candidate had served a regular apprenticeship. Otherwise, they should have walked the wards for two years and done a year's practical pharmacy.   [31] TNA, WO25/3909, fo. 49.

[32] TNA, WO25/3911, fo. 13.

[33] See, for example, Lane, 'Role of Apprenticeship', 65, 72; Lawrence, *Charitable Knowledge*, 112–13; Rosner, *Medical Education*, 88. Campbell, *London Tradesman*, 52, advises that apprenticeship should start at either age 15 or 16.

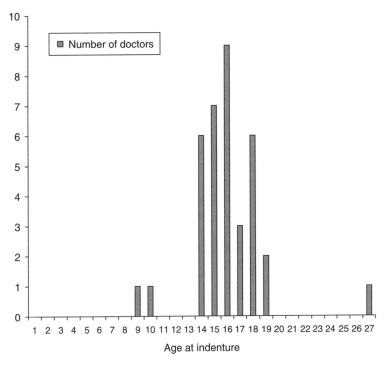

Figure 3.1. Age at Indenture

Source: Doctors' Database: Tables: Doctors; Apprenticeship.

for whom both date of birth and the year in which they were indentured are known, the youngest to have become an apprentice was Thomas Jackson at the age of 9, whilst Samuel Jeyes was remarkably old at 27 and much more so than the next eldest; 16.7 per cent were aged 14, 19.4 per cent were 15, but the largest percentage (25) was formed by those aged 16. The rest, apart from Jeyes, Jackson, and another boy, who was indentured at the age of 10, were 17, 18 or 19. Similarly, the typical period of indenture agreed upon by the masters and fathers conforms with the estimates of historians such as Lawrence that the norm was to serve something between five and seven years (Figure 3.2).[34] The majority of the contracts for which full details have been gathered, totalling thirty-nine, specify periods of either five (41 per cent) or seven years (43.6 per cent).

However, the information gathered also shows the frequent discrepancy between these figures and the period of time actually served with the master. Of those thirty-nine for whom full details of their contracts have been ascertained, at least thirteen served between one and three years less than had been stipulated, whilst

[34] Lawrence, *Charitable Knowledge*, 112. Also see Lane, 'Role of Apprenticeship', 72, and Fissell, *Patients, Power and the Poor*, 49.

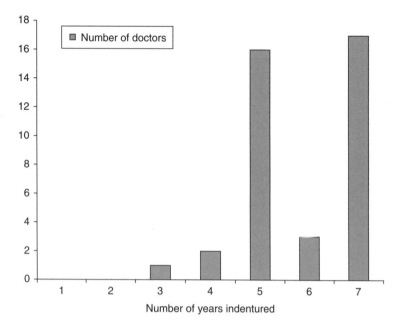

Figure 3.2. Number of Years Indentured
Source: Doctors' Database: Table: Apprenticeship.

two stayed with their master for a year longer than was technically required. Indentures were not cast in stone and disruptions could and did occur, whether due to the desertion of the apprentice or the master's inability to retain his services. Michael Gallagher felt compelled to explain why he had undertaken no less than three apprenticeships. He wrote on his service return that his first master, a man named Gallagher in Limerick (presumably a relation), had become a paralytic and that his second indenture to Drs Allen and Campbell, two surgeon-apothecaries in County Longford, had ended when their partnership had been dissolved. He had then completed his early training with Francis Smuth, an apothecary in Dublin.[35] In some instances, surgeons were less honest about broken indentures and brief apprenticeships for professional reasons, complicating the data gleaned from their service returns. For example, Lesassier recorded on his return that he had spent five years with Joseph Collier, a Quaker surgeon in Manchester, and had undertaken a further period of apprenticeship with his uncle, James Hamilton.[36] He failed to note that he had broken his indenture with Collier after escalating rows. A stroll with Collier's daughter had resulted in Lesassier being thrown out of the house for two days before he began an affair with one of the servants in the kitchen, risking being obliged 'to board & lodge

[35] TNA, WO25/3910, fo. 62.   [36] TNA, WO25/3905, fo. 85.

somewhere else'. Things came to a head when Lesassier became great friends with another medical student, named Joseph Jordan, and the two rented a cottage for anatomical dissections. Collier frowned on both their relationship and their activities, disapproving of Lesassier's late hours and concerned that his student would filch his supplies. A row led to Lesassier taking 'the bold decisive step' of leaving his master for good. Equally, although Hamilton had provided accom-modation, forwarded money, and given general support whilst his nephew had been in Edinburgh, he had never been his master. Lesassier was presumably prompted to conceal the truth after both the Army Medical Board and Royal College of Surgeons in London had expressed surprise at the brevity of his educa-tional experience when enlisting him into the army. In a meeting preliminary to his first exam, the clerk of the inspector-general of hospitals wanted to see the indentures of his apprenticeship and then, to Lesassier's consternation, asked how much of the period he had served. He had to admit that it had only been about a year and a half, but, rather than confess to a breakdown of relations, claimed that 'my master left town & my father would not allow me to follow him'.[37]

Lesassier had been indentured to Collier at the age of 16 for five years, costing his uncle the sum of £100.[38] Prices paid by the forty doctors in the cohort for whom the price of their indenture is known vary widely, from a few pounds to some hundreds of pounds (see Figure 3.3). The largest group paid £50 or less for their indenture (40 per cent) and the next largest was charged between £51 and £100 (32.5 per cent). This is not dissimilar to the findings of Joan Lane, who noted that most eighteenth-century masters charged between £60 and £84.[39] A number of our surgeons were apprenticed to members of the Royal College of Surgeons in Edinburgh, a privilege that usually cost either £50 to £60 for five years or £30 to £50 for three years.[40] For example, James Buchan paid William Inglis £50 for five years of training in 1786; John Carnegie was charged £60 by John Bell for the same period ten years later; whilst Adam Neale's three-year apprenticeship to James Russell (1754–1836), starting in 1792, cost £31. However, there were some masters who could charge extremely large premiums, particularly if they held positions at important hospitals in London.[41] In 1834, Sir Astley Cooper (1768–1841), surgeon at St Thomas's, suggested £500 to £600 as a suitable fee for an apprentice lodging and boarding in the house of a surgeon to a hospital for six or seven years and between £300 and £400 if not resident.[42] The conclusion may be drawn that the doctors in this cohort were apprenticed to well-established and respectable but not the most expensive masters, confirming the conclusion of the previous chapter that they came in the main from the lower middling sort. Only three paid £200 or more for their apprenticeships. The most costly indentures were entered into by Titus Berry of Halesworth, Suffolk, who

[37] Rosner, 16–20, 27–8, 34.　　[38] Rosner, 15.　　[39] Lane, 'Role of Apprenticeship', 70.
[40] Rosner, *Medical Education*, 88.
[41] Loudon, *Medical Care*, 42; Lane, 'Role of Apprenticeship', 71.
[42] Cooper cited in Lane, 'Role of Apprenticeship', 82. Also see Cameron, *Mr Guy's Hospital*, 146.

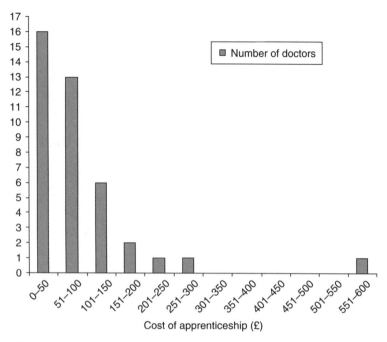

Figure 3.3. Cost of Apprenticeships
Source: Doctors' Database: Table: Apprenticeship.

was apprenticed for seven years to the London, and half-pay army surgeon, Thompson Forster (1748–1830), at a charge of £600 in 1795.[43]

On occasion, fees could be circumvented by a deal arranged to the mutual benefit of both parties. Charles Boutflower's master was his eldest brother, John Johnson, who had been apprenticed in his youth to one Francis Weaver Watkins of Wellingborough. In return, as was seen in Chapter 2, Watkins had sent his son, William, to be instructed in languages by John's father.[44] Some surgeons in the cohort may have been the beneficiaries of deals similar to that arranged for William Ross, son of an Aberdeen weaver, who was indentured in the city to Dr William Chalmers for five years. In return, Ross's father supplied Chalmers with shirts, stockings, and washing. It was also agreed that default on either side of the bargain would merit a penalty of ten pounds.[45] The cost of an indenture could also be affected by the master's personal relationship with the boy and his family. One way of securing a relatively inexpensive apprenticeship was to be indentured to a relative.[46] The eighteen fathers cited as masters to men in the cohort would have

[43] Drew, no. 841.   [44] Boutflower, *Story of a Family*, 87, 93. See Ch. 2, p. 73.
[45] McGrigor, 17.
[46] Lane, 'Role of Apprenticeship', 63, 69–70; Lawrence, *Charitable Knowledge*, 112; Loudon, *Medical Care*, 41–2.

mostly provided their services free of charge, drawing up legal contracts for their sons to produce at later examinations. Whilst Thomas Hughes Ridgway stated that his seven-year apprenticeship to his father in Pembroke had cost £5, this was a nominal amount to give the indenture the stamp of legitimacy.[47] William Williams was extremely unusual in being contracted as an apprentice to his father, Daniel, in 1774 for seven years at the reasonable price of £84. The six uncles, four brothers, and twenty other masters who had the same name as their apprentices and so were presumably related in some way would have probably provided a reduced rate of charge. Being indentured to a relative was often flexible and could mean a shorter period of training. Of the eighteen doctors who specified that their apprenticeships had been informal, seven had served a father, uncle, or a man of the same surname. It also made considerable sense to be indentured to a member of the family in the case of those fortunate enough to have well-placed relatives. Robert Keate's master was his uncle, Thomas Keate, surgeon at St George's hospital, whilst William Henry Young was apprenticed to his father, John, a Nonconformist who held the position of senior surgeon at the General Infirmary in Hull.

Details of both county of birth and county of apprenticeship(s) are known for 244 surgeons in the cohort (54 per cent). Of these, 128 (52.5 per cent) were only apprenticed in their region of origin, thus either staying within the same town or only travelling a limited distance from home. However, the remaining 116 (47.5 per cent) travelled beyond the boundaries of the county in which they had been raised in order to serve suitable masters.[48] This substantiates Lane's findings that, in the eighteenth century, a considerable number of medical apprentices were indentured outside the county in which they had been born.[49] Presumably some of those who travelled to take up apprenticeships were going where familial associations, personal ties, and recommendations required. For example, James Stuart travelled from Dumfriesshire to North Berwick to be apprenticed to his brother, George, and Robert Keate went from Laverton in Somerset to London in order to be indentured to his uncle. Others who made the trip to a major city such as London were rather seeking impressive masters in notable medical communities, important for their future career prospects. Whilst only nineteen men in the cohort were born in Edinburgh, no less than forty-five were apprenticed to surgeons in that city (see Table 3.1). Notably, eight of those were indentured to one of the members of the partnership created by Benjamin Bell (1749–1806), Andrew Wardrop (1752–1823), and James Russell. As Lisa Rosner has shown, although most masters would only take five or six students in the course of their careers, these three men took 36 per cent of the total number of Edinburgh apprentices booked between 1780 and 1815.[50] Of the other individuals in the cohort who served apprenticeships, 51 were indentured in Dublin as opposed to 17 born there, 41 in London compared to 23 who were initially from that city,

[47] TNA, WO25/3906, fo. 120. Presumably the sum covered the stamp duty.
[48] Of these, 10 (4 per cent) were apprenticed both in their county of origin and in another county.
[49] Lane, 'Role of Apprenticeship', 74.   [50] Rosner, *Medical Education*, 97–8.

Table 3.1. Place of Apprenticeships

England		Wales		Scotland		Ireland	
Berkshire	2	Camarthenshire	4	Aberdeenshire	19	County Antrim	6
Buckinghamshire	1	Glamorganshire	1	Angusshire	4	County Armagh	3
Cambridgeshire	1	Pembrokeshire	2	Argyllshire	1	County Cavan	2
Cheshire	2			Ayrshire	2	County Cork	3
Cornwall	2			Banff	5	County Donegal	6
County Durham	4			Berwickshire	1	County Down	4
Cumberland	2			Bute	1	County Dublin[b]	54
Derbyshire	1			Dumfriesshire	4	County Galway	3
Devon	6			East Lothian	2	County Limerick	3
Dorset	4			Fife	4	County Londonderry	10
Essex	1			Inverness-shire	1	County Longford	4
Gloucestershire	4			Lanarkshire[a]	20	County Louth	1
Hampshire	2			Linlithgowshire	1	County Mayo	5
Herefordshire	1			Midlothian[c]	48	County Monaghan	5
Kent	8			Morayshire	2	County Roscommon	3
Lancashire	7			Nairnshire	2	County Sligo	2
Lincolnshire	1			Orkney	2	County Tipperary	3
London	41			Perthshire	8	County Tyrone	8
Middlesex	1			Roxburghshire	3	County Waterford	3
Norfolk	3			Selkirkshire	1	County Wexford	1
Northamptonshire	2			Stirlingshire	2		
Northumberland	2						
Nottinghamshire	2						
Shropshire	1						
Somerset	1						
Staffordshire	1						
Suffolk	2						
Surrey	1						
Sussex	7						
Warwickshire	3						
Wiltshire	6						
Worcestershire	3						
Yorkshire	9						

[a] Of which 20 were apprenticed in Glasgow.
[b] Of which 51 were apprenticed in Dublin.
[c] Of which 45 were apprenticed in Edinburgh.

Source: Doctors' Database: Table: Apprenticeship.

and 20 in Glasgow where only 6 grew up. This reinforces the point that many of the cohort moved from provincial areas to major cities in order to be apprenticed to particular individuals. Training in such locations also, of course, had the advantage of allowing simultaneous access to the medical faculties of the universities and important hospitals. However, very few were apprenticed outside the country that they were born in. The Scot, Alexander Lesassier, was indentured in Manchester but only because his father had moved south to Rochdale shortly before he was born.[51] Only six of the cohort, moreover, were apprenticed outside Britain and Ireland, and two of those had been born in the countries in which they were indentured. Cases such as that of George James Hyde, originally from London but apprenticed in Paris, or Peter McLachlan, born in Renfrewshire but indentured to a master in Heemskerk in the Netherlands with the Scottish name of James Millar, were rare.

An apprentice would have been obliged to live in the house of his master, keep his trade secrets, not waste or lend his goods, and conduct himself in a moral fashion. It would be a common experience to be confined to menial tasks and running errands for at least the first few years of an apprenticeship and longer if the master was not particularly concerned with providing instruction.[52] Alexander Lesassier had initially been delighted at news of his apprenticeship to Collier and moved into his master's household in 1803 with great alacrity. However, things soon declined and one of his particular causes of resentment was the pecking order by which an older apprentice, Joseph Brown, also in the cohort, was given more interesting jobs whilst he was relegated to basic chores, including the 'slavish task of carrying out all the medicines'. According to (the admittedly not always reliable) Lesassier, Brown continually pulled rank as the senior apprentice and it was not until he left to study at Edinburgh that things improved: 'I began to discover his [Collier's] character, & was as familiar with him as Brown had ever been.' Collier also took on a small boy at this time to take over some of the more menial tasks.[53] Lesassier's view of the drudgery of apprenticeship was echoed by George James Guthrie, who had been apprenticed to Dr Phillips, a doctor in Pall Mall, and Dr Hooper, a surgeon at the Marylebone Infirmary, in London for four years. He gave a particularly negative account of the system to the Select Committee on Medical Education in 1834. In this, he related an encounter with a former student who had settled in the city and had announced himself desirous of securing an apprentice with the words, 'then I should want somebody to answer the door, and receive messages that may be sent to me; and if I have anything to do, to make up medicines, and in fact to answer any purpose which may be desired of him.' Guthrie informed the Committee that such men would go on to take further apprentices, thereby loading the system with 'for the most part, in regard to their preliminary education, unqualified people'.[54] However, for most medical practitioners, apprenticeship was undoubtedly a crucial stage in their medical training, the necessary precursor to future experiences in the wards of teaching hospitals and university auditoriums. Some masters were certainly more diligent than others and some apprentices clearly completed their indenture in possession of more knowledge and experience than others, but apprenticeship remained a key element of medical education throughout the eighteenth century and into the first half of the nineteenth.

[51] Rosner, 6 ff. Lesassier's mother stayed behind in Edinburgh to give birth.
[52] Lane, 'Role of Apprenticeship', 58; Rosner, *Medical Education*, 89.   [53] Rosner, 16–17.
[54] Guthrie quoted in Loudon, *Medical Care*, 42–4.

LECTURES AND CLASSES

The service returns at the National Archives reveal that the cohort took full advantage of the expanding opportunities for medical students in late eighteenth- and early nineteenth-century Britain. They also provide an invaluable insight into the way in which those students negotiated their way through the various classes on offer. Whilst university records are usually incomplete and it is difficult to track the exact paths of individuals, this source allows recreation of complete educational profiles. One of the most notable results of this research is evidence of the variety of institutions attended by the surgeons. Many moved around the British Isles over the course of their educational careers, sometimes seeking out famed lecturers, sometimes choosing the cheapest place to live, and sometimes deciding on a location in which contacts or family could provide assistance. Certainly, of the 432 doctors for whom information on this aspect of their education is available, the largest number (48.1 per cent) only studied in one location (Figure 3.4). However, 37.3 per cent attended lectures in two places, 12.3 per cent in three, 1.8 per cent in four, and 0.5 per cent in five. For example, John MacGregory Mallock studied in Edinburgh for four years, between 1805 and 1809. In 1815, he attended further classes on surgery, anatomy, physiology, and pathology in

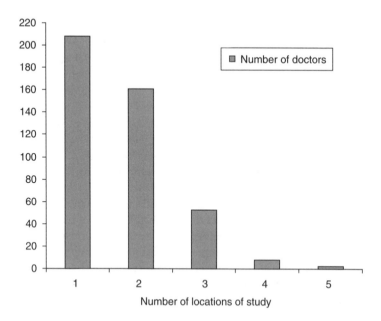

Figure 3.4. Number of Locations where Lectures were Attended

Source: Doctors' Database: Table: Lectures/Courses.

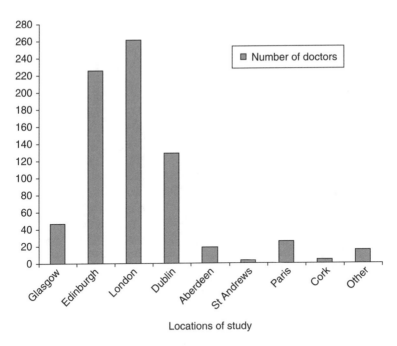

Figure 3.5. Locations where Lectures were Attended
Source: Doctors' Database: Table: Lectures/Courses.

London, before moving to Dublin and continuing his studies in that city. It was clearly an accepted practice to move around in this fashion. Both Glasgow and Edinburgh stipulated three years of study as requisite for an MD, but specified that only one of those years had to be spent at the institution awarding the degree. In the case of the 1783 statute at Edinburgh, this was in order 'that the Professors may be acquainted with [the students'] character, conduct, and diligence in prosecuting their studies'.[55] In her study of medical education at Edinburgh, Rosner groups 64 per cent of the students in her cohort under the heading of 'Occasional Auditors', denoting those who came to study at the University but left without any formal qualification. She also emphasizes that such students, attending for a year or so to follow a limited number of courses, were not potential graduates who dropped out but were rather following a particular method of training.[56]

Of the locations where doctors in the cohort studied, London was the singularly most popular (Figure 3.5): 261 went there to take full advantage of the lectures available in the great teaching hospitals, to gain experience in anatomy and dissection, and to hear talks by stars of the lecturing circuit. The vast majority of this number travelled there as only twenty-three of the cohort were actually from that

55 Rosner, *Medical Education*, 63.   56 Ibid. 104, 114–15.

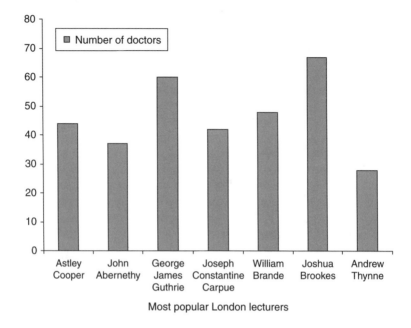

Figure 3.6. Most Popular Lecturers in London
Source: Doctors' Database: Table: Lectures/Courses.

city. Sixty-seven were present at Joshua Brookes's (1761–1833) private lectures on anatomy, given at his home in Blenheim Street, and at least sixty of the cohort attended the classes of the former army surgeon, George James Guthrie, mostly hearing him speak on the subjects of surgery and diseases of the eyes (Figure 3.6). William Brande's (1788–1866) lectures on chemistry were also very well attended, forty-eight of the doctors in the cohort being present at his classes between 1808 and 1829. The vast majority of these would have been taught by him at the Royal Institution where he succeeded Sir Humphry Davy as professor of chemistry in 1813. The lectures of the famous Sir Astley Cooper were heard by forty-four of the cohort whilst Joseph Constantine Carpue, another army surgeon, was also well favoured, with forty-two present at his classes between 1801 and 1827. Carpue began private teaching while attached to the York Hospital in the 1800s. Eventually, he established a private school of anatomy in Dean Street, where, until he retired as a teacher in 1832, he gave three courses of lectures on anatomy a day, charging 20 guineas to those attending his frequently overflowing classes. In addition, he lectured twice a week in the evenings on surgery.[57] John Murray from Turriff attended his classes during his period of study in London from 1804 onwards and

---

[57] *Plarr's Lives of the Fellows*, i. 197; Blomfield, *St George's*, 49.

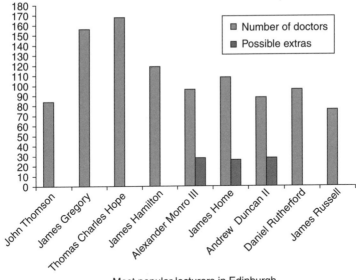

Most popular lecturers in Edinburgh

Figure 3.7. Most Popular Lecturers in Edinburgh

Source: Doctors' Database: Table: Lectures/Courses.

found him to be a 'good, honest, worthy and attentive teacher'. Indeed, Carpue even coached Murray for his army exam at the College of Surgeons.[58]

Coming a fairly close second to London in terms of popularity, Edinburgh clearly deserved its reputation as one of the most important centres for medical instruction in this period. Indeed, the two most favoured lecturers were based in Edinburgh and the largest number of classes was taken in that city (see Figure 3.7). Professor Hope's talks and demonstrations on chemistry were the most singularly well attended, attracting no less than 168 of the cohort. Rosner has shown that, after Hope took over the chair in 1798, the number of students opting to take chemistry rose to an average of 81 per cent of every year-group at the University.[59] His reputation at the time was noted by Alexander Bower, author of *The Edinburgh Student's Guide*: 'This great man may be considered as one of the chief causes of the rapid progress of chemistry of late years, both by the brilliant discoveries which he made in the science, and his popularity as a public lecturer.'[60] James Gregory (1753–1821) was another favourite teacher in the city, with

---

[58] SNA, GD1530/1, fos. 5, 19–20, 31: Murray's letters home. Carpue was attached to the York Hospital from 1799 to 1811 as a staff surgeon. He then retired from the army because he did not want to go abroad.   [59] Rosner, *Medical Education*, 50.

[60] A. Bower, *The Edinburgh Student's Guide* (Edinburgh, 1822), 42.

156 doctors from the cohort attending his classes. Although Gregory was appointed as professor of institutions of medicine in 1778, he took over the chair of medical practice on the death of William Cullen (1710–90) and it was in this capacity that most of these doctors heard him lecture. These findings show the great importance of Hope and Gregory as influences on a generation of medical practitioners, providing statistical evidence that they were amongst the most, if not *the* most, well-attended professors lecturing on medicine in this period. It is difficult to know who should be ranked third amongst the Edinburgh lecturers, largely due to confusion over names resulting from the fact that so many successive lecturers came from the same family. James Hamilton (1767–1839), lecturer in midwifery, was certainly favoured, as were James Home (1760–1844), professor of materia medica and later medical practice, Daniel Rutherford (1749–1819), lecturer in botany, and Alexander Monro tertius (1773–1859). Trying to ascertain the number of doctors who attended the latter's classes on anatomy and surgery as opposed to those of his father, Monro secundus (1733–1817), previous holder of the chair, is particularly difficult as twenty-eight only specify a 'Monro' and do not provide dates. However, at least ninety-six of the cohort studied with a Monro after 1798, the year the son took over from his father. The popularity of Monro tertius must be explained by the importance of his subject matter as he was a notoriously bad speaker.[61] Indeed, many responded to the poor quality of his classes by turning to private teachers outside the university, such as John Barclay (1758–1826), a lecturer on anatomy, who was attended by seventy-four of the doctors in the cohort.

Whilst private and hospital lecturers dominated in London and most students in Edinburgh attended university teachers, the most favoured tutors in Dublin, the third most common place to study, were from the Royal College of Surgeons. Fifty-eight of the cohort heard Richard Dease (*c*.1774–1819) lecture and fifty-five went to Abraham Colles's (1773–1843) classes, the two sharing instruction in anatomy and surgery. Glasgow was ranked next, its advantages as a cheaper place to study probably undermined by the problems created by ructions between the University and the Faculty of Physicians and Surgeons of Glasgow over the right of students to walk the wards of the Royal Infirmary. One upshot of this persistent friction was an absence of lectures in clinical medicine as the Faculty or corporation controlled access to the hospital.[62] James Jeffray's (1790–1848) lectures on anatomy and surgery were the most well attended by the cohort in this city, attracting thirty-eight students. Next in the pecking order was Robert Cleghorn (1755–1821), professor of chemistry, who was heard by thirty of the doctors under study.

[61] J. D. Comrie, *History of Scottish Medicine*, 2 vols. (London, 1932), i. 493.
[62] M. S. Buchanan, *History of the Glasgow Royal Infirmary, from its Commencement in 1787 to the Present Time* (Glasgow, 1832), 17; Coutts, *History of the University of Glasgow*, 556–61. For the Faculty of Physicians and Surgeons in Glasgow, see J. Geyer-Kordesch, *Physicians and Surgeons of Glasgow: The History of the Royal College of Physicians and Surgeons of Glasgow, 1599–1858* (London, 1999); A. Duncan, *Memorials of the Faculty of Physicians and Surgeons of Glasgow, 1599–1850* (Glasgow, 1896).

It is clear from all these statistics that anatomy, surgery, and chemistry were the staples of the trainee doctor's education. Although the first two were firmly established as the foundations of study, the prominence of chemistry and the fact that Hope's lectures were the best attended at Edinburgh is a little more surprising. Chemistry had long been established as one of those medical courses that attracted a fashionable and general audience in addition to those studying to be doctors, and Hope's dramatic demonstrations were purportedly geared towards a broad clientele.[63] Bower at the time observed that Hope's chemistry lectures 'are attended not only by medical students, but by every gentleman who is inquisitive after general knowledge'. Aesculapius similarly emphasized the subject's status 'as an elegant accomplishment, and almost necessary to the character of the gentleman'. However, crucially, Aesculapius also believed chemistry to be invaluable to the medical practitioner for professional reasons, and the popularity of the discipline amongst the doctors in the cohort implies that it was considered to be a more vital part of medical training than has sometimes been suggested.[64] A considerable number of medical students would have gone on to become surgeon-apothecaries, all practitioners would have required some expertise in pharmacy, and any wishing to undertake scientific research would have needed training in chemistry. Thus, as Rosner has argued, many would have felt the need to take classes in this subject as an important field not covered by apprenticeship.[65]

These statistics give a very good idea as to who were the most important tutors in medicine in this period, informing medical students about popular theories and their implementation. However, assessing the actual numbers of courses taken by the doctors in the cohort is much more difficult. Many service returns provide confusing dates that make it unclear whether a course was taken more than once. For example, if a doctor states that he studied anatomy in '1812, 1813', he could mean either that he studied it once, in the winter term of 1812, or that he took the course in two consecutive years. Many students did take the same course more than once, progressing to a higher level each year. Even information as to the number of months of study is of limited use as it can often be unclear as to how long an individual course lasted, particularly in the case of those offered by private lecturers. Looking at the number of different subjects taken is a little easier, although still problematic in that some of the cohort amalgamate these on their service returns whilst others cite the same topics individually. Therefore, any calculations can be at best impressionistic. A detailed analysis of the subjects taken by one doctor in every five, omitting those for whom there is insufficient information, gives some indication of the surprising number of subjects studied by the cohort (see Figure 3.8). The largest number of this selected group studied nine subjects, not dissimilar to the average of 8.4. William Macartney, for example, took two courses each in anatomy and surgery, chemistry, and medical practice,

63 Rosner, *Medical Education*, 50, 104–5.
64 Bower, *Edinburgh Student's Guide*, 42; Aesculapius, *Hospital Pupil's Guide*, 68–9.
65 Rosner, *Medical Education*, 111.

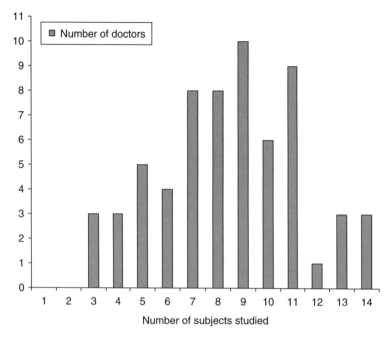

Figure 3.8. Number of Subjects Studied

Note: Beginning with the first doctor in the cohort (DID 3), one in every five was selected for analysis of the number of subjects studied. Those doctors for whom there was insufficient information to calculate this figure were omitted. This resulted in a total of 63.

Source: Doctors' Database: Table: Lectures/Courses.

one each in medical theory, materia medica, military surgery, midwifery, and botany and attended two courses of clinical lectures in Edinburgh between 1805 and 1808. On the other hand, some of the cohort took as few as three lecture courses whilst a small group, consisting of Thomas Hall, Charles St John, and Alexander Browne, attended classes on fourteen different topics.

Anecdotal evidence as to the cost of such education shows that the required outlay was substantial. As well as the expense of lodgings, books, and clothes, there was the price of courses themselves. The letters of William Dent give a good indication of the cost of studying in London. Dent wrote home to his mother in October 1808 to describe the lodgings he had just acquired. He was sharing a sitting room and bedroom with two other students at six shillings a week per head and had decided not to board at the greater price of eight shillings and sixpence: 'we thought as being three of us we could live cheaper by only lodging in the house and find ourselves of everything we wanted . . . ' He expressed his concern that his mother might think him 'very extravagant' before telling her that he had paid upwards of £70 for hospital lectures, £5 for books and a set of pocket instruments, and £10 for a new suit of clothes and boots. He also warned her that he was going to need another £15 to enable him to get into a club, presumably with the hope of supplementing his attendance at lectures with some networking with an eye on his future career.[66] Just over a month later, he was still concerned that she might consider his expenses too great: 'I dare say that you will think I am very careless, and dont care what becomes of my Money, but however I can tell you, that I am really as careful as I possibly can ... I assure you when I came away, I had no idea, that I should put you to so much expense ... '[67] The following February, having purchased a watch, a pair of pantaloons, a hat, a pair of shoes, a neckerchief, and some pocket handkerchiefs, Dent calculated that he had spent a total of £155 since arriving in London.[68]

Life as a student in Edinburgh was not much less expensive. Courses there mostly cost three guineas each and Alexander Lesassier had to pay out £18 in advance for classes on his arrival in the city.[69] When Andrew Duncan junior (1773–1832), professor of materia medica at Edinburgh University, was asked by the Royal Commission in 1826 to describe a typical medical student's expenses at that institution, he replied: 'I have known instances of students getting through the winter on less than £10; I have known other medical students spend almost £500 or £600.'[70] In November 1771, Thomas Ismay, a student not destined for service in the armed forces, informed his father that his board and lodging in Edinburgh, barring washing, cost him £10 a quarter and could have been as much as £12: 'Things of all kinds are very Dear in the Place ... The greatest Economists we have who take a Room, and live in a handsome manner but no ways extravagant, cannot Live under 16 pound the Half year, and have everything to seek [buy?] in.'[71] The accounts of students such as Dent and Ismay should of course be treated with a certain amount of scepticism as they were undoubtedly concerned to justify their expenses to their parents. However, they do give some idea of the outlay required for even a short period of training.

William Gibney's account of his studies provides an invaluable insight into the experiences of such students. He arrived in Edinburgh in 1810 to pursue his medical education and took lodgings with a lady named Mrs Jobson. Once settled,

66 WL, RAMC 536, letters of William Dent (1808–24), no. 1: Dent to his mother, London, 30 Oct. 1808; see also no. 2, Dent to his mother, London, 5 Dec. 1808. Aesculapius, *Hospital Pupil's Guide*, 27–8, conversely advised students to board and lodge during their studies. John Murray of Turriff's lodgings in London cost a similar amount to those of Dent, six to seven shillings a week: SNA, GD1530/1, fo. 4.

67 WL, RAMC 536, no. 2, William Dent to his mother, London, 5 Dec. 1808.

68 WL, RAMC 536, no. 4, William Dent to his mother, London, 17 Feb. 1809.

69 Rosner, 27. See also 'Letter from Thomas Ismay, Student of Medicine at Edinburgh, 1771, to his Father', *University of Edinburgh Journal*, 8 (1936–7), 57–61, 59–60.

70 Quoted in Rosner, *Medical Education*, 31.

71 'Letter from Thomas Ismay', 59. Ismay's figures are substantiated by the fact that another medical student, again not destined for the army, Thomas Parke, paid £12 a quarter for board and lodgings in the same year. See W. J. Bell, 'Thomas Parke's Student Life in England and Scotland, 1771–3', *Pennsylvania Magazine of History and Biography*, 75/3 (1951), 237–59, 247. By this date, as noted by Comrie, *History of Scottish Medicine*, i. 431, there was virtually no college residence available in Edinburgh.

he established a routine, attending lectures on chemistry, anatomy, and materia medica. He was impressed by the dynamic lectures of Hope but, like so many others, was not very taken with Professor Alexander Monro tertius. He therefore supplemented Monro's instruction by attending the private lectures of John Gordon (1786–1818) on anatomy and physiology and John Barclay's classes on anatomy. He noted that 'Dr. Gordon's private lectures on anatomy never would have had so many attendants, had the University Chair been properly filled.' He also made occasional visits to the Infirmary and spent the evenings reading, writing up lectures, or engaging 'in a little musical recreation and mutual instruction' with his housemates. Although he rarely went out, he did join the Royal Medical Society, a student body, listening to papers being read on suitable topics and engaging in the debates that followed.[72]

Having spent one academic year at Edinburgh, Gibney then returned home to Dublin and continued his studies at Trinity College. He was advised, for the time being at least, to 'confine myself to a repetition of anatomical lectures, clinical lectures, demonstrations on, and dissections of, the dead body'. He found Dr William Hartigan (*c*.1756–1812), professor of anatomy, a great improvement on the inadequacies of Professor Monro, whilst Francis Barker (1771/2–1859), 'although a most philosophical chemist', could not live up to the performances of Hope. Gibney was not alone in finding Barker's stilted delivery and sometimes unsuccessful experiments tiresome: 'towards the end of his course the benches were all but deserted.' In general, he was struck with the small number of pupils at Trinity and gained the impression that the ones attending all the lectures were doing so in order to become eligible for the degree. He noted that the Royal College of Surgeons provided far more popular classes, even though 'perhaps the Professors were not superior in point of talent to those at the University'.[73]

Gibney continued to work hard at his studies, but was relieved when the time came for him to return to Edinburgh for the summer season, arriving in time to attend the three-month courses of Professor Rutherford on botany and Professor Hamilton on midwifery. This time, he decided against staying in a boarding house and took a couple of private rooms, 'well-furnished and at a reasonable rental' for the duration of his stay.[74] He remained in Edinburgh for the start of the new academic year in October 1812, watching the students flooding in 'from all parts of the globe' and observing: 'The University was in the zenith of its fame, especially as regards the practice of medicine and the knowledge of chemistry.' Anatomy was still a deficiency in the faculty and Gibney again noted the stiff competition presented by private practitioners, 'listened to and appreciated by many who could not find sound and efficient instruction elsewhere'. Being concerned to make the most of his final year of study, he signed up for lectures by James Home on materia medica, Andrew Duncan (1744–1828) on medical jurisprudence, and

[72] Gibney, 11–12, 22–9. See D. Guthrie (ed.), *History of the Royal Medical Society, 1737–1937* (Edinburgh, 1952).   [73] Gibney, 48–9, 50–1.
    [74] Ibid. 57–8, 62.

James Gregory on medical practice, arranged to walk the wards at the Royal Infirmary, and attended meetings of the Royal Medical Society. His new regime required him to rise long before daybreak and continue working for ten or twelve hours a day at 'lectures, hospital practice, and private studies... denying myself all gaieties and enjoyments, even necessary exercise'. However, he deemed the sacrifice worth the achievement of getting 'through the whole routine or curriculum of my medical education as quickly and economically as possible, though with credit to myself'. For, as noted above, Gibney was not from a particularly affluent background, his father having died when young and his widowed mother having to fund his education with limited means. When he finally graduated with his MD, having written a thesis entitled *De coeli calidi imperio*, he proclaimed himself 'supremely delighted... and I trust that I was not ungrateful to God for having brought me thus far upon the threshold of independence, to be the forerunner of my own fortunes, and for the prospect of being no longer a tax on the very limited income of my widowed mother.'[75]

Alexander Lesassier was similarly from a family of relatively meagre means but had the advantage of being the nephew of James Hamilton, professor of midwifery at Edinburgh University. When Hamilton invited Lesassier to lodge in the family home, his nephew pronounced himself 'both amazed & delighted'. He was keenly aware of the opportunities that this arrangement would afford him in terms of both the company he would meet and the money he would save; 'lodgings in this town, I understand are very dear.' Despite having been a rather unruly student up until this point, he apparently applied himself to his studies and established a rigid routine:

I rise in the morning at 8, finish breakfast, & get seated in Dr Gregory's Class room by 9—from 10–11—I hear Dr Hope on Chemistry—From 11 to 12—Dr Barclay on Anatomy—Then from 12 till 1 I attend the Infirmary. From 1 till 2 the famous Dr Monro—from 2 to 3 I go home and take a basin of soup—from 3 till 4 o'clock my Uncle's lectures on Midwifery—then from 4 to 5 Dinner from 5 till 1/2 past 6 studying & reviewing what I've heard during the day—Tea over by a little past 7 & I go to the Infirmary... quarter past 9 supper & to bed by 1/2 past 10.

However, his diligence began to wane in the spring and, like many others, he did not bother to stay in Edinburgh for the summer session.[76]

James McGrigor was a third student from our cohort who attended lectures in Edinburgh despite fairly limited means. In his autobiography, he records that he began his studies as an apprentice to Dr George French, surgeon at the Infirmary in Aberdeen and professor of chemistry at Marischal College. He attended the few lectures at that time available in the city and then proceeded to Edinburgh on foot, 'a very agreeable' tour that took about a week. There, he attended James Gregory's classes on medical practice, went to the private demonstrations of Andrew Fyfe (1752–1824), dissector and assistant to both Monro secundus and

---

[75] Ibid. 66–9, 72, 86.   [76] Rosner, 26, 28, 30, 32.

tertius, and studied anatomy at the University. He was lucky enough to hear the lectures of Monro secondus rather than those of his son. In the Christmas vacation he went to Glasgow, where he attended further classes. These included those of Hope on chemistry, given before he took up the chair at Edinburgh vacated by Joseph Black (1728–99). Like so many others, McGrigor noted Hope's skill as a lecturer, observing that he 'performed the experiments with singular success, never failing in one'. He then returned to Edinburgh and, like Gibney and Lesassier, threw himself into his studies, to the point of making himself ill for several months.[77]

WALKING THE WARDS

Of the cohort under scrutiny, 93.6 per cent (425) gave some details of hospital experience. Although, as with the lectures taken by these doctors, ascertaining the amount of time spent walking the wards is fairly complicated, a similar detailed analysis of one in five of the cohort, omitting those for whom there is insufficient information, again helps to provide a rough estimate (Figure 3.9). This shows that the largest number of doctors spent twelve months in hospitals and that the average was 23.8 months (including time spent concurrently at different institutions).

London offered the greatest opportunities for ward walking and of the 425 doctors who recorded that they had attended hospitals, 244 (57.4 per cent) went to institutions in this city (Figure 3.10). Hospitals had laid down quotas for the number of pupils that could be accepted, but these were increasingly ignored from the 1770s onwards and students flooded the wards.[78] Whilst Lawrence has shown that Guy's was the most popular place for ward walking in this period, St George's was by far the most well attended by our cohort, attracting sixty-three doctors (see Figure 3.11).[79] Before and during the French wars this was most likely due to the presence there of three key figures in the army medical corps: John Hunter (1723–93), surgeon-general of the army and later inspector of hospitals; John Gunning, made surgeon-general on the death of Hunter; and Thomas Keate, surgeon-general from 1798. Presumably medical students already envisaging a career in the army believed that they would enhance their chances of getting on if they had studied with members of the Army Medical Board.[80] Most students either attended the hospital for six or twelve months, although some spent considerable periods of time there. Charles Ferguson Forbes, who despite his name was a nonconformist from Great Coggeshall, Essex, attended

---

[77] McGrigor, 29–30.
[78] Lawrence, *Charitable Knowledge*,135. For another example of this, see McInnes, *St Thomas's Hospital*, 76–8.   [79] Lawrence, *Charitable Knowledge*, appendix II.
[80] For the factors pushing medical students towards the army, see Ch. 2, 'Entering the Service'. For the role of patronage in the army medical service, see Ch. 4, *passim*. The physician-general, Sir Lucas Pepys, also held an appointment at St George's, as did Keate's nephew, Robert, one of the cohort, who was surgeon at the hospital 1813–53.

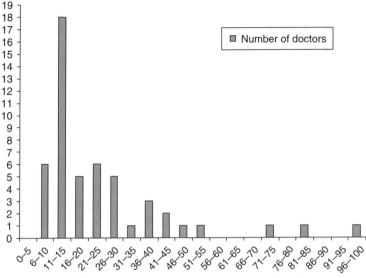

Figure 3.9. Number of Months Spent in Individual Hospitals

Note: Beginning with the first doctor in the cohort (DID 3), one in every five was selected for analysis of the number of months spent walking the wards. If two or more hospitals were attended during the same period, then the amount of time was duly multiplied. Those doctors for whom there was insufficient information to calculate this figure were omitted. This resulted in a total of 51.

Source: Doctors' Database: Hospitals.

St George's hospital for thirty-seven months, spread out over the period between 1795 and 1803. St Thomas's and Guy's, which closely cooperated until 1825, were also well attended, attracting a total of thirty-five of the doctors from the cohort. Dent was a student at Guy's during his stay in London and he informed his mother that the lodgings he had secured were ideally situated 'only a few Doors' away from the hospital, allowing him and his two fellow co-habitants to get there quickly and easily when accident victims were brought in.[81] In 1812, James Barry, the doctor later to become notorious once it was discovered upon 'his' death that he was actually a woman, arrived in London to attend St Thomas's after three years spent at Edinburgh. He became a pupil dresser, a student of Sir Astley Cooper and walked the wards for six months.[82] A pupil at St Thomas's or Guy's would pay 24 guineas for twelve months or 18 guineas for six months. However, a more senior student might attain the position of 'dresser', allowing him to assist in operations and to treat patients in the absence of his master.

[81] WL, RAMC 536, no. 2, William Dent to his mother, London, 5 Dec. 1808.

[82] June Rose, *The Perfect Gentleman: The Remarkable Life of Dr James Miranda Barry, the Woman who Served as an Officer in the British Army from 1813 to 1859* (London, 1977), 27–9; McInnes, *St Thomas's Hospital*, 80; Parsons, *History of St Thomas's Hospital*, ii. 224.

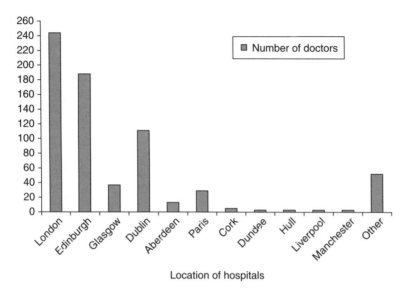

Location of hospitals

Figure 3.10. Location of Hospitals
Source: Doctors' Database: Hospitals.

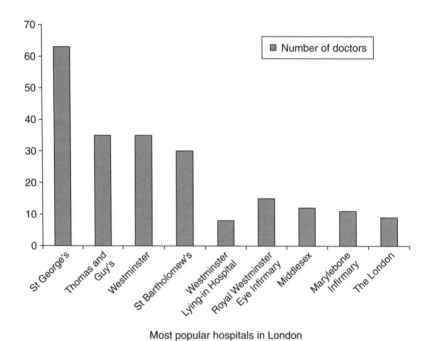

Most popular hospitals in London

Figure 3.11. Most Popular Hospitals in London
Source: Doctors' Database: Hospitals.

To enjoy this status at either of these hospitals would cost £50 for a year.[83] The Westminster was as equally well attended, whilst St Bartholomew's was the next most favoured institution, providing practical experience for thirty of the doctors from the cohort. Some of these surgeons went on to secure positions at those hospitals after they had served in the armed forces. William Bewicke Lynn spent three years at the Westminster between 1806 and 1809 and, after a period as an assistant surgeon in the army, went on to become assistant surgeon to the hospital in 1834 and surgeon in 1853.[84]

The vast majority of the 188 doctors who gained hospital experience in Edinburgh, the next most popular place, attended the Royal Infirmary (133, 70.7 per cent). Tickets for walking the wards, allowing access between the hours of 12 and 1, cost two guineas for apprentices at the Royal College of Surgeons and three guineas for all others.[85] Thirty-nine doctors walked the wards at the Lying-in Hospital, established by Alexander Hamilton (*c.*1739–1802) 'for the purpose of affording relief to the wives of indigent tradesmen'.[86] Before moving to London, Barry had taken full advantage of the hospitals in Edinburgh as well as attending lectures at the University and the private dissections of Fyfe. In 1811, he had been a perpetual pupil at all three of the key institutions; the Royal Infirmary, the Dispensary, and the Lying-in Hospital.[87] Other students gained practical experience in patient care by different means. Gibney in 1812–13 found himself in the fortunate position of being appointed a clinical clerk at the Edinburgh Infirmary. Since 'it was a great object among the students to obtain the situation of clinical clerk, or to be an assistant to any of the Professors whose turn it might be to deliver lectures at the Infirmary', such positions were in great demand. As Gibney noted, they were usually allocated by the professor in question to 'some friend from the more advanced students'. He applied to both Rutherford and Duncan, little hoping for success, but to his great delight was taken on by the former for the following quarter. His duties were to write out all the cases in a concise form and to treat them until Rutherford was able to attend to them himself. Gibney greatly valued this experience: 'I found actual practice gave me a greater insight into disease than can be obtained by months of hard reading or attendance at lectures.'[88]

The large number of hospitals in Dublin also provided opportunities for students in that city to walk the wards, attracting 111 of the cohort (Figure 3.12). In descending order of preference, students attended the Westmoreland Lock (for venereal disease), Dr Steevens's Hospital (a small hospital near the army infirmary at Kilmainham), Jervis Street Hospital, the Meath, the Lying-in Hospital,

[83] McInnes, *St Thomas's Hospital*, 80; Parsons, *History of St Thomas's Hospital*, ii. 183; iii. 9–10; Wilks and Bettany, *Biographical History of Guy's Hospital*, 173; Cameron, *Mr Guy's Hospital*, 146–7. Lawrence, *Charitable Knowledge*, 109, table 4.1, corroborates these figures.
[84] Humble and Hansell, *Westminster Hospital*, 134.
[85] Logan Turner, *Story of a Great Hospital*, 150; 'Letter from Thomas Ismay', 60.
[86] Comrie, *History of Scottish Medicine*, i. 304.   [87] Rose, *Perfect Gentleman*, 22–3, 26.
[88] Gibney, 68.

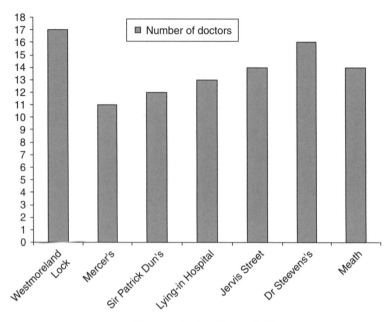

Most popular hospitals in Dublin

Figure 3.12. Most Popular Hospitals in Dublin
Source: Doctors' Database: Hospitals.

Sir Patrick Dun's Hospital, and the Mercer's.[89] They seem to have moved quite freely between these establishments. John Frederick Clarke, for example, noted that he had attended Steevens's hospital and the Lock for sixty months each, 'attending and dressing the patients of Dr Hartigan', as well as spending six months at Sir Patrick Dun's.[90] Similarly, Charles Clarke wrote on his return form that he had 'occasionally visited Madame Steven's Hospital [in central Dublin] and others; and when Operations were to be performed or any remarkable case to be seen I was generally present'.[91]

Glasgow was rated fourth, only thirty-seven of the students attending the hospitals there. As in Edinburgh, the choice was more limited, twenty-seven walking the wards at the Glasgow Royal Infirmary and ten gaining experience in the Lying-in Hospital. Alexander Dunlop Anderson started his hospital training early

[89] D. Coakley, *Doctor Steevens's Hospital: A Brief History* (Dublin, 1992); T. P. C. Kirkpatrick, *The History of Dr. Steevens's Hospital, Dublin: 1720–1920* (Dublin, 1924); P. Gatenby, *Dublin's Meath Hospital, 1753–1996* (Dublin, 1996); T. P. C. Kirkpatrick, *The Book of the Rotunda Hospital: An Illustrated History of the Dublin Lying-in Hospital from its Foundation in 1745 to the Present Time* (London, 1913); T. Gillman, *A Short History of Sir Patrick Dun's Hospital* (Dublin, 1942); J. B. Lyons, *The Quality of Mercer's: The Story of Mercer's Hospital, 1734–1991* (Dublin, 1991).
[90] TNA, WO25/3908, fo. 37.   [91] TNA, WO25/3904, fo. 37.

as apprentice to his uncle, Alexander Dunlop, a surgeon at the Glasgow Infirmary. He then walked the wards in that hospital for twelve months in 1811 and 1812 before spending three months at the city's Lock (again for venereal disease) in 1813. It may well be that such family networks were often behind choice of institutions.

QUALIFICATIONS

Although the vast majority of the doctors in the cohort attended lectures at universities, only 184 (40.5 per cent) went on to gain a degree. Of those who did so, more than half (102) acquired the MD from Edinburgh University, one of the most demanding and rigorous medical qualifications on offer (Figure 3.13). Students had to prove that they had studied anatomy, surgery, chemistry, botany, materia medica and pharmacy, medical theory and practice, and attended clinical lectures. They also had to show that they had spent three years studying medicine in a university faculty (although not all the time at Edinburgh), pass written and oral exams, and compose and publicly defend a thesis in Latin.[92] Moreover, the sixteen men from the cohort who acquired their Edinburgh MDs from the mid-1820s onwards had extra requirements to meet as the University increasingly tightened up its regulations in response to criticisms of the perceived laxness of the Scottish institutions.[93] An Edinburgh degree was expensive in time and money, even if the fee for taking the exam was only £5.

Far fewer of the cohort held MDs from the next most popular institution at which to graduate. Only twenty doctors acquired degrees from Glasgow between 1791 and 1839. As at Edinburgh, the senate at this University also became increasingly concerned with tightening its regulations. New ordinances published in 1802 stipulated three years of study, a similar list of subjects to those required at Edinburgh, oral exams in Latin, and a minimum age of 21.[94] However, as there was no thesis requirement, this was still less rigorous than the demands of Edinburgh, except in the regulation regarding age. When the senate at Edinburgh University refused to admit Barry to the degree examination due to the fact that he was supposedly only 12 years old, his patron, David Erskine, earl of Buchan, was able to point out that there was nothing in the statutes that stipulated a minimum age requirement for graduates.[95] In 1817, Glasgow instituted a degree in surgery, but only one of our cohort, Crawford Dick, attained it. For his CM, awarded in 1823, he would have been required to have spent two years in a university, undertaken two courses of anatomy and surgery, one each of materia

---

[92] Grant, *University of Edinburgh*, i. 329–32. For a first person account of the process of taking a medical degree at Edinburgh, see B. Cozens-Hardy, *The Diary of Sylas Neville, 1767–1788* (London, 1950), 217–26. [93] Rosner, *Medical Education*, 173–4.

[94] Coutts, *University of Glasgow*, 541.

[95] Rose, *Perfect Gentleman*, 27. She was, of course, *c.*17: see Ch. 2, pp. 102–3.

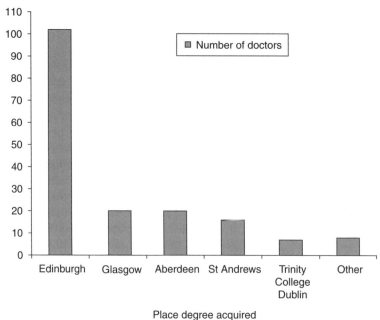

Figure 3.13. Places Degrees Acquired

Source: Doctors' Database: Table: Degrees.

medica and pharmacy, chemistry, medical theory and practice, midwifery, and the principles and practice of surgery, and to have walked the wards in a hospital for at least twelve months.[96]

Sixteen doctors gained their degrees from St Andrews whilst twenty acquired MDs from Aberdeen, seven from King's College, and thirteen from Marischal. These degrees were considerably easier to come by and suffered in reputation as a result. All that was required was the payment of a fee and the recommendation of two colleagues, making them an attractive proposition for those lacking the standard requirements and concomitantly unattractive for those who sought a qualification that would testify to years of study.[97] Unsurprisingly, only eight of the cohort had degrees from Trinity College Dublin. As the university officially only awarded MDs to students who had previously taken a BA at Trinity, the college only produced two graduates per year on average in the early years of the nineteenth century.[98] Equally unsurprisingly, only one of the doctors gained a medical degree at Oxford and one at Cambridge. Both institutions were confessionally restricted, required seven years' studying for a BA and then an additional four for the MD, and provided lectures that were generally recognized to be inferior to those on offer

[96] Coutts, *University of Glasgow*, 545–6
[97] Loudon, *Medical Care*, 38; Dow and Moss, 'Medical Curriculum at Glasgow', 238.
[98] McDowell and Webb, *Trinity College Dublin*, 88, 144–5.

elsewhere. However, the contacts that could be made at Oxbridge were thought by some to make up for deficiencies in teaching. In 1806, William Baillie advised the mother of a Glasgow medical student to send her son to Oxford to attain polish, connections, and professional advancement, but admitted that the quality of instruction would not be of the highest standard; 'his medical education will not be improved by this plan, for there are no lectures of reputation upon any branch of medicine given at Oxford.'[99]

A small number of medical graduates also became fellows of the three royal colleges of physicians and the Glasgow Faculty of Physicians and Surgeons (see Figure 3.14).[100] Technically, full fellows of that in London had to have degrees from Oxford or Cambridge, but the college exercised considerable discretion in this area. This explains why, despite the fact that only two of the cohort had Oxbridge degrees, nine were fellows of the college. In addition to George Paulet Morris, who had a Cambridge degree, one had an MD from St Andrews, three from Aberdeen, one from Glasgow, and three from Edinburgh.[101] A further fourteen of the cohort held the position of licentiate of the London college, a status open to those with degrees from other institutions.

The Royal College of Physicians in Edinburgh stipulated that those with MDs from Scottish universities could become fellows without examination.[102] It is unsurprising in consequence that, of the nine of the cohort who became fellows there, all had degrees from universities in Scotland. It is more unexpected to find that only three of those were from Edinburgh whilst two had been awarded by Aberdeen and no less than four by St Andrews. It may have been that the poor reputation of the latter two degrees prompted their holders to seek additional sources of status. The Faculty of Physicians and Surgeons at Glasgow, where fellowships were restricted to those with degrees, attracted little interest.[103] Alexander Dunlop Anderson and Robert Andrew McMunn, both with MDs from Edinburgh, and William Richardson Gibb, in possession of a degree from Glasgow, were the only fellows. McGrigor held an honorary position. Even fewer had any contact with the College of Physicians in Dublin. Luke Kelly became a member and McGrigor was again awarded the status of honorary fellow.

A larger number of the cohort attained membership of one of the three royal colleges of surgeons than attained a degree (see Figure 3.14): 240 (52.9 per cent) had a membership diploma from one of the colleges, of whom 93 were also medical graduates. In addition, 21 of the 240 held a separate midwifery diploma, principally gained from the Dublin Lying-in Hospital or Edinburgh University.[104]

[99] Baillie cited in Rosner, *Medical Education*, 16, 23.
[100] For the Royal College of Physicians, see Sir George Clark, *A History of the Royal College of Physicians of London*, 3 vols. (Oxford, 1964). See also Rosner, *Medical Education*, 22; Lawrence, *Charitable Knowledge*, 77–8.
[101] Benjamin Haywood Browne, who had an MD from Oxford, was not amongst this number.
[102] Rosner, *Medical Education*, 22. [103] Ibid.
[104] One member of the cohort had a midwifery diploma and a degree but no qualification from a surgical college.

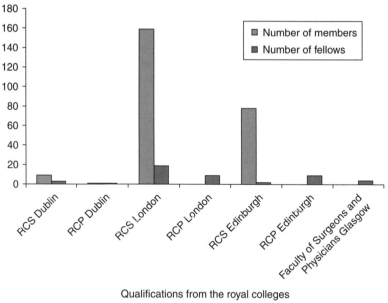

Qualifications from the royal colleges

Figure 3.14. Qualifications from the Royal Colleges
Source: Doctors' Database: Table: Degrees.

In other words, 331 of the 454 surgeons in the cohort eventually had a more prestigious qualification than the basic army diploma, which remained throughout our period the only official examination requirement of entrants to the army medical service.[105]

Significantly, well over half of the number who were members of a royal college of surgery (159) attained their qualification from the college in London, almost as many as those who gained degrees from any university in the British Isles. The cost of gaining this qualification was considerably more than the fee charged for the simple army diploma. During the French wars the cost of the army examination in the London College rose from 1*s*. 1*d*. to 2*s*. 2*d*. for an assistant surgeon's diploma and from 3*s*. 3*d*. to 5*s*. 5*d*. for a surgeon's licence. Over the same period, the price of becoming a member steadily rose from £13 18*s*. in 1800, to £15 15*s*. in 1802, £16 8*s*. in 1804, £16 10*s*. in 1805 and £22 in 1810.[106] The examination would also have been much more onerous. Nineteen of the cohort went on to become fellows of the London institution. Of these seven specified that they had become 'fellow by election' in 1844. These individuals were

---

[105] See Ch. 1.
[106] Royal College of Surgeons, London, Examination Books: RCS 1745–1800; RCS 1800–20; RCS 1820–30. William Dent paid £22 when he took the membership exam in 1810: see WL, RAMC 536, no. 12, Dent to his mother, London, 22 Apr. 1810.

beneficiaries of the new charter established the previous year that permitted the creation of fellows, several hundred of which were nominated by the council without being required to undertake an examination.[107]

Seventy-eight of the cohort had a general diploma from the Royal College in Edinburgh and, from 1816 onwards, these men were entitled to call themselves 'Licentiates'.[108] To qualify, they had to have studied 'in some University of reputation, or under teachers who are resident fellows of the Colleges of Physicians or Surgeons, of London, Dublin, Edinburgh, or of the Faculty of Medicine and Surgery of Glasgow'.[109] Until 1804, no specific course of study was specified, between 1804 and 1808 candidates were required to have attended lectures in anatomy, surgery, and medical practice, and from 1808 an increasing number of subjects was added to the list. The student also had to translate part of a Latin medical text into English. From 1777, there was no link between the diploma and a right to practise in the area and so it became an entirely formal qualification.[110] Only David Maclagan went on to become a full fellow whilst McGrigor was again appointed honorary fellow in 1824.

Only nine of the cohort earned their letters testimonial (later called the licence) from the Royal College of Surgeons in Dublin. This required a fee of ten guineas and proof of study of anatomy, physiology, surgery, and surgical pharmacy. This qualification pronounced them 'duly qualified to practise Surgery, and to be elected a Member of this College'. Three of the cohort went on to become members, equivalent to a fellowship, and would have paid an additional fee of 20 guineas for the privilege. Two were elected as honorary fellows.[111]

Finally, four non-graduate surgeons of the cohort also became extra-licentiate members of the Royal College of Physicians of London. This was a qualification designed for provincial practitioners and required recommendations, an oral exam which might or might not be in Latin according to the candidate's abilities, and certificates of either one year spent at a university, one year walking the wards in London, or two years' attendance at a provincial hospital with certificates of attendance at lectures on anatomy and physic. As noted by Lawrence, few seem to have thought the status of this qualification worth the bother of application.[112] The Glasgow Faculty of Physicians and Surgeons offered a similar facility for non-graduates and two members of the cohort, Gideon Dolmage and John Murray Strath, became licentiates there.

---

[107] Cope, *Royal College of Surgeons of England*, 70. Cope, 73, notes that McGrigor asked that a list of medical officers the Army Medical Board had selected be granted the fellowship but the Council refused.

[108] C. H. Creswell, *The Royal College of Surgeons of Edinburgh: Historical Notes from 1505–1905* (Edinburgh, 1926), 186.

[109] *Laws of the Royal College and Corporation of Surgeons* (Edinburgh, 1816), 44.

[110] Rosner, *Medical Education*, 140–5; *Laws of the Royal College*, 47–8.

[111] *By-Laws, Ordinances, Rules, and Constitutions of the Royal College of Surgeons in Ireland* (Dublin, 1785), 6–7; Widdess, *Royal College of Surgeons in Ireland*, 16–17; Cameron, *History of the Royal College of Surgeons in Ireland*, 146, 173.　　　　[112] Lawrence, *Charitable Knowledge*, 78.

EDUCATION POST-ENTRY INTO THE ARMY

The overall impression arising from this analysis of the education and qualifications attained by the cohort is of a relatively learned body of men. However, an important aspect of this subject not yet explored is at what point they attended these lectures, walked the wards, and attained their degrees and diplomas. Analysis of relevant dates shows that they appear to have been well educated before sitting their first exams at the Army Medical Board. Returning to the sample of sixty-three medical practitioners used in Figure 3.8, the average doctor studied seven subjects before enlisting. On the other hand, half the cohort took at least two or three courses afterwards, whether repeating the same topics or studying new ones (see Figure 3.15). Isaac Cousins, an Irishman, is fairly typical in this regard. Between 1807 and 1811, he studied anatomy and surgery, materia medica, chemistry, botany, midwifery, and medical practice, and went to clinical lectures at Glasgow University. In May 1811, he became a hospital mate and went on to be promoted to hospital assistant in February 1816. From that date until July the following year, he was on half-pay and took the opportunity to return to Glasgow and attend James Jeffray's lectures on anatomy, the former army surgeon Robert Freer's (d. 1827) on medical theory, Robert Cleghorn's on chemistry, and James Towers's on midwifery.[113] The case of Cousins is also typical in demonstrating some key distinctions in the timing of the study of certain subjects. Core topics, such as anatomy, were usually taken before signing up (and possibly afterwards as well) whilst others, such as midwifery, were much more likely to be studied later in a career, almost certainly with a view to its utility in future civilian practice. Hospital experience also appears to have been mostly gained prior to receiving an initial appointment in the army (Figure 3.16). James Kennedy, who spent a year at the Infirmary in Edinburgh before becoming an army doctor, and William Lempriere, who walked the wards at the London for twelve months in 1787 prior to becoming a surgeon's mate the following year, were entirely characteristic.

   Some of those who took extra classes later in life used the opportunity to qualify for an MD. Indeed, considerably more than half of those who attained a degree did so after joining the army (Figure 3.17). Analysis of those for whom both the date they were awarded a degree and that of their first army appointment are known shows that a total of 109 became MDs after they had entered into service compared to twelve who were awarded degrees in the same year and fifty-one who acquired them before. Most of the number who earned degrees after their initial army exam did so between six and fifteen years later. The educational system at the time permitted such accumulative study. Whilst graduates from Edinburgh and Glasgow had to have studied for at least three years, those years

---

[113] Drew, no. 887: Robert Freer.

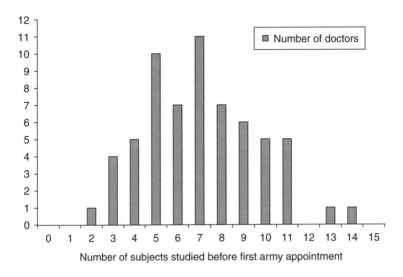

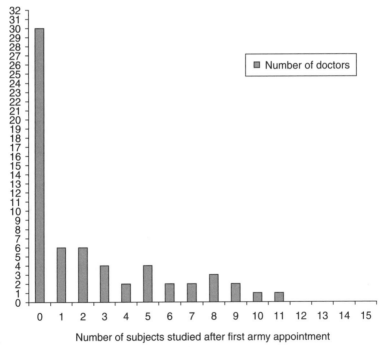

Figure 3.15. Number of Subjects Studied before and after First Army Appointment

Note: This Fig. is based on the same sample as in Fig. 3.8.

Source: Doctors' Database: Table: Lectures; First Army Appointments.

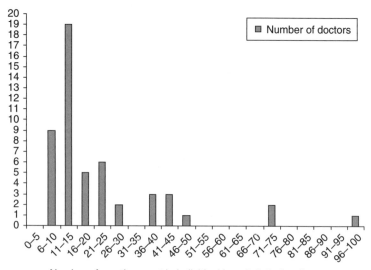

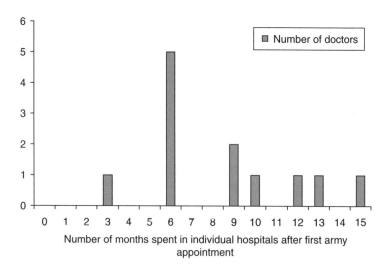

Figure 3.16. Hospital Experience Gained before and after First Army Appointment

Note: this table is based on the same sample as Fig. 3.9.

Source: Doctors' Database: Tables: Hospitals; First Army Appointment.

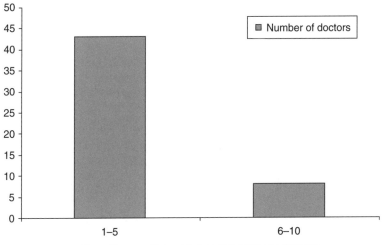

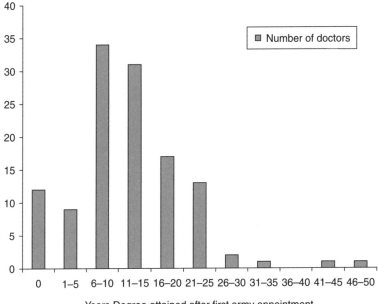

Figure 3.17. Degrees Gained before and after First Army Appointment

Source: Doctors' Database: Tables: Degrees, First Army Appointment.

did not have to be consecutive unless, in the case of Glasgow, the student held a University bursary.[114]

Alexander Lesassier was one of those who improved his learning after a period in the army and went on to be awarded a degree. When he was placed on half-pay at the end of the war, he initially tried to set himself up in practice in Viana in Portugal where he was stationed at that time. Unsuccessful, he travelled back to England and was invited by his uncle to return to Edinburgh and continue his studies. He attended four lectures every day, read widely, and studied the classics, qualifying for his degree, 'the highest academical dignity' he had ever hoped to attain, in 1816.[115] When George Gordon McLean was placed on half-pay, he also set off for Edinburgh. He had already taken courses in Aberdeen and London before entering the service but wanted an MD. Unfortunately, he was then recalled to his regiment but, according to a note made on his service return, was allowed to finish his current session at the university on the condition that he pay for a physician to take his place.[116] Similarly, John Scott noted on his form that he had arrived back in England in 1818 'to continue my professional studies' and had been 'employed in attending medical classes'. He had already studied at Edinburgh from 1810 to 1813 but, between 1818 and 1819, he took further classes in natural history, chemistry and pharmacy, clinical medicine, materia medica, botany, midwifery, and medical practice in that city. He also studied botany and anatomy and attended dissections in London and was rewarded with an Edinburgh MD in 1819.[117]

John Hennen had already had an extensive and illustrious career in the army before he, too, decided to take further classes with a view to getting an MD. He had been educated under his father in his native town of Castlebar, County Mayo, and had walked the wards in the County Hospital in 1792. Between 1796 and 1798 he had studied anatomy, surgery, chemistry, and medical practice and attended clinical lectures in Edinburgh. He became assistant surgeon to the Shropshire Militia in 1798 and worked his way up through the ranks, being appointed deputy inspector of hospitals in 1815. In 1817 he returned to Edinburgh for three and a half years and 'continued to prosecute his studies with no ordinary zeal'. He supplemented his army experience by attending Thomson's lectures in military surgery and studying materia medica under James Home and medical theory with Andrew Duncan senior. After writing a thesis entitled *De sanitate militum tuenda*, he received his degree from the university in 1819, just over two decades after beginning service in the armed forces.[118]

In contrast, many more surgical diplomas were awarded either before surgeons entered the army (88), or in the same year that they joined up (96), than after they

---

114 Rosner, *Medical Education*, 63; Dow and Moss, 'Medical Curriculum at Glasgow', 240.
115 Rosner, 125–33.   116 TNA, WO25/3910, fo. 98.
117 TNA, WO25/3906, fo. 123.
118 J. Hennen, *Principles of Military Surgery, Comprising of Observations on the Arrangement, Police, and Practice of Hospitals, and on the History, Treatment and Anomalies of Variola and Syphilis* (London, 1829), pp. vii–xi.

had spent a period in service (56). Although, as we saw in the previous section, a London diploma was quite expensive, those who took the examination early in their career seem to have felt it was a good investment. One such was John Murray of Turriff who became a member of the London College in 1804. In a letter home he explained his decision to do this rather than sit the army qualifying examination on grounds of its greater value.

Those who pass for a diploma have a peculiar advantage and are looked upon in a much more honourable light. They undergo a more serious examination, they become members of the Royal College of Surgeons, and they can go into any service they like whatever without undergoing any more examinations in the way of surgery and anatomy at least.[119]

In a nutshell, possession of the diploma brought exemption from the army surgical examination. On the other hand, given that more than 50 per cent of the cohort did not hold a college diploma when they entered the army, it would seem that many of Murray's peers were not convinced of the need to subject themselves to a more demanding exam. There seems to be no obvious factor linking the lives of the minority who took a college diploma later in their career. One who took the London diploma after serving for some years was the well-connected Alexander Dunlop Anderson, who joined the army in 1813 but only became a member of the London College in 1816. Another was an Irishman about whom next to nothing is known of his origins, Henry Hart, who became a hospital mate in 1809 but only submitted himself to the London College exam in February 1815, three days before going on a short period of half-pay. Anderson does not seem to have felt the need to take any refresher courses before undergoing the ordeal. Hart in contrast was more circumspect. Although he had attended a number of courses in London in 1806–9 and did a stint at the Middlesex Hospital, he took no chances in preparing for the exam. In the previous year he had once more put himself to school and sat at the foot of Carpue (for the third time), John Pearson (surgeon to the London Lock Hospital), and Thynne.[120]

    Bell claimed that this apparent desire of army medical practitioners to go back to the hospitals and universities after a period of service was due to realization of 'the defects of their original education': 'they return to the various schools of medicine to have knowledge and professional learning grafted upon experience, because they were hurried into the world too early to have their experience founded on previous knowledge.'[121] As it has just been demonstrated that most of the cohort's training was taken before their first army appointment, this was clearly overstating the case to make the political point that any army medical college was desperately needed. However, this said, it is likely that the men in our cohort, from less than affluent backgrounds, had not had sufficient money, time, or opportunity to undertake all the education they desired before signing up. As well

---

[119] SNA, GD1530/1, fos. 17–18. It gave him the freedom, if he chose, to enter the navy and the East India Company's medical service as well as the army. [120] TNA, WO25/3904, fo. 70.
[121] Bell, *Memorial*, 6.

as being able to exploit the opportunities offered by leave on half-pay or being stationed in one of the three capital cities, a period of service would have allowed them to save a reasonable sum of money to pay for further classes. In addition, they would have been able to take advantage of the fact that some lectures, such as those given by Guthrie and by John Halahan and Dease at the Royal College of Surgeons in Dublin, were free to those in the armed forces.[122]

Such further study was presumably undertaken by some with a view to smoothing a future transition to civilian practice. This was sometimes even true for those who had already obtained a degree. Between 1805 and 1810, William Richardson Gibb attended classes at Glasgow University, including Professor Jeffray's lectures on anatomy and Robert Cleghorn's sessions on surgery. He also spent eighteen months at the Royal Infirmary and a year at the Lying-in Hospital before qualifying for an MD in 1811. That year, he was commissioned as a hospital mate in the army. However, he returned to his studies during a period on half-pay in London in 1816; studying anatomy with Dr Abernethy (1764–1831), attending Dr Brande's lectures on chemistry, and walking the wards in the Eye Infirmary. In 1818 he went back to Glasgow and reacquainted himself with the faculty, studying chemistry with Thomas Thomson (1773–1852), surgery with John Burns (1774–1850), and revisiting Jeffray's classes on anatomy and surgery. Presumably this helped him to obtain the illustrious position of one of the four surgeons to the Glasgow Infirmary in 1821 and again in 1822.[123]

However, whilst many were intent on gaining certificates and qualifications that would further their civilian careers, others were more concerned with their position within the army. Even before the end of the French wars, study leave periods of six or twelve months could be granted to those desirous to improve or revise their medical and scientific knowledge. In 1814, Edward Johnston was given leave of absence by the director-general to go back to Edinburgh where he had studied almost a decade previously, to take further courses and obtain an MD. This was with a view to promotion within the ranks as the director had promised to place him 'on the list of Physician to the Forces as a reward for my service'.[124] From the beginning of the McGrigor era, army surgeons seeking further training were given official encouragement. 'Gentlemen already in the service are earnestly recommended to avail themselves of every opportunity of adding to their knowledge by attending universities or schools, for which purpose every facility will be afforded by the Director General'.[125] By the 1840s a degree had normally become de rigueur for the higher reaches of the service.[126]

---

[122] Drew, p. 137; Pettigrew, *Medical Portrait Gallery*, iv. 8; *Plarr's Lives of the Fellows*, i. 483; Royal College of Surgeons, Dublin, Arch/10/c/1a, 'An Account of the Class of the Royal College of Surgeons under Mr Halahan and Dr Dease', 1800.
[123] Dow and Moss, 'Medical Curriculum at Glasgow', 247.
[124] TNA, WO25/3910, fo. 80.   [125] TNA, WO30/139, fos. 228–9: qualifications 1826.
[126] TNA, WO25/3923–43: Candidates for Commission as Surgeons 1825–67, changing details on the pro forma. See Ch. 1, n. 133.

The ambitious responded accordingly. Thomas Rolston's service return of 1818 contains a covering letter to McGrigor explaining why he had not yet taken a doctorate. He had lost his left foot and part of the leg whilst attending the wounded on the field at Tarragona five years previously. When he had returned to England, he had considered going to Edinburgh to get a degree with the hope of becoming a physician to the forces, a post 'less exposed to the vicissitudes of the service'. However, John Weir, the previous director-general, had advised him of 'his entire satisfaction with his qualifications' and against spending 'so much money in so unnecessary a manner'. Whilst Rolston had taken the advice, he was now concerned, presumably in light of McGrigor's apparent concern to improve the standard of the army medical corps, that his lack of a degree would hinder his advancement. He thus concluded: 'Should you consider my taking out a degree in medicine or becoming a member of any of the colleges indispensably requisite towards my future advancement in the service, I have most respectfully to solicit your advice relative to the most expeditious.'[127]

TRAINING AND PATRONAGE

The degree to which the men in the cohort expanded their medical knowledge whilst in service, becoming well qualified and experienced by the time they retired, is one of the most notable findings of this project. As we have seen, many doctors took lecture courses during periods of leave and half-pay, and men such as Isaac Cousins both expanded their knowledge and gained expertise in fields not previously studied. Many used this additional experience to acquire an MD; some looking ahead to a future civilian career, others more concerned with the security of their positions and the possibility of promotion within the armed forces, once McGrigor had taken control.

However, this chapter has also shown that, whilst McGrigor encouraged these doctors in service to expand their training, they had mostly been well educated before ever sitting an exam at the board. Although very limited information on the cohort's schooling is available, the data would suggest that a grammar school background was fairly typical. Over 80 per cent of the cohort went on to serve an apprenticeship, mostly being indentured between the ages of 14 and 16 for a period of five or seven years. The vast majority also took classes at the universities and colleges and attended private lectures and demonstrations. One particularly important aspect of this data is the number of subjects that they studied, averaging seven before entry and nine altogether, and the degree to which they travelled around the British Isles in the process of their training, the largest number

---

[127] TNA, WO25/3904 fo. 144. At this juncture Rolston was living in Chester. He was still on active service, for according to the *Army List* he served 1815–26, when he died in Malta, as an assistant surgeon on the staff. He never took a degree.

studying in two or more cities. Although London was the most popular place for these students, the most well-attended lecturers, Thomas Charles Hope and James Gregory, were based in Edinburgh. Such information allows us to identify the key figures in medical training at this time. Alongside such classes, most of the cohort also walked the wards in at least one hospital. Again, London was the most common location in which to gain such practical experience, with St George's hospital attended by the greatest number of doctors.

The level of education that the cohort achieved prior to joining the army, mostly in the 1790s and 1800s, raises two important issues. First, it gives the lie to the idea that the army medical corps was transformed after 1815 from an unregulated conglomerate of poorly educated men into a group of highly trained and well-qualified individuals. It seems that McGrigor rather enforced and built on much that was already common practice, promoting a rhetoric of improvement to bolster the standing of the corps (not to mention his own reputation), whilst largely placing a stamp of approval on the qualifications that most army doctors already had to offer. Equally, John Bell's claim that most of those becoming army doctors in 1800 were more notable for their ability to learn by rote than for their training and medical knowledge had much more to do with his desire to promote the idea of a military school than with the actual status quo.

This in turn suggests that by 1800, institutionalized training in the country's medical schools and hospitals had become a commonplace. If recruits to the army—a service with very limited appeal—had received a medical education far in advance of the official requirements, then this can only mean that nobody at the turn of the nineteenth century was taken to be acceptably trained in medicine who had merely received an apprenticeship and read a few books. Formal learning of one or two years had become the norm. By extension, this means, too, that the vast majority of general practitioners, in England especially, would have experienced much the same *cursus* as their army brethren, if it is improbable that such a large proportion—nearly half—already had a university degree or a licence from one of the royal colleges of surgery when they started their active medical career.[128] Presumably, many army surgeons perceived that this additional investment would smooth their passage into the service, even if there was no official pronouncement to this effect before the McGrigor era.

Second, the sophistication of the cohort's early training raises the key question as to how those from the relatively modest middling backgrounds examined in the previous chapter were able to spend so much time and money on their education. If a student arriving in Edinburgh in the early nineteenth century decided to sign up for four lecture courses, he would have to spend £12 4s. immediately. In addition, to obtain a ticket to walk the wards at the Royal Infirmary would require an extra outlay of £3. Taking board and lodging in the city, following the prices

[128] Much the same conclusion is asserted in Lawrence, *Charitable Knowledge*, chs. 4–5, and Loudon, *Medical Care*, ch. 2, but no one has hitherto demonstrated it to be the case.

recorded by Thomas Ismay, could easily cost him another £36 for a nine-month stay. These figures add up to more than £51 and do not make any allowance for books, clothes, instruments, and other incidental expenses. A year in London, where again lecturers charged about 3 guineas per course, would have been just as expensive. If basic living expenses seem to have been less, gaining hospital experience as a pupil or full dresser was costly—at least £25. If Dent's experience is any guide, then even a careful student could easily have spent £100 in a year. Given that the average army surgeon had taken seven courses before joining the service and that many had spent upwards of two years in hospitals, most must have had about £250 invested in their education, including their apprenticeship fee. In many cases, this would have been equivalent to the family's annual income and explains why poorer families could only afford to place one son in the professions.[129]

Doubtless, the money was usually found by the immediate family scrimping and saving, and probably borrowing. But it is also evident that many of the cohort owed their education to outside help. Most frequently, this must have been provided by richer or less burdened relatives, for it was a commonplace at the turn of the nineteenth century for the successful or single to give a leg-up to less fortunate members of their extended family (as indeed some members of the cohort were to do themselves).[130] Of the twenty-five relatives gratefully acknowledged for their assistance in the dedications to the Edinburgh theses penned by the cohort, only nine were fathers: the rest were uncles, brothers, and brothers-in-law.[131]

John Davy's dissertation, for instance, was dedicated in 1814 to his brother, Sir Humphry, who at the very least had made his three years in Edinburgh comfortable ones. When John had arrived in the Scottish capital in October 1811, he had brought with him a fistful of letters of introduction to the great and good in the city, notably one to the novelist, Henry Mackenzie, author of 'The Man of Feeling'.[132] Humphry had also promised to give him £40 per annum above what John would receive from his mother, to ensure that he could board with a respectable family.[133] Not surprisingly, John was effusive in his brother's praise: 'Through your precepts and example, you have led me in the paths of knowledge; you have been the stimulus of my labours and opened up to me the delights of philosophy and the marvels of nature ... I freely confess that above all mortals I owe you the most; to you therefore, dear brother, I dedicate this experimental endeavour.'[134]

---

[129] See Ch. 2.
[130] See Ch. 6. Nelson's concern for his sisters' children was typical in this regard. See Roger Knight, *The Pursuit of Victory: The Life and Achievements of Horatio Nelson* (London, 2005), 424.
[131] There were probably other relatives among the dedicatees whose relationship to the graduand was not specified: e.g. the Irishman Charles Farrell dedicated his thesis to a Roger O'Farrell, gentleman of County Longford, and a Gerald O'Farrell, a barrister, of County Dublin.
[132] see *DNB*, *sub nomine*.
[133] John Davy, *Memoirs of the Life of Sir Humphry Davy*, 2 vols. (London, 1836), ii. 431–2.
[134] John Davy, *De sanguine* (Edinburgh, 1814).

A year earlier, in contrast, William Gibney dedicated his Edinburgh thesis to his paternal uncle, John. John Gibney, a Brighton physician and friend of the prince regent: had looked after William's well-being since the early death of his father: 'He was my guardian, and had the general superintendence of my education, and being a man of strong mind and literary habits, together with my mother resolved that my education should be thorough and liberal.' He also entertained the young William in Brighton during the vacations and steered him towards a medical career: 'I had accompanied him frequently on his visits to patients, more particularly to those in the country round, and observed how much he was respected and appreciated for his abilities, urbanity, and skill; and, having always a hankering after physic...I at once informed him that it was my fixed resolve to follow his profession and qualify at one of the universities.' As John Gibney also presumably paid for William's medical studies in Edinburgh and Dublin, the graduand was duly appreciative.

Dearest uncle, I have primarily prepared this dissertation in order to give you thanks. I confess it is not very well done for I have only been able to draw on a few things from my own experience. I dearly wish it were more perfect. But, albeit imperfect, I hope these first fruits of my studies will be acceptable to you as testimony to a grateful mind. It is my deepest vow that you may live and flourish long and always do honour to everything you take part in. Farewell.[135]

It was an uncle, too, who helped Lesassier enter the medical profession. Lesassier's father was at no point of much utility in his son's training. Pierre Lesassier had eloped with the daughter of Alexander Hamilton, professor of midwifery at Edinburgh University, whilst he was a student in that town. Her family accepted the marriage and they had held a second ceremony in their church, the New Episcopal Chapel. Alexander had a close relationship with his maternal grandparents as, after his mother died from consumption in 1790, he went to stay with them until he was old enough to be returned to his father and attend school. In 1802, his grandfather died and left him the sum of £200 in trust with his uncle, James Hamilton. It was this Hamilton who was ultimately responsible for his future career as a doctor. He forwarded the money for Lesassier's apprenticeship to Collier and later saved him from an abortive attempt to set up in practice in Rochdale. Hamilton pointed out that Lesassier 'was too deficient in point of medical knowledge to fill my present undertaking', and suggested he come to Edinburgh where he would advance more money from the inheritance to enable his nephew to attend medical lectures. Alexander lived with the family, was provided with money, and had nothing more required of him than 'application to my studies'. He was suitably grateful for his uncle's support, asking: 'What can be more nobly generous than my uncle's behaviour towards me—Supporting me in his own family, & advancing money for my education—What should I have been but for his assistance!'[136]

[135] Gibney, 4–5, 7–8, 74; William Gibney, *De coeli caldi* (Edinburgh, 1813).
[136] Rosner, 2–4, 6–7, 11, 15, 24–8, 32.

On the other hand, some fortunate surgeons gained their education thanks to the help of family friends or patrons. John Murray of Turriff was fortunate in having the patronage of the earl of Fife whilst studying to become a medical practitioner. Fife was his father's landlord and presumably spotted talent: he supported him throughout his education at Marischal College, Aberdeen, and his subsequent studies in London. Murray senior seems to have had only to keep his son in food, sending off to the capital frequent supplies of dried haddock and cheese.[137] The son of a London surgical goods manufacturer, George James Guthrie, was equally lucky in having the support of an influential figure, in his case John Rush, inspector-general of army hospitals, 'whose care he had been under for a serious accident' in 1798. It was thanks to Rush that the young Guthrie was articled with the Pall Mall surgeon, Mr Phillips, and became the particular pupil of Dr [Joseph?] Hooper at the Marylebone infirmary.[138]

It is also clear that such patrons could be directly responsible for the tyro surgeon's decision to join up. Either from a sense of realism or a sense of duty, they were not usually proferring their money and influence to increase the number of civilian practitioners. Lord Fife did not order Murray into the army medical corps, but he intended him to choose between the armed forces, the navy, or the East India Company and was clearly ready to support his application to the first even though he was under age. Rush, as a member of the service, was less accommodating. His assistance in getting Guthrie a medical education was dependent on his entering the army 'promising him an appointment as soon as he was capable of holding it'.

In other words, the relatively disadvantaged medical student did not necessarily choose to enter the army medical service but was sometimes compelled to enter. Even close relatives could make it clear that their bounty came to an end once their charge's education was complete. James Hamilton, who had to pay for the education of a younger brother and place another in the East India service, besides looking after his own children, had no intention of setting Lesassier up as a doctor in Edinburgh. Instead, he told him that he should look for a situation in the army and offered to use his influence to ease his passage. Once Lesassier's father had agreed to the plan, Hamilton approached Thomson, recently appointed as professor of military surgery; 'requesting Mr. T would have the complaisance to employ his interest for a situation for me in the Army, as Dr H. said he considered me fully qualified for it. There was a compliment.' Hamilton also ensured that Lesassier had the necessary documentation to present to the Army Medical Board and then personally put him on the coach to London, doubtless anxious to get rid of an expensive and troublesome nephew.[139]

John Gibney similarly decided to place his nephew in the army as William's studies drew to a close. There was apparently no negotiation between the two,

[137] SNA, GD1530/1, fos. 8, 16, 18–9
[138] Pettigrew, *Medical Portrait Gallery*, iv. 2–3; *Plarr's Lives of the Fellows*, i. 483.
[139] Rosner, 31–3. Hamilton's much younger brother, Henry Parr, was educated at Cambridge and eventually became dean of Salisbury.

although the elder Gibney did woo the Edinburgh student with the promise of a decent position. 'About this time I received the gratifying news from my dear uncle at Brighton, now knighted and appointed physician to the court, that he had succeeded in obtaining for me from the authorities the promise of an assistant-surgeoncy in the cavalry so soon as I should be qualified.' William's decision to take his degree in June 1813 rather than later on in the year was to take full advantage of this: 'I should have preferred deferring the degree until later on in the autumn, but my uncle had set his heart on my going up at midsummer.'[140] Archibald Arnott was also sent into the army on a patron's say-so, but in his case it was because an opportunity unexpectedly presented itself. Having provided his son with a medical education, George Arnott of Kirkconnel Hall was concerned that Archibald should be placed in a position worthy of his social status. He seems to have written for advice to a distant relative, Lord Lindores, who suggested that his fifth son become a medical officer: 'Would yr youngest son like to be employed with the Army on the Continent, and be able to procure sufficient certificates of his abilities to attend the hospitals? If so I will not only use the freedom to write to Sir Wm. Erskine myself, but will do my utmost to furnish him with other recommendations.'[141]

Patronage in some form or other, therefore, played an important facilitating role in recruitment to the army medical service, if one that can never be quantified. This was inevitable given the fact that the Army Medical Board clearly expected its entrants to have as good a medical education as any civilian practitioner. Since joining the army had limited attractions to the well-placed medical student, the majority of recruits were certain to come from the more disadvantaged families of the middling sort, however much they have may have been propelled into the service by patriotism as much as need. These families, though, whatever their aspirations for their children, would often have lacked the means to give their sons a decent medical education without additional help from their extended family or patrons. Patrons were thus essentially facilitators. They allowed many ambitious parents who might otherwise have lacked the means to take advantage of the window of opportunity offered by the French wars to place their sons in the army (or navy) medical service. At the same time, their generosity helped to ensure that the service received the recruits that it required. The patron played a key social function in an era in which medical education was undergoing a sea-change. By the end of the eighteenth century, only practitioners who had had one or two years' institutionalized training were considered properly prepared for any branch of medicine. In the absence of state-funded bursaries or free tuition, there was no way of meeting the temporary needs of the dangerous and less glamorous part of the profession without the help of benefactors. Patronage and philanthropy were

---

[140] Gibney, 74, 88–90.

[141] James Arnott, *The House of Arnott* (Edinburgh, 1918), 110–8. Erskine, later a major general, was at this point only an army captain but he was already a celebrity for saving the life of the Emperor Leopold.

indissolubly linked in the eighteenth century. Facilitating the entrance of the lower middling sort to the army medical corps was just one very minor part of a great web of enlightened charity.[142]

There again, if the facilitator could often be a dictator, the ultimate decision to enter the service had to be a personal one. Just as some recruits, such as Dent, entered the service without their family's permission, there must have been others who turned their backs on the pressure of parents, relatives, and patrons and refused to join up, whatever the consequences. Unsurprisingly, though, most appear to have bit the bullet without complaint, for an army career must have seemed to many young medical practitioners from unpromising backgrounds to offer a passport to a better future. At the very least, it presented an opportunity to repay their family and patron's investment in their training. At best, they may have dreamed of eventually joining the small band of London practitioners for whom army service had previously provided a stepping stone. If they survived the ordeal, husbanded their pay, nursed their contacts, and invested in further education, they might one day return to civilian life with all the advantages that they so obviously now lacked and become the next Pringle or John Hunter.

---

[142] D. Owen, *English Philanthropy, 1660–1960* (Cambridge, Mass., 1965); Donna T. Andrew, *Philanthropy and Police: London Charity in the Eighteenth Century* (Princeton, N.J., 1989).

4

Army Careers

GETTING STARTED

Throughout the French wars anyone who aspired to become an army medical officer had first to demonstrate orally his knowledge of surgery before one of the royal colleges and then, from 1798, his abilities as a physician before the Army Medical Board. Even those with a medical degree had to take the army surgical diploma: only those who were already members of one of the colleges of surgery by dint of their having taken its general licence were exempt.[1] Candidates could choose to be examined for a simple assistant's diploma at a cost of 1 guinea or a regimental surgeon's qualification at 3 guineas, rising to 2 and 5 respectively in 1810.[2] Obviously, those who took the former had to appear for a second time before one of the college boards of examiners if they wanted to progress in the medical corps. To be admitted to the examination in physical medicine, candidates had first to present their credentials to the board's clerk, who quizzed them on their age, apprenticeship, and formal training before allowing them to proceed. The board examined candidates on the first and third Thursday of each month, and examinees had to register the previous day. Those who took the surgical diploma in London, too, seem to have had to pass the exam in medicine before they could attend Surgeon's Hall. The right to appear before the college depended on obtaining a letter of introduction from the War Office.

Very little detailed information exists about either entrance examination. The registers of the royal colleges reveal how many candidates for the army, navy, and East India Company were seen each year and how many were accepted.[3] But beyond that they are silent. It would seem, though, that the surgical examination eventually became quite demanding. The Scotsman Alexander Lesassier's appearance before the Army Medical Board one afternoon in the spring of 1806 was a relatively relaxed affair. He answered questions on various infectious diseases

[1] As John Murray of Turriff pointed out in a letter home in 1804: see Ch. 3.
[2] See Ch. 3. This was the fee in London. In Dublin the cost was a little more, initially £12s.9d. and £38s.3d.
[3] RCSE, Examination Books, 1745–1800, 1800–20, 1820–30; RCSS, 1, 7–9: College minutes, 1793–1828; RCSI, Arch/3/B/1–7: Court of Examiners Minute Book, 1785–1826. There were some failures: e.g. on 25 May 1811, the Dublin Royal College rejected one John Clogher, who had attempted to gain his assistant surgeon's certificate for the navy: see RCSI, Arch/3/B/5, *sub dato*.

including smallpox and cholera and was duly certified competent. His appearance at Surgeon's Hall the following day, however, was a different experience. Early in the evening he joined a group of thirty who sat in an agitated state in an anteroom waiting to be interviewed.[4] Six or seven candidates were summoned at a time into the presence of thirteen examiners who sat on either side of a table and were then assigned an individual interrogator. Lesassier, called at 8.15 p.m., was given to David Dundas (later Sir David, 1749–1826), one of London's leading surgeons, who spent the next hour demonstrating the examinee's limited acquaintance with anatomy and surgery, especially cases of hernia.[5] As a result, though Lesassier had hoped to gain the full surgeon's diploma, he was judged only proficient to serve as a hospital mate and told to return any time after six months and try again.[6]

The Irishman, William Gibney, seven years later was more successful and gained the coveted regimental surgeon's qualification at the first attempt, but he too found the surgical examination an ordeal and fell sick shortly afterwards 'with a horrible distemper, known as "sweating sickness", which almost brought me to death's door'. As a medical graduate who had already passed an examination in anatomy, Gibney was discomforted to find that the Army Medical Board expected him to take the army diploma at all. Moreover, as his surgical knowledge was rusty, he did not feel equipped to appear at Surgeon's Hall immediately. He thus spent the next fortnight in lodgings at Holborn reading voraciously and cursing his relative neglect of surgery in his last year at Edinburgh. After a fortnight, though, he felt competent to face the examiners and succeeded in passing for the surgical diploma 'most creditably'.

There were many examiners and perhaps thirty or forty students to be examined. Various questions, some very intricate, were put to the students, and success or failure in the reply at once noted. Then after a while each examiner took over one or two students for a closer examination, noting the replies as before. I was consigned to the tender mercies of a chirurgical and very eccentric knight then in great fame. He took me on a great number of subjects; and, strange to say, on the treatments of most of the cases he suggested we entirely disagreed. I had been taught otherwise. I soon discovered that the worthy knight had his own crotchets upon almost everything; but in the end we got on famously. With a smile he observed, as I stuck to my teaching, 'Yes, young gentleman, you answer perfectly as you have been taught in the schools, but on the field of battle and in most cases, if you adopt my plans you will do much better'.[7]

Once accepted for the service, about three-quarters of the cohort (341 out of 454) entered the corps as hospital mates or assistants, regardless of the diploma they

---

[4] Presumably, they were not all candidates for the army diploma but included would-be entrants to the navy and the East India Company.

[5] Military doctors were continually called on to resolve hernias brought on by carrying great weights and lugging equipment.

[6] Rosner, 35–7. Given Lesassier's truncated education as an apprentice (see Ch. 3), the judgement was just.

[7] Gibney, 88–9. He was possibly interrogated by Sir Astley Cooper, although the latter was not yet a knight.

Table 4.1. Surgeons' Rank at Point of Entry

Year/s	SM	RM	GM	HM	HA	SAS	AS	S	SS	P	D	C
1772–92	10	5		4								
1793	2	2	1	1				2				
1794	6	1		8				1	1			
1795	6			3								3
1796	4	1		3			2					
1797	1			4			3					
1798				5			2					
1799				5			2		1	1		
1800				12			3					
1801				6			1					
1802				1								
1803				13	1		6	1		2		
1804				12			4					
1805				13			3					
1806				9			2					
1807				6			5					
1808				12			3					
1809				25			4					
1810				15	1		4					
1811				22	1		3					
1812				21	3		3				2	
1813				12	26							
1814				3	9							
1815				4	20[a]		1					
1816												
1817												
1818												
1819				1								
1820–33					60	6	1					
Total	29	8	1	220	121	6	52	4	2	3	2	3

[a] Includes 1 Acting Hospital Assistant.

Key: SM: Surgeon's Mate; RM: Regimental Mate; GM: Garrison Mate; HM: Hospital Mate; HA: Hospital Assistant; SAS: Staff Assistant Surgeon; AS: Assistant Surgeon; S: Surgeon; SS: Staff Surgeon; P: Physician; D: Dispenser; C: Purveyor's Clerk or First Clerk to the Inspector-General of Hospitals.

Source: Doctors' Database: Table: First (Dated) Army Appointments.

had gained or the date of their appointment. Most of the others, particularly in the first half of the war, entered as assistant surgeons or, as they were originally called, surgeon's or regimental mates (see Table 4.1). From 1810 everyone was supposed to enter the service as a hospital mate, but this had clearly been the common practice for a decade.[8] Even in the 1790s, the possibility of entering the service at a higher level was slim. Director-General McGrigor, who bought himself a full surgeoncy in the Connaught Rangers in 1793, was always an

[8] For the 1810 regulation, see Ch. 1.

exceptional figure. In the first year of the war, only one other entrant in the cohort entered the service as a regimental surgeon. On the other hand, right through the war, there were occasional recruits who entered at an extremely high level because they were already senior medical figures. Thus, John Thomson, the Edinburgh professor of military surgery, was seconded to Wellington's HQ for a short time after the Waterloo campaign and understandably joined the service as an acting staff surgeon.[9]

In entering the service, then, the emphasis was generally laid on an individual's educational attainment and experience in deciding his rank. Background and recommendation counted for little, except when it came to obtaining the rare medical cadetship.[10] Where meritocracy often gave way to old-fashioned patronage seems to have been at the next level in the medical officer's career. Hospital mates had their feet on the first rung of the ladder and from 1804 a commission and the attractive salary of 6s. 6d. per day, rising to 7s. 6d. plus lodgings if sent abroad.[11] However, how quickly those who had qualified as full surgeons could expect to be promoted and to what sort of regiment, depended in part on their family's standing and contacts. Obviously, the pattern of promotion was governed to some extent by the availability of appointments and a mate's perceived competence. Nonetheless, the speed with which some entrants mounted the next rung of the ladder and found billets in prestigious regiments suggests that patronage was frequently an important factor in getting an army surgeon properly launched in his career.

The majority of mates attended a military general hospital for several years after entering the service before they were gazetted as assistant surgeons, ostensibly learning the ropes under the eagle eye of experienced staff officers. Some could spend several years in the wilderness. The tenant-farmer's son John Murray of Turriff joined the service in 1805 but it was 1809 before he gained a regimental appointment.[12] Those, too, who had not passed the surgeon's examination and were immediately posted abroad—as mates frequently were—found themselves in a further predicament. They could not get home to take the examination which they needed to further their career. This was the position Lesassier found himself in, having been sent to the Gibraltar garrison in May 1806. Although after nearly a year, he was appointed temporary assistant surgeon to the 42nd Foot, the Black Watch, then stationed in the port, he was unable to retain the position because he lacked the vital certificate, and another officer, Alexander McLachlan, duly arrived to fill the post. Lesassier badgered his commanding officer, Deputy Inspector Abraham Bolton (d. 1818), to give him leave, so that he could return to London, but was told in November 1807 that this was impossible, 'because he had written

[9] Matthew H. Kaufman, *The Regius Chair of Military Surgery in the University of Edinburgh, 1806–55* (Amsterdam, 2003), 69–70.
[10] For these, see Ch. 2. Lesassier was offered one by Inspector-General Knight as a favour to his Uncle Hamilton. But Lesassier declined: Rosner, 38–9.   [11] See Ch. 1.
[12] Drew, no. 2923.

Table 4.2. First Regimental Postings

First regimental posting	Number of surgeons
Assorted	65
Corps of Waggoners	1
Corps of Miners	1
Ceylon Regiment	3
Madras Army	1
Royal African Colonial Regiment	5
West Indies Regiment	12
Sicilian Regiment	2
Royal Veteran Battalion	3
Garrison Battalion	8
Battalion of Reserve	4
Private Regiments	6
Loyal American Regiment	1
Fencible or Militia Regiment	15
Volunteer Regiments	3
Line Regiment of Foot	278
90th or above	28
50th to 89th	107
15th to 49th	77
10th to 14th	28
2nd to 9th	28
1st [Royal]	10
Light Infantry	1
Cavalry: Dragoons, Hussars, Lancers, Chasseurs, Staff	35
Guards	11
Foot	2
Horse	2
Dragoons	7
Total	389

Note: Not all members of the cohort joined a regiment.

Source: Doctors' Database: Table: First and Last Regiments.

for four Hospital Mates & consequently it would be very ridiculous to send me home who am in fact the only "*disposable mate on the Rock*", as he was pleased to elegantly express himself—Damn & blast such a beggarly title.' Lesassier did finally get to retake the examination the following February or March, but he had spent two years getting into the position where he could even lobby the Army Medical Board for promotion.[13]

Furthermore, for the majority, their first appointment as assistant surgeon would be in a regiment way down the pecking order (see Table 4.2). Only 35 out of 389 who eventually joined a regiment (9.0 per cent) gained a post in the cavalry, and only eleven began in the Guards. The large majority went into foot

[13] Rosner, ch. 4, *passim*. For Bolton (not in the database), see Drew, no. 1170.

regiments, and a sizeable proportion (16.6 per cent of the total) not even into regiments of the line but into colonial or other assorted corps. The twelve who were
promoted into one of the lowly West Indian regiments drew the shortest straw of
all. Even the 'liners' did not generally receive appointments in the most prestigious
regiments. Half the contingent of 278 who joined a line regiment had to make do
with a position in the 50th Foot or above, while only 38 began their regimental
career in the top nine and only ten in the 1st Foot (the Royals). Needless to say,
John Murray, when he finally made assistant surgeon, found himself in the 67th,
while Joseph Brown, the seventh son of a bankrupt Tynside merchant, was
gazetted to the 58th and Charles Boutflower, fourth son of a Yorkshire parson of
limited means, had to make do with a post in the 40th.

Other mates, on the other hand, made assistant surgeon within a matter of
weeks and received plum appointments. Unfortunately, too little is known about
the social origins of the eighty-four members of the cohort (18.5 per cent) who
entered the top nine line regiments, the cavalry, or the guards to confirm that they
were particularly privileged as a group. They seem to come from the same mix
of professional, mercantile, and rural backgrounds as their peers.[14] Only one
definitely had a father who was close to the centre of power. This was Michael
Lambton Este, who joined the Foot Guards in 1800, and whose clergyman father
was one of the king's reading chaplains at Whitehall and a friend of Nelson.
Interestingly, though, there was a definite over-representation of Englishmen
among the group, especially in the case of those who joined the Royals or the
Guards. Given that only 28 per cent of the cohort were English, it is notable that
they comprised 14 out of the 21 who entered the most prestigious regiments (see
Table 4.3). Such a skewed pattern of intake would suggest that patronage played
some part in appointment to an assistant surgeoncy. Arguably, Scottish and Irish
recruits had to have particularly good family contacts if they were to have any
chance of an elite posting as assistant surgeon.

Two individual cases of appointments to cavalry regiments, moreover, confirm
that this was so. Archibald Arnott's father had been promised that his career in the
army would be promoted by Sir William Erskine.[15] Sir William clearly did his bit,
for Archibald effortlessly entered the 11th Dragoons on 14 April 1795 (albeit after
an eighteen month wait). William Gibney was similarly assisted by the London
society doctor and fellow Irishman, Charles Bankhead (*c*.1797–1870), physician
to the foreign secretary, Viscount Castlereagh. Gibney's physician uncle had
promised that Bankhead would get his nephew a cavalry appointment. As soon as
Gibney arrived in London, he visited his uncle's go-between, dined at his house,
then accompanied his patron to visit Director-General Weir. Although Weir made
it clear that Gibney had to pass the exam, he seems to have offered the young
graduate a position about to fall vacant in the 15th Dragoons. After Gibney had

[14] See Ch. 2 for a discussion of the social background of the cohort and the limited information
available. The father's occupation is known of only two surgeons who entered the first nine regiments
of foot, eight the cavalry, and three the guards. [15] See Ch. 3, p. 150.

Table 4.3. Nationality of Surgeons Entering Top Regiments

Regiment	England	Ireland	Scotland	Abroad	Unknown
2nd to 9th Foot	11	8	8		
1st Foot	6	1	3		
Dragoons, Hussars etc.	8	10	13		4
Guards (Foot, Horse, Dragoons)	8	1	1	1	
Total	33	20	25	1	4

Source: Doctors' Database: Tables: First and Last Regiments; Doctors 1.

spent a token six-week stint as a hospital mate at the York hospital, Chelsea, the director-general honoured his word and the Irishman was ordered to the depot at Brighton to join the 15th, even before being officially gazetted. Received graciously by the Colonel—'he was acquainted with many of my relatives'—he was at once the CO's guest in the mess and spent a rather insipid evening with a bevy of officers from his own and other regiments. 'The conversation was more lively than improving—somewhat of shop, but more about the pretty girls of Brighton...it became rather monotonous, it being clear that the fair sex and horses monopolised the chief part of my brother officers' thoughts and ideas.'[16]

Admittedly, not every desirable first appointment should be put down to family influence. William Dent, a tenant farmer's son (not in the cohort), entered the service in April 1810 and, like Lesassier, soon shipped off to Gibraltar; by early August, however, he was assistant surgeon of the 9th Foot. But Dent's good fortune seems to have been uncommon and probably reflected the fact that he had answered Astley Cooper's call to join up temporarily in 1809: presumably, the influential surgeon looked after his interests.[17] Generally, it can be assumed, the better one family's contacts, the better the position on the starting-grid. The case of Robert Keate, the surgeon-general's nephew, demonstrates this to perfection. Made a hospital mate in 1794 in due deference to the professional hierarchy, he subsequently avoided a regimental appointment and hence serious medical service altogether. He was made deputy purveyor to the forces in 1795 (a government desk job), a staff surgeon in 1798, and field inspector of hospitals in 1799.

GOING PLACES

Most recruits to the army medical service during the French war joined up in their early twenties. Once certificated, the majority could expect to remain in the corps for at least ten years and not permanently enter civilian life until their middle age

[16] Gibney, 100–1. He was not gazetted until October because he had for complicated reasons already been made assistant surgeon of the Dragoon Guards.
[17] See Ch. 2. WL, RAMC 536, no. 17: Dent to his mother, 17 Sept. 1810, on his promotion.

Table 4.4. Length of Service

Years in service	Date of entry: pre-1815	Date of entry: 1809–15
5 or less	13 (16%)	13 (44.8%)
Less than 10	19 (25.3%)	19 (67.9%)
10–14	10 (13.3%)	2 (7.1%)
15–19	16 (21.9%)	2 (7.1%)
20–29	17 (22.7%)	2 (7.1%)
More than 30	13 (17.3%)	3 (10.7%)
Total	75	28

Note: The length of service of every fifth member of the cohort who entered the army before 1815 was calculated. The table does not include periods of half-pay. Two of the thirteen who served for five years or less died in service. It will be recalled that a small proportion of the cohort entered service after 1815: see above, Introduction, p. 18.

Source: Doctors' Database: Tables: First (Dated) Army Appointments; Residence/ Service.

(see Table 4.4). The quarter who served for a shorter time and came out in their late twenties and early thirties were to be found among the surgeons who had only joined up in the last years of the war. In the years 1814–19, as we will see later in this chapter, most surgeons found themselves placed on half-pay, as the army was quickly run down on the conclusion of peace (albeit broken temporarily in 1815). Recent recruits were not peculiarly singled out for standing-down, but they were much less likely to be recalled to the colours in subsequent years or serve thereafter long spells of duty. Gibney, for instance, may have started in a prestigious regiment in 1813 but his army career lasted a mere five years. In December 1818 he was placed on half-pay and never recalled. Conversely, surgeons who entered the service at or before the beginning of the war were often only finally released when they were into their fifties or sixties. William Chambers, probably from County Antrim, entered the service as a regimental mate in 1793 attached to the 18th Dragoons.[18] He served with only one short period of half-pay in 1821 for the next thirty years, finally retiring in 1825. He never rose above the rank of surgeon, so spent the whole of his career as a regimental doctor. A few of the cohort, who landed desk-jobs in middle age, were well into their seventies or beyond when they finally retired. Director-General McGrigor had clocked up nearly sixty years' continuous service when he handed over the reins in 1851.

After the first few years of the war, virtually all surgeons began their service career in a general hospital attached to a permanent barracks in England, even if they were then quickly sent overseas. Lesassier was unusual in being posted directly to Gibraltar.[19] For most of the conflict, the most popular location seems to have been the army depot on the Isle of Wight, although towards its end the majority probably followed in Gibney's footsteps and spent their first few months attached to the York at Chelsea. Many, too, were first dispatched to Portsmouth,

[18] He was apprenticed in Ballymoney, County Antrim. [19] Rosner, 40–3.

where they served in the barracks at Gosport and Hilsea, like Dent, while others
were sent to the Channel Islands, which were used as a holding centre prior to
invasion of the continent. McGrigor's first tour of duty was in the barracks of St
Helier in the summer of 1794, where his new regiment, the 88th, was decimated
by typhus, a disease to which he himself quickly succumbed. 'I was for several days
insensible and the earliest things I recollected was great soreness from blisters
which had been applied to my head, neck and legs, together with great prostration
of strength.'[20] In the years of peace, however, the army depot was moved to
Chatham and the York eventually run down, so that members of the cohort who
joined up after the war were initiated into the mysteries of army medicine and
surgery in McGrigor's new military hospital at Fort Pitt on the Medway.[21]

Given the number of fronts on which Britain was engaged during the war, it is
not surprising that many new recruits quickly found themselves in a battle zone
once they had left the shelter of an English barracks. McGrigor's experience was
typical. He was still recovering from typhus, when his regiment was ordered to
reinforce the defence of Holland against the French. He spent the dreadful winter
of 1794–5 moving from town to town dealing with an overwhelming number of
sick and wounded, collapsed again himself, and eventually was carried to the
point of embarkation in a wheelbarrow.[22] The longest and most costly campaign,
of course, occurred in the Peninsula, so this was inevitably the theatre in which the
largest number of surgeons saw service. As Table 4.5 reveals, at least 157 of the
cohort spent some time in the Peninsula, many for the duration. For those, like
Lesassier, who arrived in Portugal in 1808–9, their life for the next five to six years
would be a hectic round of combatting epidemics and treating wounds.[23]

A respectable proportion of the cohort were also present on other shorter
campaigns. Table 4.6 details the number of surgeons beginning a tour of duty in
northern Europe during and immediately after the war. Clearly, at least forty
attended the appalling Walcheren expedition in 1809, while about fifty were on

[20] Gibney, 93–7; WL, RAMC 536, no. 15: Dent to his mother, 24 June 1810; McGrigor, 36–7.
[21] See Ch. 1. It is impossible to give precise figures about the general hospital first attended.
The information provided by the cohort's service returns frequently only gives England or a county
as the location of their first posting, while many more precise returns do not give a date. From the
information in the Project Database, 146 of the cohort passed through Chatham (all post-1815), 94
were based at Portsmouth, 90 served on the Isle of Wight, and 67 attended the York, but these totals
do not distinguish between first and subsequent postings.   [22] McGrigor, 37–46.
[23] The best accounts of military medicine in the Peninsula are Richard L. Blanco, *Wellington's
Surgeon General: Sir James McGrigor* (Durham, NC, 1974), ch. 7; Martin Howard, *Wellington's
Doctors: The British Army Medical Services in the Napoleonic Wars* (Staplehurst, 2002), *passim*; Rosner,
chs. 6–9. Of members of the cohort only Sir James McGrigor, 'Sketch of the Medical History of the
British Armies in the Peninsula of Spain and Portugal during the Late Campaigns', *Transactions of the
Medico-Chirurgical Society*, 6 (1815), 381–489, Gibney, and Charles Boutflower, *The Journal of an
Army Surgeon during the Peninsular War* (Manchester, 1912), left an account of their service in the
campaign, and Boutflower's journal says little about medical matters. Besides Lesassier's letters on
which Rosner's account is based, David Maclagan and John Murray's letters home are extremely
informative: see NLS, Acc. 11767; WL, RAMC 830. The richest source still under-explored is
McGrigor's notebooks and journals: WL, RAMC 799/6–7 (microfilm copies).

Table 4.5. Number of Surgeons Each Year Beginning
a First Tour of Duty in the Peninsula, 1807–1814

Year	Number starting
1807	2
1808	31
1809	26
1810	16
1811	16
1812	32
1813	29
1814	5
Total	157

Note: As not all surgeons recorded the date that they began to serve in the Peninsula, the above numbers are minima. Some surgeons who had been at Corunna returned for a further spell of duty.

Source: Doctors' Database: Table: Residence/Service Table.

the Waterloo campaign. Not all, though, can have been present at the battle, for only 23 appear on the Waterloo Roll Call: 4 on the staff, 7 in the cavalry, and 12 in the infantry. Their number includes William Chambers, mentioned above, John Robert Hume, who became Wellington's personal physician, and the West Indian-born, Samuel Barwick Bruce, who served on the staff and whose Waterloo medal survives.[24] (See Illustration 7.)

A few unfortunate souls saw action on a large number of fronts. Between quitting Holland in a wheelbarrow and alighting in the Peninsula in January 1812, McGrigor had taken part in the ill-fated invasion of San Domingo in 1795–6, the 1799 attack on Egypt, and the Walcheren fiasco ten years later.[25] Few members of the cohort who had been in the Peninsula also served at Waterloo, but one surgeon who did so had even been at Walcheren. This was James McDougle from Berwick-on-Tweed who joined the service in 1804 and eventually ended up as a deputy inspector. After various postings in England, Ireland, and the Channel Islands, he was sent to Walcheren, then the following year, after a spell again in Britain, to the Peninsula, where he remained for the three years, 1810–13. In 1814 he was transferred to Holland, was present at Waterloo the year after, then became part of the army of occupation in France, and only got back to England again in 1819, when he was placed on half-pay for eight years.

Even during the war, however, army surgeons frequently found themselves posted to more peaceful locations. Throughout the conflict the army had garrisons stationed in Ireland and throughout the British empire: in Canada, the West

[24] Charles Dalton, *The Waterloo Roll-Call*, 2nd edn. (London, 1971). Drew identifies 167 army surgeons who were present at Waterloo: 27 are in the cohort. Neither source mentions that Gibney was also at Waterloo but he is the one member of the cohort to leave an account of the battle: see Gibney, chs. 8–10. [25] McGrigor, *passim*.

Table 4.6. Number of Surgeons Starting a Tour of
Service in Northern Europe per Year, 1793–1818

Year	Number	Stated location (chief)
1793	—	
1794	5	
1795	2	
1796	—	
1797	—	
1798	—	
1799	11	Holland
1801	2	Copenhagen
1802	—	
1803	1	
1804	2	
1805	7	Hanover
1806	—	
1807	15	Copenhagen
1808	3	Sweden
1809	40	Walcheren
1810	—	
1811	—	
1812	—	
1813	10	Holland
1814	16	Holland, Belgium, and France
1815	49	Belgium and the Netherlands
1815	25	France
1816	7	France
1817	1	
1818	2	

Note: Since many surgeons did not provide a complete record of their
service abroad or give dates, these are minimum figures. There must
have been many more of the sample on the continent in 1794–5.

Source: Doctors' Database: Table: Residence/Service Table.

Indies, Africa, India, and Australia. Although the West Indies was involved in the
war in the second half of the 1790s and troops stationed in Canada took part in
the 1812 war with the United States, most troops based outside continental
Europe were engaged for most of the time in local policing rather than the struggle
for world dominion. As a number of new colonies were acquired in the course of
the struggle, especially from the Dutch, the number of potential imperial stations
to which an army surgeon might be sent in the long peace of the McGrigor years
was even greater.

Table 4.7 records the number of the cohort who at some time in their army
career did a tour of duty in one of the many stations around the world where
the British flag was flown in the first half of the nineteenth century, including the
continental theatre. What is immediately clear is that there was no single station

Table 4.7. Regional Postings

Region	Number of individuals (stationed in the specified location on at least one occasion)
Africa and islands	117
Africa [unspecified station]	[13]
Cape of Good Hope	[42]
Cape Verde, Madeira, Santa Cruz	[9]
Egypt	[33]
Mauritius	[17]
Morocco	[2]
St Helena	[10]
Sierre Leone	[9]
America [unspecified station]	25
Australasia and the Pacific	13
New South Wales	[12]
Norfolk Islands	[1]
Tasmania	[2]
Canada and North America	90
Amherstburg	[1]
Canada [unspecified station]	[59]
Cape Breton	[1]
Montreal	[1]
New Brunswick	[5]
Newfoundland	[8]
New Orleans	[5]
North America [unspecified station]	[13]
Nova Scotia	[30]
Quebec	[6]
Europe and the continent [unspecified]	8
France	113
Hispanic Peninsula	195
India, Ceylon, and Asia	106
Afghanistan	[1]
Bengal	[10]
Bombay	[11]
Borneo	[1]
Ceylon	[36]
East Indies	[18]
Gujarat	[1]
India [unspecified station]	[48]
Madras	[12]
Mahratta [Maratha Confederacy?]	[4]
Seringapatam	[1]
Ireland	185
Italy, the Mediterranean, and the Black Sea	166
Corsica	[1]
Gibraltar	[87]
Ionian Islands	[31]
Italy (Genoa, Leghorn, and unspecified)	[16]
Malta	[55]
Minorca	[5]

Table 4.7. (*Cont.*)

Region	Number of individuals (stationed in the specified location on at least one occasion)
Naples and Calabria	[10]
Ottoman empire	[4]
Rhodes	[1]
Sicily	[36]
Northern Europe	158
Austria	[1]
Baltic (Sweden and Denmark)	[23]
Belgium (incl. Flanders & specific towns)	[52]
Germany (unspecified station]	[9]
Hanover	[6]
Heligoland	[4]
Holland (unspecified station)	[42]
Netherlands (unspecified station)	[23]
Switzerland	[1]
Walcheren	[48]
Zealand (unspecified station)	[3]
South America	18
Buenos Ayres	[3]
Demerara	[7]
Montevideo	[1]
Surinam	[1]
West Indies and Central America	180
Antigua	[6]
Bahamas	[9]
Barbados	[48]
Bermuda	[13]
Curacao	[2]
Dominica	[7]
Grenada	[6]
Guadelupe	[7]
Honduras	[8]
Jamaica	[78]
Martinique	[15]
Puerto Rico	[1]
San Domingo	[7]
St Kitts	[7]
St Lucia	[13]
St Vincent	[9]
Tobago	[6]
Trinidad	[5]
West Indies [unspecified station]	[85]

Note: The information is taken from the service return of individual surgeons in the cohort. Some returns are much more complete and informative than others, so the values in the Table above are only approximate. None of the returns recorded service in China but two of the cohort died in Hong Kong. The sum of the number of surgeons attending individual stations in a region does not tally with the regional total since surgeons frequently visited more than one station.

Source: Doctors' Database: Table: Residence/Service.

Table 4.8. First Postings outside Great Britain

Region	Number of surgeons
Africa	17
Canada	5
Hispanic Peninsula	22
India	2
Ireland	30
Mediterranean and Italy	17
Northern Europe	20
South America	1
West Indies	28
Unknown	4
Never left Britain	2
Total	148

Note: Table based on every third member of the cohort. As surgeons did not always give the dates of their sojourns abroad, it has been assumed that the first station cited was their first posting.

Source: Doctors' Database: Table: Residence/Service.

that every surgeon could expect to pass through, however long his career. There was evidently a high likelihood of being posted to Ireland or the West Indies, which were visited by some 40 per cent of the cohort. On the other hand, there was no more than a one in five possibility of spending time in India or Canada, only a one in eight chance of enjoying the sun in the new colony of Malta, and a one in ten of seeing the Cape of Good Hope. Service in Australia was even more improbable. Only thirteen of the cohort were ever based there, twelve in New South Wales, the first, John Martyn Dermott from Wellingborough in Northamptonshire, going out with the 73rd in 1809.

It is equally clear from Table 4.8 that there was no obvious cursus. New surgeons were not blooded in a particular location outside Britain, then gradually moved round the empire in a standard order. For mates and hospital assistants, postings abroad were determined by government exigency, while assistant surgeons and surgeons inevitably followed their regiment. In consequence, some members of the cohort found themselves in exotic locations from the very beginning. William Ferguson, who appears to have come from Jamaica, joined the army in 1813 as a hospital mate and was almost immediately whisked away to fever-ridden Sierre Leone to serve in the garrison hospital. Eugene McSwyny of Cork became assistant surgeon to the 17th Light Dragoons in 1812 and departed with them to India, while Backhall Lane Sandham, probably from Brighton, was posted as a hospital mate to South America, doubtless Surinam.[26]

---

[26] McSwyney was possibly the son of the Eugene McSwiny of Cork who published Goldsmith's *Vicar of Wakefield*.

Table 4.9. Geographical Mobility of Army Surgeons

Region visited outside Great Britain	Number of surgeons
0	2
1	20
2	42
3	44
4	25
5	8
6	6
Unknown	2

Note: The table has been drawn from information relating to every third member of the cohort. The world has been divided into the following regions: Africa; Australia; Canada; Europe: Ireland, Hispanic Peninsula, Mediterranean and Italy, Northern Europe (each treated as a separate); India; North America (called America in the records); South America; West Indies and Central America. Given the incompleteness of the service returns, the numbers only indicate the trend.

Source: Doctors' Database: Table: Residence/Service.

On the other hand, in the course of a fifteen- to thirty-year career, the average surgeon could expect to see several parts of the world(see Table 4.9). Only the surgeons who joined up in the last years of the war and soon found themselves on half-pay were likely to get no further than the Peninsula and Belgium. Most surgeons could expect at least one spell of duty outside Europe and some 10 per cent would travel the world. Edward Pilkington, probably from Dublin, joined the service as an assistant surgeon of the unglamorous 5th Garrison Battalion in 1811. He avoided being sent to the Peninsula like most of his peers and spent the next two years in Ireland until transferred to the 19th Light Dragoons. He then spent 1813 to 1817 in Canada before going on half-pay for seven years. Recalled in 1824, he passed the next four years in Corfu with the 73rd and 7th Foot, then in 1828–9 was based in Sierre Leone. There next followed three more years on half-pay before he was posted to New South Wales in 1833 with the 29th Foot, where he was also a registered private practitioner.[27] He remained in Australia for six years before moving to India for a further two and finally coming home to retirement in 1841, now with the 17th Light Dragoons. He never rose above staff surgeon, a rank obtained in 1827, but his twenty-eight years in the service had taken him round the world with a variety of regiments. He finally died in 1851 in Denbighshire.

In the course of their travels, most surgeons would visit a region only once, but some could return several times. Table 4.10 emphasizes that repeat tours of the

---

[27] See the Australian Medical Pioneers Index, *sub nom.* at **www.medicalpioneers.com** (Sept. 2005).

Table 4.10. Multiple Tours of Duty

Regions visited	Once	Twice	Three times	Four times	More than four
Africa	44	16		1	1
Australia	5	2			
Canada	34	12	2	2	1
Hispanic Peninsula	56	5	1		
India	30	6	3	1	
Ireland	54	14	2		1
Mediterranean and Italy	46	18	12		
[North] America	9				
Northern Europe	60	21	4	2	1
South America	9	1			
West Indies and Central America	68	33	6	5	11

Note: Based on every third member of the cohort. Given the idiosyncracy of individual returns the table is inevitably incomplete. Many surgeons simply listed the region where they were posted and did not record whether they moved stations during their stay. Others gave precise details, listing in the case of the West Indies, for instance, every island to which they were posted.

Source: Doctors' Database: Table: Residence/Service Table.

West Indies were particularly common. If 40 per cent of the cohort were stationed in the region on one occasion, then 20 per cent visited the islands at least twice. Indeed, a small but significant percentage (7–8 per cent) must have gone there quite frequently. Some surgeons who claimed to have done multiple tours in the West Indies admittedly counted short visits to different islands as separate postings. Although Thomas Jackson (probably from Liverpool) only spent four years in the Caribbean from 1796 to 1800, he superficially notched up eight tours of duty, as in the course of his stay with the 14th Foot he visited Grenada, Martinique (twice), Puerto Rico, St Lucia, and Trinidad, and had even spent time on the mainland in Demerara. But a number of surgeons genuinely did spend many years in the region. Thomas Draper (apprenticed in Worcester) was first stationed in the West Indies in 1803–4, once more with the 14th Foot. He returned much later in his career as the inspector of hospitals for the area, residing in Barbados from 1824 to 1828, Jamaica 1828–37, and Barbados again 1837–40. Since he lived to enjoy ten years' retirement in Devon, he must have found the climate congenial. For many surgeons, as we shall see in a later section, service in the West Indies was a death sentence, but the inspector was obviously immune to the ravages of yellow fever.

Several of Draper's peers found other parts of the empire equally enjoyable and similarly thrived in a white man's grave. William Ferguson, encountered above, continually returned to Sierre Leone. His first spell of duty lasted only a year, but he was there again in 1823–9, 1830–9, and 1840–5, the three tours punctuated by short visits to England. He sealed his allegiance in 1824 by transferring to the

Table 4.11. Number of Regiments to which Surgeons Attached during Army Career

No. of regiments	No. of surgeons
0	5
1	19
2	31
3	18
4	14
5	9
6	3
7	1
Total no. of surgeons	100

Note: The information is drawn from a sample of 100 of the cohort (nos. 3–102).

Source: Doctors' Database: Table: Regiments/Garrisons Table.

Royal African Colonial Regiment. In 1845, he retired and became captain general and governor of the colony. Francis Sievewright from Edinburgh spent even longer in India. Created a hospital assistant in 1813, he eventually was gazetted to a West Indian regiment and passed the years 1815–17 in the Caribbean. From 1819, however, he was transferred to Ceylon and spent the next thirty-four years in different parts of the Indian subcontinent with the 11th Dragoons and various regiments of foot. Unlike Inspector-General Draper, his cannot have been a particularly comfortable life. He never made regimental surgeon till 1835 and, like Ferguson, never rose above the rank of staff surgeon.[28]

As so many of these examples demonstrate, many of the cohort not only spent their army service seeing the world but regiment hopping. They were engaged in a tour of the British army as much as a tour of the British empire, doubtless accumulating useful contacts as they moved around. Surgeons who were only in the service for a few years frequently stayed with the same regiment. William Gibney began and ended his short regimental career with the 15th Dragoons. But as Table 4.11 reveals he belonged to a minority. A third of the cohort passed through two regiments, such as McGrigor, who went from the Connaught Rangers to the Blues, while another third enjoyed the hospitality of three or four. One peculiarly skittish surgeon managed to put his feet up in the mess of seven. This was Andrew Browne from County Mayo, who joined the 99th Foot as a surgeon's mate in 1795. Two years later, he moved to the 39th as an assistant surgeon, before transferring again in 1801 to the 8th West Indies regiment as surgeon. He then moved a further five times between 1804 and 1819 always with the same rank, visiting the 8th Battalion of the Reserve (1804–5), the 99th Foot again (1805), the 3rd Garrison Battalion (1805–6), the 9th Foot (1806–19) and finally the

---

[28] In the years of peace this was an honorary rank: the holder still served with a regiment.

2nd Dragoon Guards. There he stayed for eleven years until made a deputy inspector. Curiously, according to his dossier, in all this time he saw precious little of the world beyond two short visits to the West Indies and precious little action.[29]

Browne's idiosyncratic career path immediately raises the question of the purpose behind such regiment hopping. Some surgeons may have sought a transfer on discovering that their regiment was bound for India or the West Indies, hoping thereby to avoid serving in an unpleasant part of the world. Others may simply have had to move in order to gain promotion. Assistant surgeons seldom had the good fortune to gain a surgeoncy in the same regiment. However, given the relatively lowly regiments in which so many of the cohort began their regimental service, it is hard not to believe that most, especially once they were surgeons, were attempting to move up. In Browne's case this is clear-cut. Having been forced into a West Indian regiment to become a surgeon, he spent the next six years manoeuvring his way into respectability before landing a post in the 9th Foot. There he stayed for thirteen years before obtaining the even more prestigious surgeoncy of the 2nd Dragoon Guards. For the son of an apothecary-surgeon from County Mayo, albeit one who claimed descent from the Montagues of Cowdray, Browne had done very well for himself during the war for a surgeon who had first entered the 99th Foot.[30]

Yet, if this were the aim of the regiment hopper, not everyone was successful. Table 4.12 charts the position of the cohort at the end of their regimental career. Put simply, upward regimental mobility was a fact but not for all. While a surprisingly large proportion of surgeons starting out in prestigious regiments traded down, at least a quarter of surgeons who entered lowly regiments ended their regimental career in the same sort of corps. Those who moved up, moreover, seldom journeyed far. None, apart from Browne and McGrigor, successfully rose from a lowly line regiment to the guards.

Similarly, as Table 4.13 confirms, there was little chance of a surgeon who had started out in a non-line regiment ever getting into an elite one. Only six of the sixty-five in this category recorded in Table 4.2 got into the top nine line regiments and none at all into the cavalry, while the four who were received into the Dragoon Guards were peculiar figures. They were not from colonial regiments, but two were from volunteer corps (the Nova Scotia Fencibles and the York Light infantry), one from the Garrison, and one from the Royal Veteran Battalion. The last, too, John Bickerson Flanagan of Somerset, had worked hard to climb the ladder, only making the Guards on his fifth move.

It would seem, therefore, that for many surgeons there was a limited chance of ascending a long way up the regimental ladder. But, as will be explained in the following sections, this reflected the reality of the army promotion system. Although

---

[29] His service record must have been filled in cursorily because his descendant, Sir Anthony Montague Browne, possesses Andrew's Peninsular medal: personal communication Mar. 2005.

[30] Browne was descended from Anthony Browne, first Viscount Montague (1526–92), who had many sons. Personal communication from Sir Anthony Montague Browne, Mar. 2005.

Table 4.12. Inter-regimental Mobility: First Regiment Compared with Last

Initial regiment	No.	No change	To (other) line regiment	To line regiment less than 10	To cavalry	To (other) guards	To other corps or regiment
West India Regiment	12	5	6	1			1
All line regiments	278	217	217	30	24	12	25
Line regiment (90th and above)	28	7	13	2	1	1	6
Line regiment (9th to 2nd)	28	10	13	10	2	2	1
1st Regiment of Foot	10	4	4	4	1		1
Dragoons	23	9	10			2	2
Guards							
Foot	2					1	1
Horse	2		1		1		
Dragoons	7	3	2	2	2		

Source: Doctors' Database: Table: First /Last Regiments.

Table 4.13. Inter-regimental Mobility: Last Regiment Compared with First

	No.	No change	From (other) line regiment	From (other) cavalry	From (other) guards	From other corps or regiment
West India Regiment	7	5	2			
All line regiments	269	219	219	12	3	35
Line regiment (90th and above)	23	6	16			1
Line regiment (9th to 2nd)	27	11	9	1	2	4
1st Regiment of Foot	13	4	7			2
Dragoons	35	9	19	4	3	
Guards						
Life	1				1	
Foot (Grenadiers)	1		1			
Horse	1		1			
Dragoons	20	3	11	2		4

Source: Doctors' Database: Table: First /Last Regiments.

advancement was supposedly based on seniority, solidly combined with merit in the McGrigor years, patronage was usually the key to going far. Reaching the upper rungs of the regimental ladder and rapid and continual movement up the table of ranks depended on knowing which army buttons to push. Those who enjoyed the greatest success in the service had often, like McGrigor himself, started with few obvious advantages beyond their medical training. They were not precluded from a stellar career, but their advance depended on their knowing how to demonstrate that they were worth cultivating and investing in. Equally, surgeons who might have been propelled into a prestigious regiment through external influence could not rest entirely on their laurels. Unless they had impeccable outside support, continued success came through working within the army's system.

MAKING A CAREER

Once an army surgeon had eventually entered a regiment, irrespective of how quickly he had got there and whether by fair means or foul, his chances of having a modestly successful army career were reasonably good (see Tables 4.14–15). Although a substantial 30 per cent of the 413 in the cohort who made assistant surgeon or its earlier equivalent never rose any higher, nearly 50 per cent of the cohort at least reached the rank of regimental or staff surgeon, and one in six would rise to the dizzy heights of the inspectorate.[31] A substantial minority, then,— including surgeons who had served for thirty years—would eventually return to a civilian life on half-pay or a pension worth at least 12*s*. 6*d*. per day (and sometimes more, if their record was judged particularly meritorious).[32] In the early 1840s there were seventy-one veterans of the French wars of the rank of deputy inspector/ physician or above still alive and enjoying the fruits of their years of service (seventeen in the cohort). The most senior was Theodore Gordon, former member of the Army Medical Board, who had been retired on an allowance of £600 per annum in July 1810. Gordon, who died on 27 January 1843, must have thought himself particularly blessed, but there can be few of his high-ranking colleagues who did not believe that their entry into the army medical corps had not been a wise move.[33]

Success was the result of a variety of factors. In the first place, since it took time to mount the ladder, promotion to the higher echelons of the service usually depended on staying in the army for two or more decades (see Table 4.18, below). By and large, the most successful in the cohort were those who avoided the massive cull of the service in the aftermath of the French wars and then managed to stay alive, healthy, and fit for duty for a considerable time afterwards.[34] Typical in this respect was the Irishman, Charles Farrell, who joined the service in 1799, departed as a full inspector in 1833, and lived in comfortable retirement until

---

[31] Although it would appear from Table 4.14 that 60 per cent of assistant surgeons became surgeons, the figure needs to be adjusted down a little: the table lists the number of the overall cohort who reached a particular rank. Some surgeons, such as McGrigor, were never assistants.

[32] See Ch. 1, Table 1.4.

[33] TNA, WO25/3897. This is a collection of service records from the early 1840s completed by officers of the rank of staff surgeon above on half-pay or a pension. There are returns from fifty staff surgeons. For Gordon, not in the database, see Ch. 1, n. 56: he was not the only highly ranked officer on half-pay to receive special treatment.   [34] For a fuller discussion, see p. 188 ff.

Table 4.14. Ranks in the Army Medical Service Obtained by Members of the Cohort

Rank obtained in service	Total number
Hospital mate	250
Surgeon's mate/ assistant surgeon	413 (91.0%)
Regimental surgeon	246 (54.2%)
Staff surgeon	153 (33.7%)
Deputy inspector (general) of hospitals	78 (17.2%)
Inspector (general of hospitals)	33 (6.6%)
Total in cohort	454

Table 4.15. Highest Position Obtained in the Army Medical Service

Rank on leaving the service	Number of surgeons
Hospital assistant/mate	18
Purveyor	5
Apothecary	12
Assistant surgeon	124 (27.%)
Surgeon	131 (28.9%)
Staff surgeon	92 (20.3%)
Physician	4
Deputy inspector of hospitals	21
Deputy inspector-general of hospitals	17
Inspector of hospitals	10
Inspector-general of hospitals	17
Director-general of army Medical Board	3
Total	454

Source: for Tables 4.14 and 4.15: Doctors' Database: Table: Army Positions.

1855. Charles started his career as an assistant surgeon in a Hanoverian regiment recruited in Germany (Hompesch's Mounted Rifles, existed 1798–1802), moved to the West Suffolk's (the 63rd Foot) in 1804, made staff surgeon in 1806, then physician to the forces in 1811, deputy inspector in 1817, inspector of hospitals in 1825, and inspector-general in 1830. He only had two short periods on half-pay—in 1802–4 (early in his career) and 1827–9—and over his thirty-year stint as a medical officer had the luck to spend a large amount of his time in the Mediterranean (1806–15 and 1829–33) and to escape unharmed and very wealthy from a twelve-year tour of duty in the tropical heat of Ceylon (1815–27).[35]

[35] Farrell became a rich Irish landowner: see Ch. 6. Presumably he was sent out to head the medical station in Ceylon at the end of the French wars. His last period of service was spent at Gibraltar, where he arrived just after the virulent epidemic which carried off the principal medical officer there, John Hennen.

Table 4.16. Number of Years Taken to Move from Assistant
Surgeon to Surgeon

Years taken to move from assistant surgeon to surgeon	Number of surgeons	Assistant surgeon 1810 or after
Less than 1	1	1
1–2	2	
2–3	2	1
3–4	7	1
4–5	8	
5–6	9	
6–7	6	1
7–8	6	
8–9	4	
9–10	1	
10–11	2	
11–12	1	1
12–13	2	2
13–14	2	1
14–15	5	4[a]
15–16	3	2[a]
16–17	2	1
17–18	1	1
18–19	1	1
19–20	1	
23–4	2	2
26–7	1	1
Total in sample	69	20

[a] joined post-1815.

Note: The sample was drawn from nos. 3–100 in the database. 24 assistant surgeons in this subgroup did not become surgeons. One got no further than hospital mate. A few also went straight from assistant surgeon to staff surgeon.

Source: Doctors' Database: Table: Army Positions.

The most upwardly mobile, too, were usually those, such as Farrell, who joined the service earlier rather than later (see Table 4.16). Medics who entered the service before 1810 were likely to make regimental surgeon within five years of becoming an assistant, and almost certainly within eight, and many could expect to end up on the staff. With new expeditionary forces continually being formed for active service in unhealthy locations, there was a rapid turnover of medical personnel at both the regimental and staff levels. From the moment Wellington took over the Peninsular campaign, however, the rate of attrition seemed to improve and the opportunities began to dry up. Those who became assistant surgeons in the final years of the war were unlikely to proceed up the ladder with any speed. With a few exceptions, it was usually ten to twenty years before they received a further promotion. One poor soul, James Smith had to wait more than twenty-six.

Born in 1785, almost certainly in north-east Scotland, Smith made a good beginning when promoted assistant surgeon to the 4th Foot (The King's Own) on 25 September 1812. He only made surgeon, however, on 15 February 1839, when he transferred to the 61st Foot (The South Gloucestershire), with whom he departed to India to meet his maker seven years later at Umballa.[36]

Nor did it make any difference how quickly a latecomer had been assigned a regiment. William Dent served as assistant surgeon of the 9th Foot for fourteen action packed years. During that time, he served in the Peninsula, Canada, and France, and was finally posted to the West Indies in 1819. He only became a full surgeon in the summer of 1824, when he was gazetted to another regiment stationed in the Caribbean, the 21st (The Royal Scotch Fusileers), on the death of the incumbent.[37]

Many army medics, furthermore, who entered in the final years of the war were destined never to rise above the rank of assistant. As Table 4.17 suggests nearly all the recruits who never made full regimental surgeon joined in the years 1810–15. In these years, 60 per cent of the intake, not the 25 per cent overall, were condemned to ending their days in the service as assistants. In part, this is to be explained by the fact that a large proportion of these surgeons died in harness before they had had time to accumulate the long years of service needed for promotion in the lean post-war period. Moreover, the chances of a further third of the subgroup were directly stymied by their being placed permanently on half-pay, when the army was quickly run down with the return of peace. This was the fate, for instance, of William Gibney, who had doubtless seen his rapid promotion to the 15th Dragoons as a useful staging-post on the road to an illustrious army career. After five years in the service and having been in the thick of the action at Waterloo, where he had to amputate the colonel's leg, he was summarily laid off in 1818 at the niggardly rate of 3/- a day.[38] But the fact that many of these assistant surgeons clearly served well into middle age without being promoted and that the lower achievers came in a peculiar high proportion from Scotland and Ireland would suggest that more partisan forces were determining their progress.

Indeed, this was true of the advancement of all members of the service. For all the rhetoric, the seniority system seems to have been honoured in the breach, especially in the era of the French wars, and entrants, early or late, could considerably improve their chances of success by skilful self-promotion. An assistant surgeon who wanted to get on would make sure his face was continually before the eyes of his medical superiors. With the rapid inflation of its personnel after 1793, the army medical service became the size of a large school: with over 1,200 officers on active service at its greatest extent, a surgeon could easily become a colourless name in a ledger. Simply keeping a clean face, obeying orders, and placing one's

[36] Smith's birthplace and country of origin is unknown, but he was apprenticed to William Watson of Keith, Banffshire.
[37] WL, RAMC 536, letters 27 Nov. 1810–9 Jan. 1826, esp. 9 Jan. 1824 relaying his promotion.
[38] Gibney, 250.

Table 4.17. Nationality and Service Record of Surgeons Moving No Higher than Assistant Surgeon

Characteristics	Number of surgeons
Year of entry	
1800–9	6
1810	5
1811	9
1812	9
1813	13
1814	6
1815	8
[1810–15]	[50] (86.2%)
1820–1	2
Total	58
Length of active service	
Less than 5 years	8 (13.8%)
5–9 years	26 (44.8%)
10–19 years	17 (29.3%)
20–3 years	3
Unknown	4
End of service	
[Permanently on half-pay from 1815–20]	[19] (32.8%)
Died in service	24 (41.3%)
Half-pay commuted *c.*1830	14
Permanently on half-pay post 1830	14
On active service after 1830	2
Unknown	4
Nationality	
England/Wales	10 (17.2%)
Ireland	22 (38.0%)
Scotland	24 (41.4%)
Abroad	1
Unknown	1

Note: The information is drawn from a sample of 198 of the cohort (nos. 3–200). Of the 198, 7 left as hospital assistants, 51 as assistant surgeons or staff assistant surgeons, while 140 made surgeon or above. 82 of the 198 joined the service 1810–15, so 61% of this subgroup got no further than assistant surgeon.

Source: Doctors' Database: Tables: Doctors1; Army Positions; Half-Pay; Service/Residence.

faith in the system was unlikely to be a sensible strategy in an age when personal contacts were still all important, all the more when many surgeons were away from England for many years and, before the McGrigor era, largely out of official contact with the board's HQ in Berkeley Street.

In the first part of the war the most unsubtle way to press one's suit once well established in the service seems to have been simple bribery. The erstwhile army surgeon, Charles Maclean, in 1810, admittedly not a highly reliable or experienced witness, claimed that William Moore (d. 1832), principal medical officer on the Isle of Wight in the early 1800s had paid Thomas Keate £1,000 for the office, and that another surgeon, John Buffa (d. 1812) had lavished the surgeon-general with presents in order to be permanently stationed at Chatham.[39] No young assistant surgeon, however, could have afforded such an outlay. The most obvious way to keep a foot in the door was to seek advancement in a suitably deferential letter. It can be assumed that the vast majority of letters which the board and chief medical officers on campaign received were personal requests for promotion. Typical was the letter sent to William Fergusson (1773–1846) by Samuel Hill (1786–1830), assistant surgeon of the 71st Foot on 21 January 1812. Fergusson had been ordered out to the Peninsula on 3 April 1808 to serve under Inspector James Franck, chief medical officer to Sir John Moore and later Wellington's army, and within a short period of time was himself head of the medical department of the Portuguese army with the power to recommend appointments.[40] Hill, after serving in Portugal, was back in Portsea convalescing and wrote seeking a place on Fergusson's staff. As a testimonial of his fitness, Hill included a certificate from Michael Balfour (d. 1824), the former surgeon of the 71st. If this was insufficient, then Fergusson should contact his successor, Thomas Macredie (d. 1856). The letter was nothing if not sycophantic.

Hope you will excuse the liberty I now take in addressing you, without having the honour of being previously introduced to you. But my wishes of becoming a candidate for the appointment of surgeon on the staff to the Portuguese forces when any vacancy may occur & being desirous of submitting my name before you as early as possible to prevent any tedious delay, will I trust plead for me as an apology. I beg leave to assure you that I shall feel much pleasure in having the honour of serving under you on the Portuguese staff, and that I shall use my greatest exertions to render myself useful & endeavour to merit your approbation.[41]

Yet, however sweetly penned, the sheer number and predicability of such missives were likely to have deadened their effect. A better tactic was to get to know one of the general officers or, on campaign, a medical officer with serious influence who would champion a surgeon's cause. This was Lesassier's ultimately successful method of getting on. Having been posted with the Black Watch to Portugal in

---

[39] Charles Maclean, *An Analytical View of the Medical Department of the British Army* (London, 1810), 118–40. Buffa excused his conduct on the grounds that he had children from two marriages to support. He had temporarily been physician to the emperor of Morocco. For Maclean's views of the Army Medical Board, see Ch. 1. For his time in the army, see p. 191. For Moore and Buffa, not in the database: see Drew, nos. 1256 and 1380.

[40] James Franck was Wellington's first Principal Medical Officer in the Peninsula. He was put on half-pay in October 1811 but continued to be paid at the full rate until he died in 1843: TNA/WO25/3897, no. 8. The Portuguese army was reorganized under the command of seconded British officers in 1809.

[41] WL, RAMC 212, assorted letters to Fergusson, no. 20. For Fergusson's life, see William Fergusson, *Notes and Recollections of a Personal Life*, ed. James Fergusson (London, 1846), pp. xi–xiv. He was the third son of a provost of Ayr. None of these four are in the database: For Hill, later an FRS, Balfour, and Macredie: see Drew, nos. 3156, 1547, and 2230.

the summer of 1809, he contrived for the first couple of years to be continually absent from his regiment attending the general hospital at Lisbon. There he made contact with a number of top medical men, including Fergusson, to whom he was introduced through the good offices of Dr, later Sir, Andrew Halliday (d. 1839), one of the first appointments to the Portuguese staff.[42] Fergusson's favour became an important patronage asset. While making it clear that there was no more space on the Portuguese staff, he did not hesitate to recommend Lesassier to the new head of the medical department of the British army in the Peninsula, James McGrigor. McGrigor particularly disliked personal approaches—he preferred applications to be forwarded by the candidate's immediate medical intermediaries, who knew their worth. Fergusson, though, was his close friend, so Lesassier was guaranteed special treatment. When he eventually called on McGrigor in June 1812, he was received affably. 'He assured me that Inspector Fergusson's letter of recommendation had prepossessed [him] exceedingly in my favour; and although there was no vacancy at present, he would embrace the earliest opportunity of serving me.' Admittedly, initially, Lesassier received nothing more than fine words. He never did get promotion in the British army. Nonetheless, a year later he was given a place on the Lusitanian gravy train: he had jumped from assistant to staff surgeon at one leap. Not surprisingly, he wrote McGrigor a fulsome letter of thanks.[43]

Only the less dedicated, however, could hover around general hospitals hoping to make contacts. And once McGrigor took over and placed the emphasis on regimental hospitals, it became well nigh impossible.[44] Another, more modern tactic, was to make a splash by demonstrating super-efficiency and medical skill. This was presumably how Guthrie rose to the top so quickly in the Peninsula. He was a superlative battlefield surgeon and an ardent supporter of McGrigor's hospital policies. Already a regimental surgeon when he arrived in Portugal with the 29th Foot in 1808, he made staff surgeon in January 1810 and deputy inspector in October 1812. In between he showed his skill as a surgeon and administrator when in charge of 3,000 wounded after Albuhera.[45] On the advance across Spain, McGrigor placed him in control of the new general hospital at Madrid which served General Hill's division. His conduct was exemplary. Insistent that regimental hospitals were set up to look after most of the sick and that surgeons supplied him with weekly returns, he excoriated those who fell short of his exacting standards. When Henry Forcade of the 83rd Foot forwarded him a private with the unfortunate name of Cane, who had received 300 lashes the previous day, Guthrie in turn whipped the junior officer with his tongue. Forcade should know that sending

---

[42] Not in the database; a voluminous author: see Drew, no. 2779.

[43] Rosner, 72–88, 97, 107. Another medical officer high in McGrigor's favour he cultivated was deputy inspector Edward Tegart (1772–1845) (not in the database), who served in the army from 1793–1824: TNA, WO25/3897, no 23; Drew, no. 1354.   [44] See Ch. 1.

[45] T. J. Pettigrew, *Medical Portrait Gallery*, 4 vols. (London, 1838–40), iv. 4: life of Guthrie. For Guthrie's contribution to military surgery, see Ch. 7.

178

such malefactors to the rear only encouraged them to shirk their duty. A punished man could march with his regiment unless severely flogged (!) or feverous as a result.[46]

McGrigor himself had relied on both strategies to ease his passage to the top. Part of the reason for his rapid rise to head of the medical service after his transfer from the Connaught Rangers to the Blues in 1804 was that he was both friendly with Francis Knight, the inspector-general of hospitals, and clearly a good administrator who could tackle waste. He had shown his abilities as a regimental surgeon and continued to do so once elevated to the post of deputy-inspector in 1805. He was someone that the board could safely send out to Walcheren and the Peninsula to head the medical staff.

McGrigor, though, as surgeon of the Blues, was fortunate to be based near London and able to remind Knight continually of his worth. It would even seem he was able to force Knight's hand. William Dundas of the East India Company, a relative of Lord Melville and another of McGrigor's friends, had offered to make the Aberdonian head of the medical service attached to a new fourth presidency of the company, which was planned in 1805. McGrigor, therefore, went to Knight and told him he intended to resign his commission, unless, presumably, he received promotion.[47] His colleagues, on the other hand, who were unable to lobby the board directly, had to think up other ways of currying favour with its members. What they could do personally to bring themselves to notice during the French wars must have been limited, but during the McGrigor era there were several ways of improving their claims.

One was to pander to the director-general's enthusiasm for lifelong learning and take refresher courses and new diplomas, whenever a surgeon found himself billeted in a city with a medical school.[48] A number of army surgeons therefore went back to college in middle age, not least Staff Surgeon Joseph Brown of North Shields, who was no sooner put on half-pay in August 1814 than he was off to Edinburgh, proposing to spend eighteen months attending lectures and then take his degree.[49] Frustrated in his intentions by the return of Napoleon and the reformation of Wellington's staff corps, he still found a way to continue his studies by attending the Paris faculty, while based in the city as part of the army of occupation after Waterloo.[50]

[46] WL, RAMC 209, pp. 1–22, paginated from the end of the book: Guthrie's letter book Oct.–Dec. 1812, esp. p. 4, letter Oct. 26. Forcade is not in the database: see Drew, no. 2278.

[47] McGrigor, 120–1, 123. McGrigor claimed he eventually decided not to take up the appointment because of political opposition to the Dundas machine and anti-Scottish feeling. William Dundas was appointed head of the fourth presidency based on Prince Edward Island. McGrigor met William in India. [48] See Chs. 1 and Ch. 3.

[49] Letters of Joseph Brown to his family in TWA, Acc. No. 1132: to his sister-in-law, 11 Aug. 1814 (transcript and photocopies of original in private hands).

[50] While Paris in the eighteenth century was renowned as a centre of surgical teaching, the new school of medicine founded by the Revolutionaries in the French capital quickly gained a reputation as a centre of the new science of pathological anatomy. Once the French wars were finally over, medical students from all over Europe, including the British Isles, flocked to Paris to sit at the feet of the

I am endeavouring to make good use of my time. The duties of the Corps being inadequate to filling it up I have entered myself to l'Ecole de Médecine here. I attend the hospital of La Charité, M. Boyer, and some other lecturers[. T]o say the very best of it, this is better than lounging about public places, and it has the important recommendation of being unattended with expense.[51]

Another tactic was to help McGrigor build up his collections at Chatham. Staff surgeon and physician to the forces, John Davy, cannot have harmed his chances of further promotion by sending the director-general interesting specimens from the Mediterranean in the late 1820s, just as Farrell undoubtedly knew what he was doing when he set up a station museum on the island of Ceylon.[52] Yet a third was to demonstrate one's commitment to medical and scientific advance by publishing articles and books on military surgery, tropical diseases, and the natural history of Britain's colonies, often fulsomely dedicated to the head of the service.[53] This was precisely the tactic which McGrigor himself had used to advance his career, when he published in 1804 an account of his encounter with the plague while principal medical officer of the contingent of the Indian army (which included the 88th) sent to participate in the Egyptian campaign of 1801. Having languished in the Connaught Rangers since 1793, he must have seen the possibility thereby of stepping out of the shadows into medical prominence, and at the first opportunity on returning to England he sought a high-placed medical patron for his embryonic manuscript.

[A]fter my return from Egypt to Bombay, having but a small charge of sick, I had much leisure time on my hands. At Bombay, as well as on my passage homewards, I employed some of that time in compiling from my notes, and from public documents to which I had access, an account of the medical transactions of the army from India to Egypt. This I did for my amusement and to pass away time. On mentioning to my friend Sir Walter Farquhar,

masters and take advantage of the easy access to bodies in the French hospitals to hone their dissection skills: see esp. E. Ackerknecht, *Medicine at the Paris Hospital, 1794–1848* (Baltimore, 1967); Michel Foucault, *The Birth of the Clinic: An Archaeology of Medical Perception*, trans. A. M. Sheridan Smith (New York, 1973); Russell Maulitz, *Morbid Appearances: The Anatomy of Pathology in the Early Nineteenth Century* (Cambridge, 1987); Caroline Hannaway and Ann La Berge (eds.), *Constructing Paris Medicine* (Amsterdam, 1998).

[51] TWA, Acc. No. 1132: to his brother, 29 Oct. 1815. He continued to study in Paris on a second visit to the French capital in the spring of 1817, although he was not impressed by French medical practice: 1132/19, to his sister-in-law, 7–8 Mar., 1817. Alexis Boyer (1757–1833) was surgeon at La Charité and a leading authority on the art.

[52] Both are among a number of surgeons praised for their scientific activities in the printed abstract of the minutes of the AGM of the Medical Officers' Society in 1829: see WL, RAMC 262/l/19: personal papers of surgeon W. Lindsay (see below). Davy, who joined in 1815, became staff surgeon in 1821, physician to the forces in 1827, and eventually deputy inspector in 1840. McGrigor circulated all foreign stations encouraging contributions to the Chatham collection in 1826: see ibid., RAMC 215, papers of Assistant Surgeon Thomas Murray (not in the database), no. 8: printed circular from the inspector's office, Kingston, Jamaica, 14 May 1826. On the development of Chatham as a teaching centre, see Ch. 1.

[53] A detailed analysis of the publications of the cohort is given in Ch. 7. Again McGrigor had encouraged this in the 1826 circular.

in London, what I had done, he expressed a desire to see the manuscript. Sir Walter showed it to the late Sir Gilbert Blane, who strongly urged me to publish it as the public had no account of it from any quarter and he said it was particularly desirable they should know what had been done at the time of the plague.[54]

Farquhar (1738–1819) and Blane (1749–1834) were useful champions of any book. Both physicians to the prince of Wales, both former medical officers of the services, and Farquhar an Aberdonian to boot, they were just the supporters a battle-worn veteran in an Irish regiment needed. The tactic seems to have worked like a dream, even before the book appeared. McGrigor had hardly rejoined the 88th in their quarters at Helsham, Sussex—he had travelled back from India separately—before he was mysteriously transferred to the Horse Guards Blue in February 1804 to fill the vacancy left by Dr William Hussey (d. 1821), promoted deputy inspector. Admittedly, Farquhar and Blane's names did not eventually appear on the dedication page—this honour went to two members of the Army Medical Board, Knight and Keate. All the same, it is difficult to believe that they were not instrumental in some way in ensuring McGrigor's elevation.[55]

Finally, the canny medical officer could always contribute with gusto to McGrigor's medical charities. Indeed, not to do so was a sure way to get a full surgeon into the director-general's bad books. In March 1824 the Dumfriesshire Assistant Surgeon William Lindsay of 36th Foot (d. 1830), serving on Corfu, was promoted surgeon. Anxious to show he was duly grateful to the father of the army medical service, when the clerk to the board asked if he would like to subscribe a guinea to have one of the prints being made from McGrigor's official portrait, he immediately agreed. Despite his higher salary, however, he did not cultivate the director-general further by sending a donation to the Widows and Orphans Benevolent Fund. As a result, he received a curt letter from his chief, dated 7 November 1826, in which McGrigor much regretted this oversight. Needless to say, two guineas were dispatched the following year.[56]

Yet, however much effort an individual surgeon might take in bringing himself to the notice of the board, it is unlikely his exertions would have reaped much reward on their own. As McGrigor's words remind us, what every surgeon needed in the service was a patron. This time, though, he preferably required a champion within the army. Civilian friends and relatives seem to have had far less influence once a surgeon had a foot on the ladder. When John Erly (d. 1844), surgeon to the

---

[54] McGrigor, 111–12. McGrigor, always a cultivator of modesty, claimed he was unwilling to publish at first because another doctor on the expedition, James Buchan, d. 1834 (not in the database; Drew, no. 2053), was more knowledgeable about the plague. In the preface to the published work, McGrigor presented it as initially a memoir for the government in India.

[55] McGrigor, 112. McGrigor just says he found life with the 88th irksome on his return. He does not explain how the transfer took place. For Hussey, not in the database: see Drew, no. 1149. For the dedication, see Illustration 15.

[56] WL, RAMC 262/1/6, 14, 17: letters 2 Aug. 1826, 7 Nov. 1826, 14 June 1827. Lindsay's promotion was welcomed by his family in ibid., 262/10/6 and 7: letters 21 June and 18 July 1824. Not in the database. For his career, see Drew, no. 2934.

1st Battalion of the Black Watch, was made physician to the forces in June 1812, assistant surgeon Lesassier appealed to his uncle, James Hamilton, to pull the necessary patronage strings to get him the vacant position despite his junior standing. Hamilton, however, in this instance proved a broken reed. Although an Edinburgh professor, he claimed to have no influence over the Army Medical Board and that his nephew would have to accept the rules of seniority and wait his turn.[57]

The best way for a surgeon to obtain a champion with clout was to cultivate his commanding officer. Although colonels or their serving lieutenants no longer had the right to nominate their own regimental surgeons from 1798, it is evident that their recommendation continued to carry peculiar weight. For the most part, military patrons either lobbied the Army Medical Board directly on the behalf of a favoured candidate—this was usually the case if they commanded a foreign station or were based at home—or, when on campaign, they approached a senior officer to push their client's claim with the head of the medical department in the field. Towards the end of the Peninsular war, it seems to have been felt necessary for applicants to get military and medical patrons to work in tandem. When the Irishman, Assistant Surgeon Robert Shekleton of the 66th Foot, sought to fill a vacant surgeoncy in the much more prestigious 3rd (the Buffs) on September 1813, he not only got two colonels, Nicholls and Leith, to sing his praises, but also Staff Surgeon Wardelo. The letters of recommendation were all sent to Inspector-General Fergusson, who then passed them on to McGrigor, accompanied by his own heart-felt pennyworth, which stressed Shekleton's medical proficiency, talent, and unexceptional conduct. Four days after Fergusson wrote his own letter, Shekleton was duly promoted surgeon.[58]

One particularly well-documented beneficiary of military patronage in the Peninsula was John Murray of Turriff. He was already not just another faceless assistant surgeon when he landed in Portugal early in 1811, in that shortly before he had left Sicily, the head of the medical department on the island, Dr (later Sir) William Franklin, had been called home to join the Army Medical Board. As Murray realized, this could only work in his favour in the long run. His precocious promotion to surgeon of the 66th Foot after barely a year in the Peninsula, however, owed everything to the army patrons he cultivated on campaign, in particular Colonel Wilson, the brigade commander, with whom he seems to have been permanently billeted.[59]

---

[57] Rosner, 95. The post was given to Alexander McLachlan. Admittedly, Hamilton may have been deliberately non-committal, not wanting to help Lesassier further. John Erly (not in the database) eventually retired as inspector in 1836 and died at Brighton on 7 Aug. 1844: TNA, WO25/3897, no. 7; Drew, no. 1700.

[58] WL, RAMC 209, Fergusson's Letter Book, p. 97: Fergusson to McGrigor, 5 Sept. 1813. For another example relating to Assistant Surgeon Joseph Brown of the 57th Foot, see ibid. 108: Fergusson to McGrigor, 2 Oct. 1813: Brown too was promoted and made staff surgeon with the cavalry. Wardelo (not in the database) does not appear in Drew.

[59] WL, RAMC 830, letters home: 24 Sept.–12 Oct. 1810; 4 Nov. 1811; 6 July 1812. For Franklin (not in the database), see Drew, no. 1126.

Unfortunately, Wilson soon died, but Murray had a stroke of good fortune, which ensured his further progress up the slippery pole. During the summer of 1813, the British invasion of France was halted by Soult and the army retreated across the Pyrenees. During the retreat, the lieutenant-colonel of the 34th was badly wounded and Murray was ordered to stay behind to look after him. He expected to be captured and his army career brought to an abrupt halt, but the French let him care for his charge, then return to the British lines. In consequence, he was able to anticipate instead a reward for his sacrifice.

I have reason to think that I shall lose nothing by it by way of promotion, on the contrary I have already had the assurance of getting the first vacant staff surgeoncy, which is a most respectable, honorable & comfortable situation, both with respect to distinction of rank and pay.[60]

On 9 September 1813 the tenant farmer's son from Aberdeenshire was duly elevated to the staff.

It might be thought that the surest way for a surgeon to ingratiate himself with his commanding officer was to prove competent at his job. The colonel's own standing with his superiors depended on having as many of his troops as possible ready for the field. Successfully curing the commanding officer himself, when sick or wounded, would have been an added bonus. But a regiment would normally have two or three surgeons striving to catch the colonel's eye, and it must have been difficult in normal circumstances to stand out. The successful, then, probably had other strings to their bow. There is no reason to believe that Murray was a poor surgeon by the standards of his time, but he definitely found favour with Wilson for other than medical reasons.[61] To start with, the colonel had a soft spot for the Scots. He had been to Scotland, liked the country and its people, and was a Burns enthusiast. More importantly, Murray had a peculiar facility: he was a born linguist. While in Sicily he had picked up Italian and was speaking it better than 'Scotch'. He had no sooner landed in Portugal than he started to learn Portuguese and could make himself understood within a month. Two years later, he claimed to be fluent in Spanish, too, and no longer needed a dictionary to write letters or translate. Such a facility must have been rare among the British officer corps, and it is not surprising to learn that Wilson used him as an interpreter and that the brigade general had him settling affairs with local magistrates.[62]

Ingratiating oneself with the commanding officer, moreover, could bring longer-term benefits if the colonel himself moved up the ranks. McGrigor's rapid elevation must have owed a great deal to the glittering career of his commanding officer

---

[60] WL, RAMC 830, letter to father, 4 Aug. 1813.

[61] Murray's letters tell us very little about his work as a surgeon. After Badajoz in the spring of 1811, he was put in charge of operating in a field hospital and claimed his amputees were doing well. A few months later he was given the chance to show his organizational ability when the regimental surgeon fell sick and he took his place. Ibid.: to his mother 2 May 1811; to his father 17 July 1811.

[62] Ibid., letters to his father 19 Feb. and 21 Mar. 1811; to his brother 13 Mar. 1813; to his mother 5 Apr. 1813.

in the 88th, William Carr Beresford, the illegitimate son of the marquis of Waterford. Beresford was McGrigor's second CO and took charge of the Connaught Rangers in 1795. At first he and his surgeon were at daggers drawn, so much so that McGrigor approached the regimental army agent, Macdonald, about an exchange, doubtless in hope of finding a more emollient patron in another regiment. The quarrel between the two, though, seems to have been quickly healed once Beresford had ensured the Scot that his department 'was the only one of which he could say anything favourable and that he had so reported to the Horse Guards. In short we became friends, warm friends, and continued so ever after.'[63] It was fortunate for McGrigor that relations thawed, for Beresford, who left the Connaught Rangers at the end of the Egyptian campaign, turned out to be one of the great success stories of the French wars. In the Peninsula from 1807, he was eventually given the task of reorganizing the Portuguese army, and unsurprisingly filled his staff corps with officers he knew. Needing a chief medical officer, he inevitably picked the man with whom he had served for a number of years in the 88th, and McGrigor, now a deputy inspector, was all set to leave for Lisbon, when he was diverted by the Army Medical Board to Walcheren to take over from the incapacitated Webb.[64] In the event, then, it was William Fergusson, as we saw, not McGrigor, who immediately benefited from Beresford's patronage.[65] But it was the Aberdonian who ultimately gained the most from the association. It is likely that Beresford's good standing in the army earlier assisted McGrigor's transfer to the Blues in 1804: his good fortune cannot all have been the result of a book![66] It is almost certain that Beresford got him the job as Wellington's medical supremo, when Franck retired through ill-health.[67] Wellington had met McGrigor once in India, but he had no experience of his abilities. It is hard to imagine that the duke would have accepted anybody the Medical Board cared to send him and much more likely that he demanded the Scot on Beresford's advice.[68]

A close friend in the officer corps was also useful when a medical officer fell foul of the Army Medical Board, as the troubled career of Robert Jackson emphasizes. Jackson was the son of a small, impoverished landed proprietor in Lanarkshire who joined the service during the American War of Independence after a short period as a locum in Jamaica.[69] In his case, his fairy godmother was

---

[63] McGrigor, 50–3. It was possible to exchange a surgeoncy for one of a similar status for a small sum of money, though how frequently this occurred is impossible to say. McGrigor may not have got on with Beresford as quickly as he recounts, since he tried to exchange again two years later, while in the West Indies, but the other party inconveniently died (see 65–6).   [64] See Ch. 1.

[65] McGrigor, 151–2, 164. McGrigor claimed to have got the position for Fergusson while he was in Holland. Fergusson retired on half-pay on 5 Sept. 1817.

[66] His transfer may also have been assisted by the commander of the Indian army in Egypt, Sir David Baird, who receives a good press in the autobiography and was later one of McGrigor's civilian patients: ibid. 87.   [67] See above, n. 40.

[68] McGrigor gives a laconic account of his appointment: a letter arrived in the post: McGrigor, 165–6.

[69] [Borland]. 'The Life of Robert Jackson', in Robert Jackson, *A View of the Formation, Discipline and Economies of Armies*, 3rd edn. (London, 1845), pp. xix–xxvii.

not the colonel of his regiment but a captain in another—Harry Calvert of the 23rd—with whom he became close. After serving as a mate in America, Jackson was stood down without pay and took up a civilian career at Stockton-upon-Tees, but when the French wars broke out, he wrote to the secretary at war asking to be given the post of physician to the forces on the strength of a book he had had published in 1791 on fevers in the Americas. Although with the help of John Hunter he secured a surgeoncy in a desirable regiment, the Buffs, the surgeon-general's successors made it clear he could expect no advancement to the post of physician since he was not a Fellow of the Royal College in London and lacked an Oxbridge degree. In high dudgeon, Jackson secured an interview with the then commander-in-chief, Amhurst, but to no avail.[70] His army career only took off when, by chance, he fell in again with Calvert, now a major, during the first Dutch campaign. Calvert was close to the duke of York, the future head of the army, and immediately informed the prince of his friend's difficulties. 'The impression this made upon the duke was so favorable, that to it Dr. Jackson ascribed his rapid promotion, notwithstanding the physician-general's opposition. Indeed, as long as the duke remained c. in c., the subject of this Memoir continued to be honoured with his countenance & protection.'[71]

Jackson was soon physician to the forces, and by the end of the campaign in charge of the whole medical department in Holland. In later years, thanks again to his military patrons, he would be offered the medical superintendancy of Abercromby's expedition to the West Indies, placed in charge of the medical arm of the military depot at Chatham, made inspector-general of the Army of the Reserve, and temporarily created chief medical officer of the Spanish army. At no time were these and other promotions supported by the Army Medical Board; rather they were usually actively opposed. Keate and Pepys loathed him and tried to have him court-martialled for negligence at the Chatham hospital in 1802. Jackson's pamphlets in favour of reform of the service in the years 1803–8 only soured relations further, which reached their nadir when the surgeon physically assaulted Keate in the street.[72] But Jackson's star waxed once more under the new Army Medical Board and he was eventually placed in charge of the West Indian station, until he retired in 1815.[73] Throughout his chequered career, Calvert, now knighted and adjutant-general (1799–1818) was his rock and shield, as he readily acknowledged.

If my labours have effected any useful change in the management of the medical department of the British army, Sir Harry Calvert may be regarded as the author of it; for had not Sir Harry been with the army on the continent, in the year 1794, and had he not been a sincere and unostentatious friend, I would have left the service, at the close of the campaign in Holland, as the simple surgeon of a regiment.[74]

---

[70] Ibid., pp. lxi–lxiv.   [71] Ibid., p. lxv.   [72] See Ch. 1.
[73] [Borland], 'Life', pp. lxvi–xc.   [74] Cited ibid., pp. lxx–lxxi.

Military patrons were still crucial in the McGrigor era, however sincere the director-general's commitment to professionalization. Indeed, with so many well-educated recruits and so little chance of advancement, patronage was probably more important than ever in fashioning a successful career. Applicants might play by the rules and only seek promotion if they were properly qualified and had served the requisite number of years in a junior post.[75] But they still relied heavily on high-ranking military officers or others with influence in the army to make their case.

Witness the tactics deployed by Sir John Hall (1795–1866) to gain his first promotion to regimental surgeoncy. Hall, the son of a Westmorland gentleman, would end his career as an inspector-general and principal medical officer in the Crimea. In 1827, however, he was languishing as an assistant surgeon in the West Indies and suffering ill-health. On 3 September he wrote to the officer commanding on the island, General Sir John Keane, a veteran of the Peninsular campaign, seeking the latter's good offices with McGrigor to get him promoted to a different station. He admitted he was not the senior assistant surgeon serving on the island but he had suffered the pernicious environment longer than anyone else.

In making this application I rest my hopes of success more on your kind recommendation than any merit or claim of my own. And I feel confident if I have overstepped the bounds of propriety in addressing you on the subject you will pardon my presumption.

Hall went on to explain there was nothing improper in his request in that he only had to serve for five years in the junior ranks before promotion and he had become a medical officer in 1815. Moreover, he had watched while others less senior than himself had been promoted to staff or regimental surgeon. Keane's protection, he insisted, would turn the key. 'I cannot but entertain hope of success if I am favoured with your patronage.'[76]

Within a few weeks, Hall had the chance to help his client. A few days later, James Dillon Tully, deputy inspector of hospitals in Jamaica, died of yellow fever (perhaps Hall knew that the Irishman was on his last legs when he penned his plea), and the general wrote to McGrigor recommending he be replaced by a surgeon Weir and Weir by Hall. McGrigor graciously accepted the recommendation and a few months later on 8 November, assistant Hall was promoted directly to staff surgeon and transferred to Barbados, a healthier location. Obviously, the director-general had not complied exactly with Keane's wishes since Hall was being moved off the island, but this suited the new surgeon even more and he was quick to offer his patron thanks.

Few people, my dear General, owe such weighty obligations to others as I do to you, and no one I am confident can entertain a deeper or more lasting impression of another's kindness than I do of yours—words, however—can convey but a faint, and imperfect

[75] For the rules governing promotion and the quality of recruits in the long period of peace after 1815, see Ch. 1.
[76] WL, RAMC 508, Hall's letter book, 2–3. Hall is not in the database: see Drew, no. 3924.

idea of the sentiment I feel, and would wish to express—but if the fervent prayer of a grateful heart for your health, and happiness be acceptable to you I tender you mine with sincerity.[77]

In fact, the general had done more than write a letter of recommendation. Hall had been given six months' sick leave by the Army Medical Board (presumably as a result of a request prior to his appeal to Keane) and he was sent home with Tully's body carrying a letter to McGrigor highlighting the deficiencies of certain other medical officers in Jamaica (none in the cohort). William Charles Callow of the 84th, the director-general learnt, would have been brought before a court martial had Tully lived; O'Halloran was a bad example to the troops: when they fell sick with fever, he would only take their pulse with an extended arm and would immediately wash his hands; while Dr William Thomas Rankin shirked work, even when the physician said he was fit. Only hospital mate Oligath deserved praise, for working like a Trojan when sick. Keane, therefore, wanted Hall back as soon as possible: 'no man could be more esteemed personally and professionally'. McGrigor was being given a steer, and Hall was now back in London to press his suit.[78]

In the McGrigor years, however, the competition was fierce and the director-general could not respond positively to all the appeals of the great and good on behalf of their clients. Keane could not help Hall further up the ladder. Rather, he had the ignominy of seeing his protégé effectively demoted. Only a year after he returned to the West Indies in the spring of 1828, Staff-Surgeon Hall was called home on half-pay against his wishes, then offered the surgeoncy of the 33rd. Keane wrote to the Army Medical Board on 10 July 1829 demanding Hall be placed again on the West Indies staff, but to no avail.[79] Hall was gazetted to the 33rd the following month and had to spend twelve years with the regiment in various stations, ever more desperate to regain his old status.[80] Finally, based in Gibraltar, he tried to find new patrons to lobby on his behalf. In April 1839, hearing that a position on the staff of the Ionian islands was about to become vacant, he approached his army agent, John Laurie, to argue his case. Laurie had already agreed to do this 'when an opportunity presents itself', and presumably

[77] WL, RAMC 508, 5, letter Jan. 1828. Weir is probably James Weir (not in the database; Drew, no. 3494), who held the rank of physician.
[78] WL, RAMC 508, end of book (reverse order), Keane to McGrigor, 8 Oct. 1827. Presumably Keane had given Hall a copy of the letter. Hall also had an ally in London, Lieut. General Conran. Initially Hall feared lest Keane's letter of recommendation should arrive too late. News of Tully's death had left Jamaica before Keane wrote and there was a likelihood that McGrigor would fill the vacancies before seeing his patron's letter of support. To obviate such a disaster, Hall sent a letter to Conran ahead of Keane's, asking him to approach McGrigor on his behalf, which the lieut. general duly did: ibid., 3–4, Hall to Conran, 14 Sept. 1827, with Hall's notes. O'Halloran's hygienic precautions were evidently seen by his superior officer as a sign of discourtesy to his men! For Callow, O'Halloran, and Rankin, none of whom is in the database, see Drew, nos. 2749, 3253, and 4139. Oligath, also not in the database, is not recorded in Drew.
[79] WL, RAMC 508, end of book (reverse order). The letter written in London was to Franklin as McGrigor was out of town.   [80] He dutifully subscribed to the Medical Benevolent Fund.

had influence with the board because his partner was McGrigor's son, Charles.[81] When this failed, Hall stepped up a gear. A year later he tried to use the good offices of Sir John MacDonald, and when even the adjutant-general received the brush-off from the director, he went straight to the top and harangued one of the war ministers, either Lord John Russell or Thomas B. Macaulay. In a long memorandum dated 29 September 1840, Hall outlined his service career and begged, if he was to be sent again to the West Indies with his regiment as McGrigor decreed, he should go as a staff surgeon. This was only fair, since one of the staff in the West Indies, Thomas Spence, had only just entered the service when Hall had first made the senior post.[82] The appeal must have done the trick, though how Hall was able to elicit support from the Melbourne ministry is a mystery. McGrigor had told Hall on 16 September that his desire for promotion would not be overlooked, but that he should expect a considerable time to elapse before it would happen. However, on 26 February 1841, merely five months later, he was duly promoted from regimental surgeon to staff surgeon 1st class on 19/- per day.[83]

McGrigor after 1830, when the medical service was slimmed down even further to cut costs, seems only to have jumped when grandees at the very top of the establishment cracked the whip.[84] Sir Charles Napier was another Peninsular veteran and a British hero for conquering Sind in the mid-1840s, but his status cut limited ice with the director-general. Writing to the general on 24 January 1844, he expressed pleasure that the conduct of an Assistant Surgeon Anderson of the 22nd had met with Napier's approbation, but insisted that the rules had to be obeyed. 'From [his] short standing in the service I dare not immediately recommend him for promotion but I have noted the strong terms in which you mention his conduct which shall be kept on record for a favourable opportunity.'[85] Four years later, McGrigor's reply similarly did no more than to keep the door ajar when approached by Napier on behalf of Surgeon Austin of the 97th.

I have lately promised him promotion specially on condition of his proceeding in the first instance to the West Indies—he has acceded to the condition and I suppose now wishes to evade it, but I cannot agree to his doing so without injury to the service.

Mr Austin is a fine medical officer for whom on account of the interest which you take in him I am ready to do anything which with propriety I can do.

81 WL, RAMC 508, 25. McGrigor Jnr split with Laurie the following year: see ibid. 37–8: Hall to Charles McGrigor, army agent, 10 Dec. 1840. For McGrigor's sons, see Ch. 6.

82 WL, RAMC 508, 32–3: McGrigor to MacDonald, 21 Mar. 1840; pp. 34–6: Hall to secretary of war, 29 Sept. 1840; as there were two war ministers, the secretary for war and the secretary at war, it is impossible to know to whom the letter was sent. For Spence, not in the database, see Drew, no. 4176.

83 WL, RAMC 508, 33, McGrigor to Hall. The director could afford to give in. He had allowed Hall to act as temporary deputy inspector of hospitals Gibraltar, when James Gillkrest (not in the database; Drew, no. 2126) was indisposed.

84 Around 1830 many surgeons were removed from the half-pay registers: see pp. 198 ff.

85 BL, Add. MSS 54552, fo. 115. This was John Anderson, not in database, d. 1851, who had only served four years: see Drew, no. 4597.

For the last 4 years the troops in the West Indies Islands have been in a very healthy state. Mr Austin's period of service there will be only 3 years and should his health fail he will be sent home to this country where I will provide a berth for him.[86]

Charles Gordon Lennox, the fifth duke of Richmond, on the other hand, who had been one of Wellington's secretaries in the Peninsula, received preferential treatment. On 20 October 1834, McGrigor wrote to the duke promising he would do all in his power to assist the progress of Surgeon Straw of the 16th. The following May a second letter informed the duke that the director had found a home posting for Dr Straw 'whose health had suffered by service in India'. At the same time his grace was assured that he would 'never find me inattentive to any Medical Officer in whom you may be pleased to take the same interest'. Then, barely five months later, the director-general informed the duke that his protégé had been transferred again.

Anxiously desirous as I ever am to meet your Lordship's wishes I have [moved] Dr Straw whose regiment the 89th is [bound] for the West Indies to the Royal Fusiliers in the Mediterranean and which will soon return to this country. I have . . . to add that I have singular pleasure in doing what may be acceptable to your Grace.[87]

And McGrigor was still singularly pleased to accommodate his lordship seven years later, in 1842, in the case of a Dr Gray, even if his promotion was covered in the fig-leaf of competence.

I have much pleasure in informing your Grace that the name of Dr Gray appeared last night for a commission in the Medical Department of the Army. Dr Gray's appointment ought to have appeared earlier as the delay rested with the War Office. I have obtained that his commission takes date from the 28th January [the letter was written on 14 March]. I have much satisfaction in stating that the reports from Chatham of Dr Gray's talents and conduct while there are most favourable and that I have to thank you for an excellent report . . . to my Department, who will never discredit your Patronage. I will ever be happy to pay all the attention in my power to any gentleman in who [*sic*] you may be pleased to take an interest.[88]

Clearly, getting on in the army medical service in the first half of the nineteenth century always remained in part a question of contacts. As Hall's chequered career suggests, even gaining entry to the top rungs of the ladder in McGrigor's years cannot simply have been a question of seniority and merit. In the thirty-five years the Scot was in charge of the medical service, he appointed forty members

---

[86] BL, Add. MSS 54559, fo. 1. Probably many other such polite refusals can be found in the uncatalogued papers of the Army Medical Board in the National Archive. Austin, not in the database, is not recorded in Drew.

[87] West Sussex County RO, Chichester, Goodward Collection, MS 1477, fo. 118: letter 20 Oct. 1834; MS 1573, fo. 558: letter 28 May 1835; MS 1577, fo. 289: letter 20 Sept. 1835.

[88] Ibid., MS 1643, fo. 1196. The letters McGrigor wrote to the duke of Richmond 1832–53 are the largest collection of his correspondence to any one person discovered. Presumably, he was equally accommodating to other prominent members of the establishment. Why this was is discussed pp. 201 ff. Neither Straw nor Gray are in the database; nor do they appear in Drew.

Table 4.18. Profile of Deputy (General) Inspectors Elevated by McGrigor

Characteristics	Number of surgeons
Date of entry	
Before 1800	17
1800–14	21
1815	2
Rank on entry	
Hospital assistant/mate	28
Assistant surgeon/surgeon's mate	5
Surgeon	2
Apothecary	1
Physician	4
Length of service before rank of Deputy inspector (includes periods on half-pay)	
Less than 10 years	1
10–19 years	3
20–9 years	22
30–9 years	6
40–9 years	2
Unknown	6
Service in the Peninsula	19
Medical doctorate	
Aberdeen	5
Edinburgh	14
Glasgow	2
Oxford	1
St Andrews	1
Trinity College Dublin	3
Total	26
Nationality	
English (including 1 from the Channel Islands)	15
Irish	13
Scots	10
Unknown	2
Social background	
Business and manufacturing	4
Church	3
Civil Service	1
Land	5 (1 gentleman farmer, 4 assumed landed)
Medicine	2
Unknown	25

Source: Doctors' Database: Tables: Army Positions; Doctors1; Degrees, Residence/Service; Relationships 1.

of the cohort to the rank of deputy inspector or its equivalent (see Table 4.18). There is nothing obviously suspicious in the fact that a few were on a much faster track than the rest, for the elevation of those with less than twenty years' service could be tribute to their talents. Only the elevation of James McDougle in 1815 after a mere seven years in the service evinces real surprise.[89] There is no evidence either that serving in the Peninsula with McGrigor was an advantage, even if those who waited longest for promotion to the inspectorate were more likely not to have done so. What is more damning is the fact that, despite McGrigor's commitment to education, only twenty-six out of the forty had degrees, and that only fourteen had taken their degree at Edinburgh, where their knowledge would have been seriously tested. Equally damning is the national profile of the group, where the English are over-represented by ten points. It is difficult not to believe, then, that in many, if not most of these appointments, patronage played more than a part in determining success, even if McGrigor can never usually have been forced into promoting anyone in whom he did not have confidence.[90]

At the very least, a patron must have considerably smoothed the path of the ambitious and talented's rise to the top. The Englishman John Hall eventually gained the promotion he craved, thanks to the good officers of a member of the government. Significantly, in all his years of lobbying to be restored to his former rank of staff surgeon, he had not felt it would improve his chances of success if he took a degree. It would be a further five years before he clothed himself in the mantle of medical respectability by purchasing a doctorate from St Andrews, the year before he finally became deputy inspector. Nor had he obviously contributed to the sum of human knowledge by publishing a book and earning McGrigor's favour through his pen.[91] He evidently had felt that the key to advancement was influence. It is a fair assumption that he would not have waited until 1840 for promotion, had he had a duke of Richmond behind his ascent from the start.

GETTING OUT

There were only five ways out of the army medical service once a surgeon had embarked on a military career. He might take French leave, be expelled after a court martial, resign, die in service, or be permanently placed on half-pay. Given our assumption that most surgeons became medical officers in order to enjoy a reasonable standard of living and better position themselves in any future return to civilian life, leaving the army under a cloud was unlikely to be a good career move. So, too, was simply resigning, since the surgeon lost his rights to half-pay and an eventual pension. Understandably, then, hardly any member of the service departed under one of the first three heads. The vast majority survived long enough to ensure either themselves or their widows reaped some material benefit from their years in the army.

---

[89] McDougle quit the service for the two years 1807–9: TNA/W025/3897, no. 43.

[90] For the peculiar case of Barry, see pp. 207–8.

[91] His only published writings were two pamphlets of 1857 and 1858 defending the army's medical officers in the Crimea.

Desertions and resignations presumably did occur from time to time—we earlier saw that McGrigor threatened to tender his on one occasion—but they have left little trace. No deserter has been found among the cohort, and only two surgeons are known to have handed in their commission: Charles Lambton Este, who resigned as an assistant surgeon in 1802 and Joseph Constantine Carpue as a surgeon in 1811. Este seems to have had little choice, given the prestige of his regiment, the Buffs, for he had married in haste his brother's wife's sister, Louise Caroline Smythe, the year before, then immediately left her on the grounds she had 'committed acts of misconduct'.[92] He then held various secretarial appointments to the great and good, including Nelson, before re-entering the service as surgeon to the 1st Life Guards in 1812, only eventually retiring on half-pay in 1835.[93]

The few surgeons who did walk out were presumably self-important hotheads, such as Charles Maclean, who thought their *amour propre* had been intolerably tweaked. Maclean was a former East India Company surgeon who was interned by Napoleon while visiting Hamburg. Returning from prison in France in 1804, Maclean, a surgeon with a high reputation now aged 40, asked to join the army medical service and be placed on the hospital staff as a mate. When the Army Medical Board expressed surprise that someone of his experience should want to enter the lower ranks of the service, Maclean purportedly claimed a desire to serve his country and a wish to use the opportunity to investigate epidemic and pestilential diseases. Within a year, though, he was fed up with seeing surgeons who entered the service after him speedily promoted regimental assistants or being given the rank without first being mates. Loath as a man of honour to offer bribes to forward his career—the only currency, he maintained, which Pepys and company understood—he deserted his post in disgust while stationed in Cork in late summer 1805. In justification, he claimed that a commissioned officer was free to behave as he wanted.[94]

Expulsions were also extremely infrequent before 1815. Even though surgeons were sometimes threatened with court martial for venality, insubordination, or embarrassing their superiors, troublesome medical officers usually escaped with a reprimand or were quietly paid off. This was what happened to John Buffa in 1805 after he had blown the whistle on the peculation of Dr Moore, principal medical officer on the Isle of Wight. Rather than risk the service's dirty linen being washed before a military tribunal, the inspector-general ordered an internal inquiry, suppressed the evidence, and had Buffa placed on half-pay.[95] It was only

[92] E. H. D. Este to Michael Moss, private letter, 13 Mar. 2003.

[93] Nelson knew and esteemed Este's father: see Sir Nicholas Harris Nicolas (ed.), *Nelson's Dispatches*, 7 vols. (London, 1846), vi. 215–16: Nelson to Este, 4 Oct. 1804. Carpue went on to a stellar career as a private anatomy teacher: see Ch. 5.

[94] Maclean, *Analytical View of the Medical Department*, 149–62. Maclean, 162, claims another surgeon, Buchannan had walked out the previous year. Maclean had been William Pitt's surgeon in 1788 and had great experience in working in tropical climates. Neither Maclean nor Buchannan (not in the database) appear in Drew. For Maclean's life see *DNB, sub nomine*.

[95] Maclean, *Medical Department*, 118–34. According to Maclean, Moore claimed he could do what he liked, for he had paid for his office: see p. 176.

once McGrigor took over, standards were tightened, and the need for surgeons was reduced that members of the service began to find themselves dishonourably discharged. The numbers, though, were always low, and only two members of the cohort, David MacLoughlin of Quebec and John Williamson, probably from Edinburgh, ended their careers in disgrace.[96]

John Williamson was a rare bird in that he served almost continuously in the West Indies from 1798 until his court martial in 1824, initially doing a fourteen-year stint and being 'fortunate enough to enjoy a less interrupted state of good health than commonly falls to Europeans'.[97] His passage up the career ladder, though, had been slow. By the early 1820s, although a graduate physician, he was still only a regimental surgeon, who for a few months in late 1823 was in charge of the regimental hospital of the 33rd on the island of Jamaica before being moved to Honduras to take over the garrison hospital. Prior to his departure, the local deputy inspector, Jacob later Sir Jacob Adolphus (1774–1845) had his accounts audited by Assistant Surgeon John Hall, who discovered £115 7s./8d. was missing.[98] Williamson's only explanation for this was that he must have been robbed. But since he promised to cover the deficit with a bill of exchange he quickly negotiated in Kingston, he was allowed to leave for his next posting. Unfortunately neither the bill nor a successor could be redeemed on presentation, so Williamson was arrested when he returned to Jamaica in October 1824, now with the higher status of apothecary to the forces.

Initially, Williamson was given the chance to avoid a court martial: Adolphus was willing to send him home so that he could plead to be placed on half-pay. But Williamson chose the martyr's route and was duly tried. The court, presided over by the lieutenant-colonel of the 91st, was asked to decide whether such culpable dishonesty 'evinces any degree of that nice feeling of honor which ought to distinguish the Gentleman and the soldier'. It had no difficulty in concluding it did not, all the more that it heard how Williamson had received £175 towards his hospital expenses only seven days before the audit, and that while in Honduras he had drawn an extra allowance from the commissariat on the grounds he held the fictitious office of acting purveyor to the forces.[99] Williamson was therefore summarily dismissed, at which point his customary iron constitution deserted him. Within a year he was dead leaving a widow and a paralysed daughter in dire straits. Refused a widow's pension, Mrs Williamson became a menial, and on

[96] MacLoughlin seems to have been dismissed for disobedience in the 1820s after a distinguished career. He was taken prisoner during the Peninsular war and helped run the French hospitals, thereby being the first Briton to gain the *légion d'honneur*. In his will, proved in 1870, he claimed to be owed £20,000 by the British government (presumably in back-pay). Two other members of the cohort were brought before a court-martial and found guilty but they were not permanently ejected: see Ch. 6.

[97] John Williamson, *Medical and Miscellaneous Observations, Relative to the West Indian Islands*, 2 vols (Edinburgh, 1817), p. vii. More will be said about this text in Ch. 7.

[98] Adolphus (not in the database) retired as inspector in 1829: Drew, no. 2178; TNA/W025/3897, no. 3.

[99] WL, RAMC 508, letter book of Sir John Hall, end, reverse order: transcription of the court martial: quotation at 5.

Table 4.19. Place of Death of Surgeons Dying on Active Service

Place of death	Born in England/Wales	Born in Ireland	Born in Scotland	Born abroad	All recorded deaths
Afghanistan			1		1
Africa	5	5	2		12
Australasia		1	2		3
Canada			1		1
Central America		1	2	1	4
Ceylon	2	2	1		5
China	1		1		2
Channel Islands	1				1
England		2	1		3
Europe		2			2
India	2	7	9		18
Ireland		3			3
Russia	1				1
St Helena		1			1
Sea passage	1	4	3	1	9
South America		1	1		3
Unknown					1
West Indies	6	4	7		23
Total	19	33	32	2	93

Note: It has been assumed that all surgeons dying in countries in italics and at sea, barring Williamson and Tully Daly, were on active service. This is a maximum figure. In the case of countries in roman the row records the number of surgeons on service who definitely died there. This is a minimum figure.

Source: Doctors' Database: Tables: Doctors; Doctors1.

5 July 1827 was awarded a £10 emergency grant by the trustees of the Medical Officer's Fund when they learnt of her plight from surgeon Andrew Anderson of the 92nd.[100]

Williamson would have done better by his wife and child had he died in service before his sins were discovered. Had he done so, he would have been in good company, for ninety-three of the cohort (20.5 per cent) were destined to end their lives in the years following the end of the French wars serving their king in various parts of the world.[101] As can be seen from Table 4.19, there was no particular white man's graveyard. The West Indies, Central America, India, Afghanistan and Ceylon, not surprisingly, accounted for more than a half of the deaths, including that of Lesassier who died at Kandahar on 4 May 1839. Part of the expeditionary force sent into Afghanistan to keep Shah Sujah on the throne, he was not a victim of the general slaughter but succumbed from heat,

[100] Ibid., RAMC 206, 68–70. Both the 91st and the 92nd Foot were in the West Indies at the time of the trial.

[101] These were all the victims of disease or accident. It should be remembered that with a handful of exceptions the cohort contains surgeons who had served in the French wars and were still alive in 1815, plus a small number who joined after that date: see Introduction.

malnutrition, and dysentery.[102] But service in the unhealthy barracks of the United Kingdom could be just as lethal, as the Irishman George Richard Melin discovered to his cost, when he expired at Coventry, one of the worst of them all, in 1836. Indeed, no station was particularly benign. Even the eastern Mediterranean was a cesspit of disease. John Davy may have expatiated from Zante on the wonders of a Mediterranean winter, but Corfu seems to have destroyed William Lindsay's health, as it destroyed many others, and officers returning from the Ionian islands had to be first quarantined for two weeks at Ancona (north-east Italy) before they were allowed to step foot on mainland Europe.[103] The simple act of travelling by sea to and from Britain was also clearly hazardous. McGrigor had several close shaves during his early career in the service and he must have lost several surgeons to the waves while director, including Dent, who drowned in the Caribbean on his way back to England from a tour of duty in the West Indies in 1826.[104]

For a few who died abroad in positions of authority, their service career might have ended abruptly but the game had been worth the candle. They had gambled their future on taking the king's shilling and good fortune (or the right mix of luck, talent, and patronage) had brought them rich rewards. Another victim of the Indian subcontinent was the tenant farmer's son, John Murray (not in the cohort), who died at Kurnaul in Bengal on 21 October 1841. He, though, did not end his days dragging his tired carcass over the Hindu Kush but enjoying a high standard of living as an inspector-general in Madras with his third wife, twenty-five servants, and an income of £2,500 per annum.[105] In one of several letters home delineating his good fortune, he expressed the hope he would be able to return to Scotland after three to four years: by which time he would have completed nearly forty years' service. This was not to be, but it is hard to imagine he did not leave a reasonable inheritance to his new wife and five daughters.[106]

For the majority of medical officers who died as assistant or regimental surgeons, on the other hand, the gamble had largely failed. Most of them had been in the service too short a time to accumulate much capital, and if they had had the temerity to marry on their expectations, they could easily leave their families little. Widows could look forward to a pension, but, where the wife predeceased the husband or quickly followed him to the grave, the future could be bleak for any children. The records of the Officers Benevolent Fund suggest there were always a

---

[102] Rosner, 199–200.

[103] WL, RAMC 262/8, no. 16: Davy to Lindsay, 15 Dec. 1824. Lindsay seems to have come home to recuperate in May 1825. When he was due to return the following March, McGrigor sent for him and pronounced him too sick to regain his post. He died in 1830: ibid., esp. no. 36, Lindsay to Captain Jones RE (with whom he was to travel), 14 Mar. 1826.   [104] Drew, no. 3179.

[105] See p. 51.

[106] WL, RAMC 830, 25 Nov. 1838. One daughter, Isabella, was already married to Mr Burgh of the Madras civil service: letter 28 Oct. 1837 (from the Cape). One member of the cohort died in India with the rank of deputy inspector. This was Frederick Albert Loinsworth, who died at Bombay in 1842 after only a few months in the presidency: see BL, Oriental and India Office, European MS D758, Loinsworth's papers: Hearst (Bombay merchant) to Captain Denny, 20 Nov. 1842.

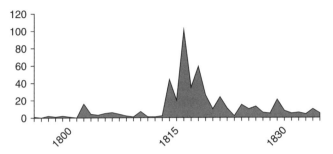

Figure 4.1. Number of Medical Officers Placed on Half-Pay, 1793–1835

These figures include those who were recalled to service and later transferred back to half-pay.

Source: Doctors' Database: Table: Half-Pay.

number of orphans in need of assistance. Assistant Surgeon James R. Morgan, probably from Camarthenshire, lost his wife as she tried to land in Ceylon. When he in turn died on the island in 1825, he left two daughters aged 6 and 4 in relative penury. In consequence, on the application of his brother, Rowland, probably a Nonconformist minister, the trustees awarded the children £10 a year for eleven years from 1827.[107]

Understandably, the members of the cohort who had the most successful professional lives were usually to be found among the 80 per cent of the cohort who safely exited the service on half-pay, as we shall see in the following two chapters. Either they quit the army with a high rank after enjoying many years on a good salary, or they left earlier enough in their life to build a substantial civilian career. The emphasis is on the verb 'exit'. In theory, a surgeon on half-pay could be recalled to the colours at any time until he had spent thirty years on active service, unless the Army Medical Board effectively granted him early retirement and pensioned him off. Figure 4.1 and Table 4.20 reveal the number in the cohort going on half-pay each year and whether this was the first or subsequent time. Evidently, more than three-quarters of the cohort (76.7 per cent) were placed on half-pay at least once in their army career, for the most part (66.9 per cent) in the years 1814–18 when the service was dramatically run down, and above all in 1816 when 101 were released, 83 for the first time. But it is clear from the half-pay registers that 170 (37.4 per cent) spent a second spell in the army, some being called up within a few months of being stood down, especially those on the staff who were put on half-pay in 1814 only to be summoned back for the Waterloo campaign. Indeed, 10 per cent of the sample

---

[107] WL, RAMC 206, 57: initial decision 5 Apr. 1827. No Rowland Morgan attended Oxbridge. Information given in a letter in TNA, WO42/34/800 suggests that Morgan's wife died after him and that a third child, a boy, had died on the voyage to Columbo. Possibly, she had initially stayed at home when he went out to Ceylon and had gone out to join him, not knowing he was dead. Morgan had a lacklustre career: he was made hospital mate in 1814 and took ten years to become an assistant surgeon.

Table 4.20. Number of Surgeons Placed on Half-Pay per Year, 1783–1850

Year(s)	Number	First time	English/Welsh	Irish	Scots	Others	Unknown
1783–1801	9	9					
1802	16	15					
1803–12	34	22					
1813	2	2					
1814	44	40	17 (17)	12 (10)	15 (13)		
1815	20	14	9 (5)	6 (6)	3 (1)	2	2
1816	101	83	36 (27)	30 (29)	26 (24)	5	4
1817	35	33	9 (7)	14 (14)	10 (10)	1	1
1818	59	42	20 (16)	25 (17)	13 (10)		1
1816–18	195	158	65 (50)	69 (60)	49 (44)	6	6
1814–18	259	212	91 (72)	87 (76)	67 (58)	8	8
	(66.9%)		(34.0%)	(35.8%)	(27.4%)		
1819	26	16					
1820	10	6					
1821	24	10					
1822	11	8					
1823	2						
1823–8	49	15					
1829	21	13					
1830–50	103	20					
Total in cohort	454	454					
Total joining the service pre-1816	387						

Notes:
Figures in brackets = number on half-pay for first time.
(66.9%): 259 as a percentage of 387.
387 of the 454 surgeons in the database joined the army before 1816. The rest joined in the 1820s. 377 were still alive in 1819. The number in service in 1814 was slightly less than 387 as several had died before 1814 and two resigned. Thus slightly more than two-thirds of serving officers were placed on half-pay 1814–18.
Source: Doctors' Database: Tables: Doctors1; Half-Pay.

definitely went back a third time and eight hardy souls returned for a fourth period of duty.

Admittedly, those who returned on more than two occasions tended to be officers who reached the top of the promotional ladder, such as Charles Farrell, and whose army career could be counted a resounding success.[108] On the other hand, for perhaps as many as a half of the second timers, returning to full pay was a death sentence. It was among this group that the majority of the ninety-three who died in service were to be found. Henry Cowen's fate was brutally typical. The Irishman from County Cavan, who had joined as a hospital mate in 1808,

[108] See pp. 171–2.

Table 4.21. Number of Surgeons Entering the Army Pre-1816 who were Placed on Half-Pay on One or More Occasion, 1814–19, and Not Recalled Thereafter

Years of service	Number entering pre-1816	Number entering 1809–15	English	Scots	Irish	Unknown
Less than 10	13	13 (46.4%)	6	1	5	1
10–19	9		1	4	2	2
More than 20	2			1	1	
Total	24 (33.8%)		7	6	8	3
Total in sample in service in 1814	71	28				
Total in sample	75					

Note: Table based on information relating to every fifth member of the cohort. A further four of the 28 entering 1809–15, although recalled after 1819, served for less than 10 years. A further two of the 28 died in service.

Source: Doctors' Database: Table: Half-Pay.

enjoyed a year on half-pay from July 1817, but was soon back in harness and sent over seas. Six years later he was dead, expiring on a passage from Rangoon to Calcutta on 18 August 1824.

In fact probably only a third of the 387 members of the cohort who joined before 1816 permanently left the army at a relatively young age and could concentrate on building a civilian career. These were chiefly the surgeons who were never recalled after 1819, however many times they had been placed on half-pay before (see Table 4.21). Usually, they had served no more than twenty years, the majority, recruited in the latter stages of the war, less than ten. The other two-thirds either died in service, served with only short periods on half-pay well into their middle age, or were called back into the service after initially setting themselves up in civil society. Further comment about how surgeons were selected for half-pay or recall will be made in the following section. Suffice it to say at this juncture that the majority of those summoned back to the colours after 1814 would have avoided the call-up if they could. If we are right in thinking that the surgeons principally used the army as a potential springboard to a civilian career, then once hostilities had ceased and they had been released fit and well after five, ten, or even fifteen years campaigning, they were unlikely to be anxious to re-enter the service. Those who did so, it can be assumed, were largely those still unable to command the standard of living they wanted in civilian life. Even those who had reached a high rank in the service must have thought twice about going back.[109]

Almost certainly, therefore, a number of the surgeons who went on half-pay and never re-entered the service were *refusniks*. At some time in their civilian life they would have received a summons to return but declined the invitation, on the grounds they had greater expectations at home. Staff Surgeon George James Guthrie for one may have had an illustrious career in the Peninsula, but once

[109] For further discussion, see Ch. 5.

having tasted half-pay in 1814, he refused to rejoin for the Waterloo campaign. 'Having hazarded nearly all he had on his success in London, he could not accept the offer made to him of employment, or the solicitations of many kind friends, high in rank, to accompany them, although he promised to join them in case of accident.'[110] Even surgeons anxious to be recruited in order to restore their financial position were known to reject a place, if the moment was inopportune. Staff Surgeon Samuel Barwick Bruce was placed on half-pay in 1816 after serving in the Peninsula, in America, and at Waterloo, and eventually established himself in Ripon. Although continually begging to be re-employed in the next few years, he was not resummoned until September 1832 when he was ordered to the West Indies forthwith. The summons could not have been more untimely. On the one hand, 'his wife at that time having been confined a few days, and then exceedingly ill, her indisposition was considerably augmented by this unexpected command'. On the other, the summons got in the way of Bruce's political activities. This was the year of the First Reform Act, which saw hotly contested general elections. Bruce had been active in support of the two losing Tory candidates in the first election and was anxious not to desert his party in the second, which was about to occur. He thus refused to go and tried to buy time by asking 'for leave of absence for three months, to settle his private and professional affairs'.[111]

Refusing to return or accompany one's regiment abroad was not necessarily a dangerous strategy in the years before 1828. Provided the surgeon agreed to stand ready to be recalled at some later date, he did not forfeit his half-pay. Guthrie certainly did not suffer. After Waterloo he went out to Brussels without pay to offer advice to the staff, then on his return lectured on military surgery free of charge at the York Hospital for a few years. As a result, even though he never again drew full pay, he was eventually raised to the rank of deputy inspector and continued to remain on the books until he died in 1856.[112] Eventually, however, the army became less accommodating. Both the Tory and Whig ministries at the turn of the 1830s were keen on retrenchment in the armed forces, and it would seem the heavy expenditure on half-pay came under close scrutiny in all departments. One way to cut the bill, it was apparently decided, was to change the rules. In future, officers ordered to return who refused would be paid off with a lump-sum in lieu of their continuing pension, on the understanding that they would never again be summoned.[113] Lesassier received such an offer in the course of 1830: either he had to go back in or accept £500 in lieu. In his case, though, he could not take the money. After being released at the end of 1814 and taking a degree at Edinburgh two years later, he had set himself up in the fashionable part of the Scottish capital.

---

[110] Pettigrew, *Medical Portrait Gallery*, iv. 6: life of Guthrie.

[111] [S. B. Bruce], *Short Memoir of S. B. Bruce Esquire* (York, 1841), 5–6. The quotations come from a letter in the *Lancet*, 1 (1834–5), 4. But it is Bruce who supplies the political information.

[112] TNA, WO25/3897, no. 36: military records of half-pay officers, staff surgeon, and above.

[113] The conclusion is a deduction from the information concerning individuals in the Project Database. No document has been found setting out the policy.

Sadly, he had not proved a success. Receiving no more than £70 per annum from his Edinburgh practice, he was in queer street, even with his half-pay, and desperate to be re-employed. He therefore rejoined, was sent out to India, and, as we have seen died during the First Afghan War, another casualty of returning to the colours.[114] Many other surgeons similarly importuned, on the other hand, were in a happier position: at least thirty-four of the cohort accepted commutation between late 1828 and early 1833.[115] The first to do so, in December 1828, was Assistant Surgeon Tully Daly, probably of County Galway, who had been placed on half-pay in December 1818 after five years' service and had never returned.[116] The last was Barwick Bruce in January 1833, whose delaying tactics clearly eventually exhausted the patience of the Army Medical Board.

Of course, the government would not have had to have stooped to such an underhand practice had surgeons resigned from the service in greater numbers. This, though, as was said at the beginning of the section, they were loath to do: the large majority, whatever their rank, seem to have been unwilling to enter civilian life without the cushion of half-pay or give it up once economically secure. This reluctance inevitably meant that the large majority only quit active service, either temporarily or permanently, when it was judged to be in the 'management interest' by the army's top brass. It was insufficient to want out: unless a medical officer was deemed unfit, useless, or superfluous to requirements, he was unlikely to be placed on half-pay, however fulsomely he pleaded his case. When Deputy Inspector John Robb of Ayr, in charge of the Cape Town station, inherited his brother's fortune in 1822, he had no difficulty in gaining his release papers. Not only was it peacetime, but Robb had served since 1796 without a break, done sterling service in the Peninsula, and headed the medical department on Sir Edward Packenham's ill-fated expedition to the United States in 1815.[117] Ten years previously, however, while the struggle with

---

[114] Rosner, 196–7. Lesassier had tried unsuccessfully to importune McGrigor for a place in the mid-1820s (182–3).

[115] This is the number recorded in the half-pay registers. There may be others. Virtually all of the thirty-four had not served since the late 1810s. Thirty-six of the cohort returned to the service in the years 1829–32: thirteen had not served for more than seven years and one for fourteen. Presumably, like Lesassier, the thirteen had been offered the same deal and been forced to accept. Thirty-nine surgeons in service were placed on half-pay in these years, twenty of whom returned to the colours after six months to two years and a further six in less than eight years, which would suggest that McGrigor did not like to keep his 'active' surgeons too long in civvy street. Thirteen of the thirty-nine seem to have retired for good, including several who had been resummoned in the years 1829–32 after a long interval and had only spent a short time back in the service before ostensibly going on half-pay again: perhaps they too commuted to get out. The medical officers who definitely commuted were those who had generally joined up in the latter part of the war and been placed permanently on half-pay with the peace, suggesting they were the target of the initiative. The half-pay bill cannot have been greatly reduced as a result. Unfortunately, no documentation has been uncovered elucidating the strategy.

[116] Daly in the 1820s was living in Chelsea. On losing his half-pay, he must have decided to emigrate for he died en route to New Holland (Australia) in 1829.

[117] WL, RAMC 506, letters of John Murray of Turriff, 11 Dec. 1821, 25 Jan., and 22 Mar. 1822: Murray was with Robb in the Cape. TNA, WO25/3897, no. 20: Robb's service record to 1841, with transcribed commendations. In 1830, while on half-pay he was elevated to inspector-general.

Napoleon remained undetermined, Deputy Inspector William Fergusson had no such joy. Although heading the medical department of the Portuguese army, he became disillusioned with the responsibility after quarrelling with his commanding officer, General Beresford, over the organization of the service.[118] His appeal to be allowed home and placed on half-pay, though, fell on deaf ears. He was transferred to Wellington's medical staff in late 1812, so was relieved of further altercations with Beresford, but he was only finally released in 1817.

There can be no doubt, too, that Fergusson's appeal did not succeed from lack of trying or lack of contacts. As a letter from Director-General Weir to his brother, James (1769–1842), member of the Edinburgh Faculty of Advocates, in October 1812 reveals, he could call on the support of the Army Medical Board as well as a galaxy of the great and good.

The long and arduous services of your brother are well known to me since he was surgeon in St Domingo.

The high esteem he is held in by his Highness the Duke of Gloucester, the Honorable General William Stuart and every officer he has served under entitle him to any indulgence that can be granted to him and now the interest of Lord Eglinton is added to that of the Galloway [Earls of] family I think there can be no doubt of Mr Fergusson gaining the point he aims at.

I beg leave to suggest that an application to his Highness the Duke of Gloucester in his favour from some of your [powerful?] friends may have great weight at this time in his getting the half-pay of an inspector; nothing shall be wanting in my part to second his views.[119]

Perhaps Weir was being disingenous and had no intention of pushing Fergusson's case, but it looks as if his release was blocked at the very top—by Gloucester's brother, the commander-in-chief, the duke of York. Whatever the truth of the matter, one thing is clear. The power of patronage could oil your passage through the army medical service, but it was less effective at getting you out!

PATRONAGE VERSUS PROFESSIONALIZATION

Throughout the French wars, even before the Army Medical Board was reconstructed in 1810, promotion within the service was supposedly linked as much as possible to seniority and merit. Once McGrigor took over in 1815, the commitment was stressed ever more strongly, with the added insistence that promotion

[118] The quarrel seems to have been over the deployment of regimental hospitals. There is a lot of material on this in Fergusson's papers in the RAMC collection in the Wellcome Library. But see especially the letters home in his letter book: RAMC 208.

[119] Ibid. 81: James Fergusson to William Fergusson, Oct. 1812: a copy of Weir's letter was enclosed. Stuart (usually Stewart) had been James's colonel when he served with the 67th and was MP for Wigtonshire 1796–1814. He was the younger son of the earl of Galloway. James Fergusson acted as Stewart's electoral agent in the 1802 election: ibid. 15–16: William Stewart to William Fergusson, 22 Sept. 1802. Fergusson had been placed on half-pay in the May of that year, then gone off to St Petersburg in the entourage of the duke of Gloucester, doubtless thanks to Galloway patronage.

would also be determined by educational attainment.[120] From what has been said in the previous sections, however, it is quite clear that throughout the first half of the nineteenth century patronage, whoever was in control, continued to play a major role in a surgeon's progress through the hierarchy from the moment he entered as a hospital mate. In other words, if the army medical service certainly experienced professionalization in the course of this period, it was never, before the Crimea, a modern profession. It was a profession tempered by personality.

It is not difficult to see why the board lent a sympathetic ear to patrons within and without the service who wanted their clients to jump the queue. The board members themselves were the beneficiaries of patronage. Not only had they received help in gaining their lofty position, but they continued to look to patrons to give them an entrée into the wider and social and cultural world. Britain in the late Georgian and early Victorian eras was a society in which gaining a knighthood, being elected to the Royal Society, or simply obtaining a ticket to the annual Caledonian Ball depended on contacts. Unless, the members of the board wanted to spend their professional lives in honourable obscurity behind the shutters of their headquarters in Berkeley street, they had to join the patronage game. And patrons, however intimate, did not offer their services free. They expected their clients to provide reciprocal favours when called on to do so.[121]

McGrigor was no more aloof from the game than his predecessors. In early Victorian hagiography, he was presented and, doubtless wanted to be seen, as detached from the world of favours. The surgeon and antiquarian, Thomas Pettigrew, in his biography of Guthrie has the director-general sending his subject away with a flea in his ear, when, on finding his civilian career not prospering as he had hoped, he had the temerity to ask for his post back, a few years after refusing to join the staff for Waterloo.

His kind friend, Sir James McGrigor, on his mentioning it to him, said, 'My good friend, if I do this for you, it will be called a job, and no one will be more sorry than yourself. I will answer for it you will not fail of success, and you will not long want the money.'[122]

But McGrigor was not the enemy of jobbers and jobbery he pretended and was perfectly ready to lobby the great and the good on his own behalf. His willingness to play the game was all the greater in that his appetite for social and cultural renown was particularly huge, and his patron and friend of the Peninsula, for whom he was undoubtedly indebted for his position as director-general, had snubbed his wider social ambitions.[123]

---

[120] See Ch. 1.

[121] Before 1870 patronage still continued to determine progress in the civil service, despite the 1853 Northcote-Trevelyan report. In the first parliamentary election after reform, some 60–70 MPs, including Gladstone, owed their seat to old-fashioned borough patrons: see Eric J. Evans, *The Forging of the Modern State: Early Industrial Britain, 1783–1870* (London, 1983), 215–16, 285–7.

[122] Pettigrew, *Medical Portrait Gallery*, iv. 7. Instead McGrigor allowed Guthrie to work without pay at the York hospital for two years.

[123] McGrigor gradually accumulated a clutch of honours and honorary offices: see Ch. 1.

McGrigor seems to have returned from the Peninsula expecting to be honoured by a grateful prince regent. Either he was peculiarly arrogant or peculiarly naïve as to the openness of the British establishment, but he seriously believed that the head of Wellington's army medical department would be given a baronetcy.[124] When the duke informed him that he was to get only a knighthood, he expressed dismay and declared he believed he was worth something more permanent. The duke, presumably flabbergasted by the chutzpah of the Aberdonian merchant's son, quickly put him in his place and icily replied, 'You are the best judge of what you will take, but I would recommend your taking the knighthood in the meantime.' McGrigor demurred but inwardly seethed.[125]

Thereafter, he worked tirelessly to gain the honour he desperately wanted. Early in 1826, for instance, McGrigor asked his commander-in-chief, still the duke of York, to support his claim with the then prime minister, Lord Liverpool. His argument was twofold. Earlier holders of the post of physician-general had been made baronets for their services and the office of director-general was a much more onerous one than theirs.[126] York graciously did the director's bidding, but Liverpool once more gave him the cold shoulder, even though his suit was now supported by Wellington.[127] The prime minister sympathized with McGrigor's case, but had recently decided that baronetcies would only go to those who held a certain amount of land. McGrigor replied through the duke of York's aide-de-camp, Sir Herbert Taylor, expressing his understanding of the conditions but hoping that in his case an exception might be made. Had he been permanently pensioned in 1814 and gone on to build up a large private practice, he would easily have met this qualification. As it was, he had sacrificed wealth for the public good.

With the utmost deference, and respect to the First Lord of the Treasury, I would humbly appeal to his Lordship's well known sense of justice, if I should be permitted to suffer for my adherence and devotion to the public good . . . Although my qualifications of landed property be but small, I have ever found that in Scotland personal influence and connections carried with me as much sway and ascendancy as some who could boast of a large rent-roll . . . . [I]n a recent occasion, without solicitation and even without my knowledge, I have been elected almost unanimously Lord Rector of the Marischal College and University of Aberdeen, where I received my early education, and when Lord Arbuthnot and Mr. Hume were candidates for the Office. As this honour has been conferred on individuals of Rank, I owe my elevation to the favourable opinion entertained of my

---

[124] At this date there were only two medical baronets extant: Sir Lucas Pepys, created in 1784 and Sir Everard Home (1756–1832), surgeon at St George's, elevated in 1813. A few years later, Hardinge, Wellington's aide-de-camp at Waterloo, also only received a knighthood, so McGrigor could hardly claim he had been ill-done-by.

[125] McGrigor, 241–2. McGrigor must have been still seething when he came to write his memoirs. This is the only passage in the book implicitly critical of the duke.

[126] BL, Add MSS 38301, fos. 123–4: McGrigor to York, no date. Presumably McGrigor was thinking of Sir John Pringle, baronet in 1766, and Pepys, although the latter was elevated ten years before he became physician-general.

[127] University of Southampton, Wellington Papers 1/848/20: Wellington to Liverpool, 2 Feb. 1826.

Public Services; and I would presume to say that should my principals be graciously pleased to bestow on me the honour of Baronet, it would be considered as conferring an honour on the University in which I hold a distinguished rank.[128]

However, the good lord was unmoved. Neither the thought of the Scottish votes that McGrigor might bring his way nor the good opinion of the students of Aberdeen caused him to change his mind.[129] Rebuffed once more, the director played his final card: he would do his best to acquire the necessary property as soon as possible and buy his way in.[130] But even grovelling compliance was of no avail. The door to the baronetcy remained firmly shut while the Tories remained in power. McGrigor would only get his dearest wish in 1831 with a new king and a Whig ministry, presumably more sympathetic to his merits.

A director-general who blew his own trumpet so stridently for social gain and marshalled the highest in the land to fight his corner hardly occupied the moral high ground. McGrigor was too deeply mired in the mud of patronage himself to turn his back on the requests of the great and powerful. In his case, moreover, the professionalized career structure that he claimed to uphold was further undermined by the fact that he had little idea how to appoint objectively in any modern sense. Decisions about promotion, reduction, and reappointment, particularly in regard to senior positions, seem to have been heavily influenced by his personal prejudices as much as any external pressure upon him. McGrigor was never a modern meritocrat.

The director-general, especially in his first years in office, seems to have been reluctant to appoint anyone to a senior position whose abilities he had not personally witnessed. As McGrigor had had many years' experience in the field, both at home and abroad, he had encountered in the course of his career a large proportion of the serving and half-pay officers by 1815. It is evident, too, that when assessing a candidate for promotion, he did not have to rely on his memory. From the moment he became an inspector in 1805, he kept meticulous records of the qualities of the surgeons under his supervison, especially in the Peninsula. By the time of his own elevation, therefore, he had marked the card of many of his junior colleagues. Those he admired, he was anxious to favour; those he did not were prime candidates for half-pay or to rise no further in the service.

One surgeon who benefited positively from the director's approval was John Robb of Ayr. In his journal, McGrigor described Robb at the siege of Badajoz in April 1812 as 'indefatigable in his superintendance' and in the course of the Peninsular campaign wrote him two personal letters of thanks for his efforts in

---

[128] Ibid., fo. 120: McGrigor to Taylor, 15 Mar. 1826. Taylor, later known as the King's Tailor, became William IV's private secretary: he was well connected with the aristocracy. John Arbuthnot, 8th Viscount Arbuthnot, was the unsuccessful candidate in the 1826 election. Joseph Hume, the radical MP, had been elected in 1824 and 1825, but was defeated by McGrigor in 1826 and 1827.

[129] In a further letter McGrigor went on to suggest that his elevation might help the prime minister in calming the ructions at Aberdeen university: McGrigor to Taylor, 20 Mar. 1826: ibid., fo. 140.

[130] McGrigor to Lord Liverpool, 11 July 1826: ibid. fo. 265.

looking after the medical needs of the light division and administering a number of general hospitals.[131] Understandably, then, Robb never went on half-pay until he requested it. McGrigor was presumably happy to see Robb taken off to America by Packenham (before he actually became director), and even happier to place him in charge of the Cape Town station when he returned.

Another veteran of the Peninsula who was peculiarly favoured was the Irishman, John Hennen, renowned for always having a cigar in his mouth. He entered the service in 1800 and served virtually continually until his death. On the staff from 1811, then put on half-pay in late 1814, he had hardly settled in Dumfries before he was called back in for the Flanders campaign. After Waterloo he had sole charge of the wounded of the general staff and in September 1815 was promoted deputy inspector of hospitals. Back in Britain, he was made principal medical officer of the army medical service in Scotland in 1817 before being put in charge of the Mediterranean theatre in the 1820s. He eventually rose to the rank of inspector, in which position he died in Gibraltar in 1828, victim of the particularly virulent epidemic which struck the garrison town in that year.[132]

McGrigor, too, was reluctant to let go of surgeons he had grown to admire. The Scot, John Schetky (not in the cohort) had been assistant surgeon to the 3rd Dragoon Guards in the Peninsula from 1809 until 1812. With the support of the colonel of the regiment, Sir Granby Calcraft, he had then been promoted to the position of staff surgeon to the Portuguese forces under Marshal Lord Beresford, with whom McGrigor had served in the Connaught Rangers. Although Beresford had made it clear that Schetky was 'one of those whom his Lordship wished to retain in that service', he could not initially be re-recruited once the Portuguese staff was dissolved. According to his biographer, he wanted to return to Edinburgh 'to enjoy for a time the society of his aged father and affectionate family, and to renew those liberal studies both general and professional . . .' McGrigor, however, eventually got his man. A distinguished water-colourist and anatomical artist, Schetky was enticed back into the service in 1819 to produce drawings at McGrigor's Museum of Medical Anatomy in the General Hospital at Fort Pitt, Chatham. He was rewarded by promotion as deputy inspector of hospitals on the African Coast, where he died in 1823.[133]

Surgeon Edward Walsh, in contrast, was a different story. McGrigor crossed swords with the Irishman early in his career as an inspector, when Walsh's regiment, the 62nd, was in barracks at Winchester. On 15 September 1807—and not for the first time—Walsh was accused of failing to produce weekly returns of the sick,

[131] WL, RAMC 799/6, McGrigor's journal (microfilm), n.p., *sub* Apr. 1812; TNA, WO25/3897/20: Robb's service record, early 1840s.
[132] John Hennen, *Principles of Military Surgery, Comprising of Observations on the Arrangement, Police, and Practice of Hospitals, and on the History, Treatment and Anomalies of Variola and Syphilis*, with life of the author by his son, Dr John Hennen (London, 1829), pp. x–xi. There is a memorial to him in Gibraltar.
[133] [David Maclagan], *Biographical Sketch of the Late John Alexander Schetky* (Edinburgh, 1825), 1–3.

then the following December, having grudgingly obeyed, he was chastised for returning them incorrectly. At the same time, he was in trouble with McGrigor for passing Surgeon Turley of the Bedfordshire militia, 'variolous matter' rather than vaccine for inoculating his men against smallpox.[134] Just as understandably, therefore, Walsh was quickly put on permanent half-pay in 1816 once McGrigor was director, despite his status as a Waterloo veteran and his rank of physician to the forces.[135]

On its own, admittedly, McGrigor's prejudice in favour of those of whom he had personally formed a positive opinion could scarcely be called unjust. It was an approach, though, which inevitably prejudiced those who did not know him personally. It might well be the case that the hapless Williamson did not take the chance to return to London and plead his cause before the director-general in 1824, because, having nearly always been in the West Indies since 1798, he was well aware that McGrigor hardly knew him from Adam.[136]

Medical critics of the director-general, moreover, thought that when hard choices had to be made as to whom to retain, place on half-pay, or recall, he was peculiarly solicitous of the welfare of his fellow countrymen to the detriment of the English. When the Ripon surgeon, Samuel Barwick Bruce, was forced to accept commutation in the early 1830s, his case was taken up by that scourge of Old Corruption, the *Lancet*. An apoplectic letter written in 1834 insisted that Bruce had had a shabby deal throughout the director's rule. Despite his record of exemplary service, he had been placed on half-pay after Waterloo and his post given to someone who had never been at the battle. 'Because why? The Doctor was a Scotchman.'[137]

In this particular case, there was more than a kernel of truth in the accusation. Bruce's 'replacement', according to the *Lancet*, was a Dr Murray. This was John Murray of Turriff, Aberdeenshire, an army surgeon in the McGrigor era on whom the sun always smiled. Murray, a staff surgeon at the end of the Peninsular campaign, had been placed on half-pay in September 1814, after politely refusing General Hill's invitation to join his mooted expedition to America. But he was soon back in the service and given a desk job.[138] Once the fighting was over, moreover, Murray was transferred to the staff in Paris in December 1815, where he remained for three years, always avoiding being placed once more on half-pay

---

[134] WL, RAMC 799/3, McGrigor's letter book, 1805–9 (microfilm), fo. 167. The army was a major vehicle for the promotion of Jenner's new technique of smallpox vaccination, a much safer method of producing immunity than the previous one of introducing a small amount of matter from a smallpox pustule into the blood.

[135] Admittedly, Walsh was getting on in years, but he could have been promoted. The surgeon may have been on the campaign, but not at the battle. Drew accredits him with being there, but he is not on Dalton's roll. He was a colourful character with literary and radical pretensions in his youth: see Ch. 7.   [136] McGrigor had only been in the West Indies in 1796 with Abercromby.

[137] *Lancet*, 2 (1834–5), 27–8. Bruce, of course, was born in the West Indies and was only English by place of residence once he came out of the army.

[138] WL, RAMC 306, esp. letters 2 June and 7 Aug. 1814 (on Lord Hill's invitation); 26 Aug. 1814 (half-pay rate); 28 July 1815 (his work in Aberdeen).

until the army of occupation withdrew.[139] Bruce, meanwhile, another Peninsular veteran who had served on the staff at Waterloo, was released from the service as early as March 1816 in the first wave of cut-backs. Arguably, he had the right to feel that it was unfair that Murray had been brought across to France to strengthen the staff on the eve of a reduction, and to have wondered how Murray survived until 1818, while many of his seniors were placed on half-pay.[140] It certainly must have looked as if McGrigor was protecting a fellow Scot from Aberdeenshire, all the more when Bruce was passed over year after year while Murray was back in again in December 1819 and posted to another desk job at Chatham.[141]

On the other hand, there is no hard statistical information to confirm that McGrigor favoured Scotsmen. They were not grossly under-represented among surgeons first placed on half-pay in the first three years of McGrigor's period of office, forming 27.8 per cent of the total as against 29.7 per cent of the whole cohort. Nor were they recalled in peculiarly large numbers, for 24 per cent of the Scots reduced on one or more occasion in the years 1814–19 would never see service again, while only 32 of the 93 surgeons who died abroad after 1815 were north Britons (see Tables 4.19–21). In fact, in the promotion stakes, the Scots were disadvantaged: 41.4 per cent of members of the cohort who never rose above assistant surgeon were Scottish—a completely disproportional number— while only 25 per cent of those elevated by McGrigor to the deputy inspectorate were his fellow countrymen (see Tables 4.16–17). If anything, as has already been noted, it was the English who seemed to have the better chances of getting to the top in the McGrigor era, a tribute perhaps to their better connections.[142]

It is much more likely in consequence that Murray rose because he was a surgeon who had won the director-general's approval in the Peninsula, while Bruce languished because he had not. It cannot be coincidental that Murray appears in a highly positive fashion in the Aberdonian's autobiography, applauded for his surgical skill and gentlemanly conduct, when imprisoned by the French after being left behind on McGrigor's orders with the wounded.[143]

This is not to say that McGrigor's readiness to bow to patronage pressure or favour surgeons he knew was necessarily detrimental to the health of the service. In a period when every recruit was well educated and most, after a few years, presumably competent medical officers, it probably made little difference who was appointed. The massive recruitment during the French wars and the quality of the recruits also made it difficult to separate them out on grounds of seniority or merit. Some mechanism would have had to have been found for making promotions, especially above the regimental level. In a world still dominated by

---

[139] WL, RAMC 306, esp. letters: 30 Dec. 1815 (first from Paris)–20 Dec. 1818 (first from London): esp. 23 May 1816, 13 Feb. and 1 Mar. 1817 (on his good fortune in avoiding reduction).

[140] The reduction of the staff seems to have begun with the most junior.

[141] From there he was sent to the Cape in 1821.

[142] Only 17 per cent of English recruits left as assistant surgeons (see Table 4.17); however, since many, if not most, Englishmen in the cohort had reached a higher rank before McGrigor took charge, he can hardly be accused of favouring Sassenachs at all levels.   [143] McGrigor, 231–2.

patronage and place, it was scarcely surprising that personal preference and recommendation oiled the promotional wheels. Before the invention of internal examinations and staff assessment, there was no other way of making them turn.

There again, the significance of personal factors in a surgeon's advancing up the professional ladder made for some peculiar success stories. James Barry, who joined the service as a hospital assistant in 1813 and retired as a deputy inspector-general in 1859, had the most implausible career of all. Not only was Barry a woman with a slight figure and high voice, but she was tetchy, difficult, and insubordinate, perhaps not surprisingly given the strain she must have been permanently under. An early clash with her superiors came as an assistant surgeon serving in the Cape in 1819, when she fought a duel with the governor's aide-de-camp, Captain Cloete, after the captain had pulled her rather long nose for the disparaging remarks she had made about a local lady. But this was only the first of many signs that she had little sense of rank or propriety. Wherever she was stationed she quarrelled with the military or civilian authorities over their neglect of the soldiers or her own inadequate pay and conditions. In Corfu, towards the end of her career, now a deputy inspector, she supposedly horse-whipped Colonel Denny of the 71st for drilling his regiment in the full glare of the sun.[144] On one occasion, while serving on Mauritius as a staff surgeon, she even took French leave and came back to England and dared McGrigor to do his worst.

'Sir', said Sir James McGrigor, 'I do not understand your reporting yourself in this fashion. You admit you have returned without leave of absence. May I ask how this is?'

'Well', said James, coolly running his long white fingers through his crispy curls, 'I have come home to have my hair cut'.[145]

The director-general, however, never took action, but steadily allowed her to scale the promotional ladder. Possibly, she was forgiven because of her commitment to troop welfare, but this is unlikely. A much more plausible explanation for his leniency lies in the protection she was given by the Beaufort family. On her first posting to Cape Town, she became close to the governor of the province, General Lord Charles Henry Somerset, second son of the duke. It is possible he learnt her secret and she became his mistress, or he may simply have employed her to minister to his family, and found her a congenial and successful doctor. Whatever the truth of the matter, so close did their friendship become that it was rumoured they had a homosexual relationship, a factor which played some part in Somerset's recall in 1825. The governor's disgrace, though, did not undermine her standing with the family, and when Lord Charles died in 1831 she was taken up by his younger brother Lord Fitzroy Somerset. Wellington's aide-de-camp in the Peninsula and his brother-in-law, a Waterloo hero, secretary at Horse Guards,

---

[144] June Rose, *The Perfect Gentleman: The Remarkable Life of Dr James Miranda Barry, the Woman who served as an Officer in the British Army from 1813 to 1859* (London, 1977), 44, 133. Duelling was not unknown in the British army, of course, but this is the only example uncovered of a duel fought by a medical officer, who was supposed to save life not take it.   [145] Ibid. 92: source unclear.

then commander-in-chief in the Crimea from 1852 as Baron Raglan, Fitzroy's influence ensured she was untouchable. Only when Fitzroy died in 1855 did her star in the service wane, by which time McGrigor, who must have secretly loathed her, had himself retired.[146]

MAKING MONEY

The small percentage of army surgeons who reached the highest rung of the service ladder must have accumulated an enviable nest-egg by the time their career came to an end. John Murray in India in the late 1830s enjoyed a salary in present-day values of £146,000 without tax.[147] Even though he died in office, his wife and children must have received a large inheritance.[148] New recruits were well aware of the financial heights to which they might soar in their chosen profession, and many in their early days must have imitated Joseph Brown in tempting relatives nervous of their choice with the prospect of riches to come. Writing from the army depot on the Isle of Wight in 1806, the Tyneside surgeon reassured his sister-in-law that he had a patron in the service and a lucrative goal.

From Dr [George Paulet] Morris, the Inspector, I receive great attention and frequent invitations. He was at Shields in 1795. He often speaks of his intimacy with the Miss Hutchinsons. His pay is 3 guineas per diem, besides great allowances; his rank that of Brigadier General. From this you will perceive that Inspector of Hospitals is one of the good things the King bestows.[149]

Such a good was obviously not to be cast off lightly. It was for this reason that William Fergusson's mother cautioned patience when he expressed the desire to give up his post in the Portuguese army, and his brother reminded him he had obtained the best appointment he had ever had. He must learn to trade 'a few years absence from his family' for 'a comfortable independence at last'. A retired army surgeon friend, Thomas Christie, was just as bemused to learn that Fergusson had accepted a transfer back to the British army. In that he had received double pay from serving with the Portuguese, he should have stuck it out and got home to his family all the sooner.[150]

[146] Ibid. 35–85, *passim*; 93, 135, 140–1. Needless to say, as Raglan's client, Barry berated Florence Nightingale when she visited the Crimea. The *Lancet* queried Barry's promotion shortly before it defended Bruce, claiming s/he had refused to perform surgical operations while in Jamaica: *Lancet*, 1 (1834–5), 792.

[147] **www.eh.net/hmit/ppower/bp**: University of Miami prices index (Jan. 2006).

[148] Unfortunately, we have not located his will or a valuation of his estate. For his pay in India, see p. 194.

[149] TWA, Acc. No. 1132/5: letter 24 Feb. 1806 (photocopy of original and transcription).

[150] WL, RAMC 208, nos. 71, 75: John Fergusson to William Fergusson, 17 Mar. and 14 Sept. 1812; no. 87: Christie to Fergusson, 7 Jan. 1813. Christie, not in the database, does not appear in Drew.

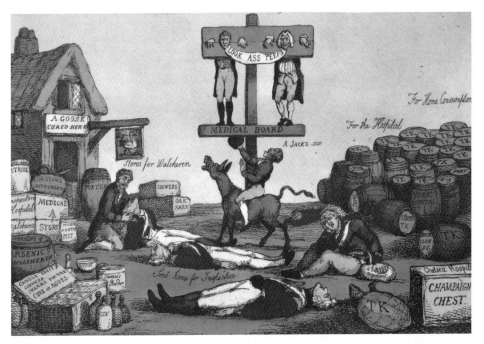

1. Thomas Rowlandson, *Winding up the Medical Report of the Walcheren Expedition* (1810) [Engraving by Courtesy of the British Museum]. In the aftermath of the disastrous Walcheren campaign in the summer of 1809, where the troops were decimated by fever, Physician-General Pepys and Surgeon-General Keate were heavily criticised for their inadequate medical preparations. Rowlandson, in a cartoon that appeared at the end of March 1810, literally placed them in the pillory, looking down on the dead and dying, while one of the Army Medical Board's chief critics, Robert Jackson, mockingly rode past on a donkey.

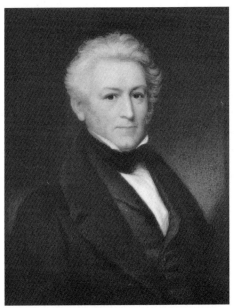

2. R. Easton, *George James Guthrie* (n.d.) [Oil Painting: By courtesy of the National Portrait Gallery, London]. Guthrie (no. 255 in the database), the son of a London surgical goods salesman, was the most famous military surgeon of the first half of the nineteenth century who honed his operative skills in the Peninsula. After leaving the army in 1814 as a deputy inspector he spent most of the rest of his life as a surgeon to Westminster Hospital.

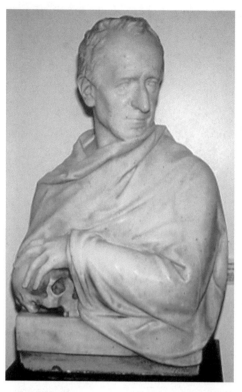

3. William Belnes, *Joseph Constantine Carpue*
[1847] [Marble Bust: by courtesy of St George's
Hospital, London]. Carpue (no. 294) came
from a London Catholic family. He was one of
the few surgeons in the cohort who never went
abroad but spent his army service attached to
the York Hospital. From the mid-1800s until
his death in 1846, he ran a very successful
private anatomy school in the capital.

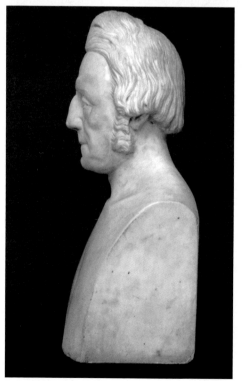

4. A. R. Fry, *Joseph Brown* (1886) [Marble Bust:
By courtesy of the Tyne and Wear Museums].
Brown (no. 6) was the son of a Quaker merchant
from North Shields. After the French wars he
settled in Sunderland where he became senior
physician at the local infirmary and a member
of the city corporation.

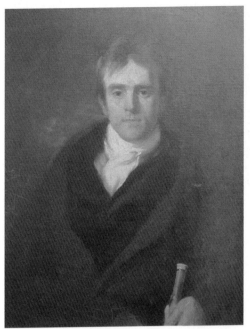

5. Anon., *David Maclagan as a Young Man* (n.d.) [Oil Painting: Photograph by Ben Morris. By courtesy of the Maclagan family]. Maclagan (no. 106), an Edinburgh episcopalian by origin whose father had been a bank-teller, was one of the most successful Scottish recruits to the Army Medical Service during the wars. On retiring on half-pay, he set up his plate in Edinburgh New Town and enjoyed a lucrative career as a private practitioner. The portrait was possibly a gift to his new wife before he left for the Peninsula. Unusually he was a prominent Whig and a close friend of the Broughams, Cockburn and Jeffrey.

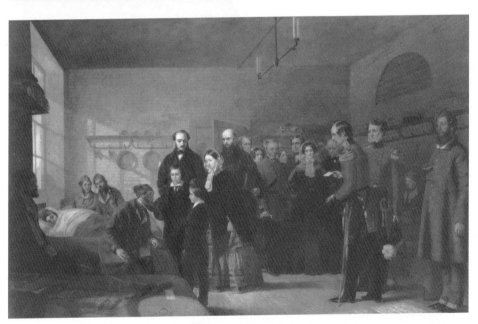

6. Jerry Barrett, *Queen Victoria's First Visit to Her Wounded Soldiers* [1856] [Oil Painting: By Courtesy of the National Portrait Gallery, London]. Towards the end of the Crimean War, the royal family paid a morale-boosting visit to recuperating soldiers in the hospital at Fort Pitt, Chatham. The visit gave belated royal recognition to McGrigor's army medical service at a time when it was coming under attack for its shortcomings. The medical officer third from the left is the Irishman, George Russell Dartnell (no. 199) from Limerick, who joined the army medical corps after the French wars and rose to the rank of Deputy Inspector General of Hospitals. He was an accomplished watercolourist who retired to Hampton-in-Arden, Warwicks, in 1857 and set up an asylum for the insane.

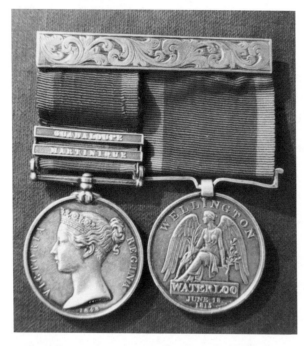

7. Samuel Barwick Bruce, Waterloo Medal [By courtesy of David Hurst]. Bruce (no. 72) came from Barbados. After the French wars he settled in Ripon, Yorkshire, where he was the local government inspector of mills and prisons. He was one of the cohort forced to exchange his right to half-pay for a lump sum when he refused to re-enter the service in the early 1830s. He was a staff surgeon at Waterloo, one of 23 members of the cohort who were definitely present at the battle.

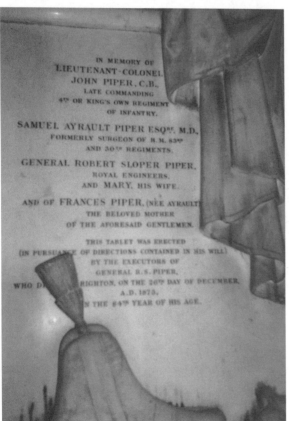

8. Memorial to the Piper Family, Colyton Church, Devon [Authors' photograph]. Samuel Ayrault Piper (no. 220) was one of the few members of the cohort who belonged to a military family. His father was an army captain who settled in Devon, where Samuel was born, while two of his brothers became senior officers. He himself had a long career in the army medical service, but never rose above the rank of surgeon.

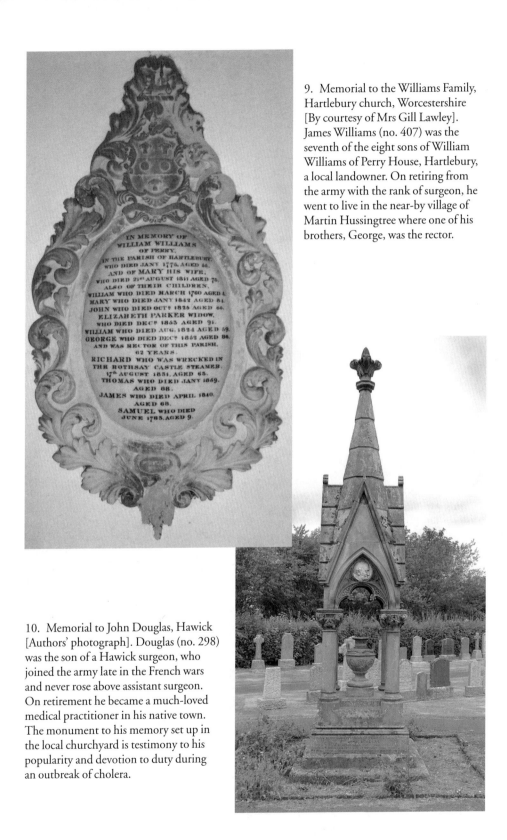

9. Memorial to the Williams Family, Hartlebury church, Worcestershire [By courtesy of Mrs Gill Lawley]. James Williams (no. 407) was the seventh of the eight sons of William Williams of Perry House, Hartlebury, a local landowner. On retiring from the army with the rank of surgeon, he went to live in the near-by village of Martin Hussingtree where one of his brothers, George, was the rector.

IN MEMORY OF
WILLIAM WILLIAMS
OF PERRY,
IN THE PARISH OF HARTLEBURY,
WHO DIED JANY 1776, AGED 44.
AND OF MARY HIS WIFE,
WHO DIED 21st AUGUST 1811 AGED 79.
ALSO OF THEIR CHILDREN,
WILLIAM WHO DIED MARCH 1760 AGED 4
MARY WHO DIED JANY 1842 AGED 84
JOHN WHO DIED OCTr 1825 AGED 66.
ELIZABETH PARKER WIDOW,
WHO DIED DECr 1853 AGED 91.
WILLIAM WHO DIED AUG. 1824 AGED 59.
GEORGE WHO DIED DECr 1852 AGED 86.
AND WAS RECTOR OF THIS PARISH.
62 YEARS.
RICHARD WHO WAS WRECKED IN
THE ROTHSAY CASTLE STEAMER,
17th AUGUST 1831, AGED 65.
THOMAS WHO DIED JANY 1859,
AGED 68.
JAMES WHO DIED APRIL 1840,
AGED 68.
SAMUEL WHO DIED
JUNE 1785, AGED 9.

10. Memorial to John Douglas, Hawick [Authors' photograph]. Douglas (no. 298) was the son of a Hawick surgeon, who joined the army late in the French wars and never rose above assistant surgeon. On retirement he became a much-loved medical practitioner in his native town. The monument to his memory set up in the local churchyard is testimony to his popularity and devotion to duty during an outbreak of cholera.

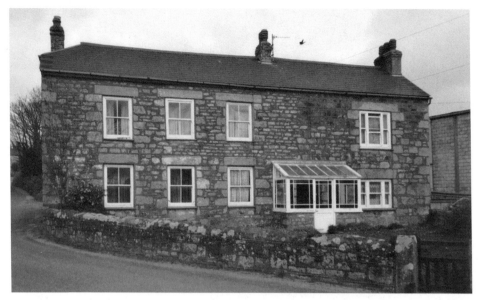

11. Varfell Farm, near Penzance, Cornwall [Authors' photograph]. John Davy (no. 196) was the younger brother of the scientist, Sir Humphry. His father owned a small farm in the village of Ludgvan, where John was raised. John entered the army a few months before Waterloo and had a highly successful career. On retiring as an inspector general, he went to live in the Lake District and was Wordsworth's physician in the poet's last years.

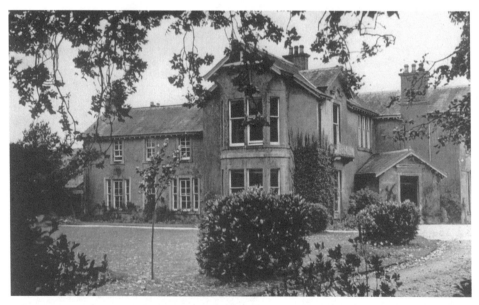

12. Langlands, near Twynholm, Galloway [Photograph by kind permission of the present owner Peter Murray Usher]. Dr Alexander Browne (no. 358) was the son of a small Scottish landowner who owned an estate in Kirkudbrightshire. Browne inherited the estate in 1823, but he did not leave the army until 1850, even though he never rose above the rank of surgeon. He retired to Langlands and died in the house in which he was born in 1872.

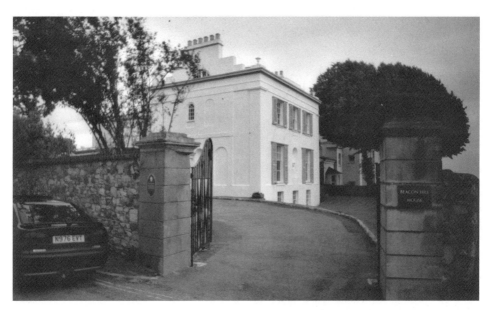

13. Beacon House, Exmouth, Devon [Authors' photograph]. William Henry Burrell (no. 9) was born in Edinburgh. After long years of service in the army where he made deputy inspector, he retired to Exmouth and bought Beacon House, a building of considerable architectural interest. The probate value of his estate in 1866 was £6,000. This was a fashionable street, looking out across the sea, where Nelson's widow, Fanny, spent her declining years.

AVUNCULO SUO

JOANNI GIBNEY, M. D.

&c. &c.

DE BRIGHTON.

Charissime Avuncule, ut tibi grata facerem, hanc Disputationem primùm suscepi ; rem non benè tractatam fuisse omnino fateor, nam paucissima ex propriâ experientiâ dicere potui. Libenter eas perfectiores esse optarem ; sed quamvis imperfectas, te has studiorum meorum primitias, animi gratissimi testimonium, accepturum esse spero. Diu vivas et valeas, et omnibus amicis multos annos decori intersis, ex imo pectore voveo. Vale.

14. William Gibney, *De coeli caldi* (1813) [Edinburgh doctoral thesis, dedication page: By courtesy of Edinburgh University Library]. Gibney (no. 24) was from County Meath, Ireland, the son of a small landowner distantly related to the Wellesleys. Unlike most of his army colleagues, he had a medical degree before he entered the service. His dissertation was dedicated to his uncle, John, a Brighton medical practitioner in the Prince Regent's circle, who had looked after his education on his father's early death. Gibney retired from the service to Cheltenham where he became a physician to the dispensary and helped promote the town as a spa resort.

15. James McGrigor, *Medical Sketches of the Expedition to Egypt from India* (1804) [Dedication page: By courtesy of the Wellcome Library, London]. McGrigor wrote up his account of the Egyptian campaign on his way back from India, then submitted it for approval to two of the physicians to the Prince of Wales on his return, presumably in the hope they would push his case for promotion. The gambit worked for he was quickly transferred from the 88th to the Horse Guards Blue, even before the book appeared. The dedication of the work to the three general officers of the Army Medical Board was a way of politely thanking them for acceding to the solicitations of his patrons.

16. George James Guthrie, *Lectures on the Operative Surgery of the Eye* (1823) [Dedication page: By courtesy of the Wellcome Library, London]. Apart from being a great military surgeon, Guthrie was also an expert on eye-diseases who co-founded the Royal Westminster Ophthalmic Hospital. Like many ex-army surgeons who went into print, he dedicated his lectures on the subject to the Duke of Wellington. Since the duke was the president of the new hospital, this was a mark of respect, but the dedication also ensured that the book would be received respectfully by readers.

The large majority of army surgeons, however, were never in the happy position of making a fortune out of army service. This is not to say that the average medical officer did not receive from the moment he joined as a hospital mate a reasonable salary, nor that he did not set out with the best of intentions. Lesassier was cock-a-hoop with his original pay of 6*s.*/6*d.* per day. 'I am now handsomely independent of anyone', he wrote in a letter home, '& may with care not only keep up appearances & live like a gentleman but may also save money.'[151] The problem, as Lesassier and countless others found, was that army service was expensive. It was not just the temptations of the mess: a careful officer could avoid the gaming-table and excessive drinking.[152] It was rather the welter of hidden costs that entrants quickly discovered.

At the outset, the new surgeon had to provide himself with a uniform, boots, and camping equipment which he had thereafter to keep in a respectable condition. Joseph Brown in the letter cited above estimated the cost at £50, which would have been about sixteen weeks' wages. But full ceremonial rig in a prestigious regiment would have been much more expensive, so much so that when William Lindsay's friend, Richard Webster, a married officer, was gazetted to the 8th Hussars from the 51st Foot in 1826, he viewed his promotion with alarm.[153] Purchasing the uniform, however, was only the beginning for thereafter the new surgeon would have to pay an annual standing charge to support the mess and the regimental band, and in the McGrigor era subscribe to the director-general's charities. Lindsay may have been reluctant to contribute to the Orphans' Society, but even as an assistant surgeon he paid an annual five-guinea sub to the Widows Fund on top of mess and band charges of £16 per annum.[154]

On campaign, where the medical officer needed a horse, the outlay grew even heavier. Although officers were given free forage, they received no allowance towards purchasing their mounts. One horse, too, was not enough. As Assistant Surgeon William Dent explained to his mother, writing home from the Peninsula in February 1813, he needed two animals to keep up appearances: one to ride and one for his baggage. He therefore requested urgently that £20 be deposited with the army agent, James Window, so that could set himself up properly.[155] Horses, too, on campaign, frequently needed to be replaced, as Acting Surgeon Joseph Brown, with an equine retinue of four to maintain, informed his sister-in-law in another letter six months later.

I have at present charge of the Regiment and to this acting situation some emolument is attached and I had been pleasing myself with the idea of returning to England somewhat

[151] Rosner, 37.   [152] On the temptations, see Ch. 1, p. 48.

[153] WL, RAMC 262/8, no. 29: Webster to Lindsay, 7 Feb. 1826. At this moment Webster (not in the cohort) was burdened by heavy investment in his sons' careers: see Ch. 6. It would be interesting to know how McGrigor afforded the dress uniform of the Horse Guards Blue. Drew says Webster transferred to the 4th Dragoon Guards in 1826: no. 2144.

[154] WL, RAMC 262/7, no. 14: Lindsay's bank statements from the agents, Greenwood and Cox, 1822–7.   [155] Ibid., RAMC 536, no. 24: letter 17 Feb. 1813.

richer than I left it, perhaps worth several hundreds [,] but the loss of two horses the one by death, the other by theft compell me to deduct at least £20 from my dream of wealth. The sums I have mentioned will, I am sure, appear very insignificant to commercial folks, but to us who live from hand to mouth, they are very important. When it is considered that in general we receive from the Commissary as much bread, meat and wine as we could consume, it may be a matter of surprise, that we fail to save a little out of the pittance we get in this country, but it is thus, that it is spent in loss of animals or in the wear and tear of attending them. I have restored my establishment to its primitive strength of four, and I could not part with one of them without most materially abridging my comfort.[156]

The expense of campaigning, moreover, rose as the officer advanced up the scale and keeping up appearances became more demanding. John Murray at the same date must have felt himself peculiarly privileged when, as a newly promoted staff surgeon, now allowed forage for two horses and three mules, he was given a superior mount worth 40 guineas by a Colonel Fenwick. But the gift was particularly timely, for he had spent heavily in kitting himself out for his new position and establishing a mobile household. Most medical officers seem to have hired a local inhabitant as a batman, but Murray considered that his new position demanded two man servants, a boy and a cook, which would set him back £50 per annum out of his pay of 18/- per day.[157] Writing from Toulouse the following spring with the campaign running down and about to depart for a ball in honour of the duc d'Angoulême, he painted a picture of a man living in style but barely making ends meet. When he had entered the service and had earned less than half his present salary, he had used to save a little; now, he admitted, his salary went as quickly as it came in.[158]

The problem of keeping afloat at the beginning was only aggravated by the fact that the British army usually paid its officers three months in arrears. Although a travelling allowance was provided to get the officer to his garrison or point of embarkation, this was often all he received for a considerable time. The tyro army surgeon therefore frequently had to go into debt in order to join his hospital or regiment. When Joseph Brown departed for the Isle of Wight in 1806, he was allowed five guineas for the cost of travelling from Edinburgh to London (presumably he took the surgeons' exam in Scotland) and £3 11s./6d. to get him from the capital to Newport.[159] Neither sum, though, was given in advance, and the prudent Quaker had to borrow £10 from his brother William and £5 from a family friend in London, John Beaumont, in order to get to the Army Depot.[160] And debts, once

[156] TWA, Acc. No. 1132/12: letter 5 Sept. 1813.

[157] Under the 1804 regulations, he received 15/- per day basic, plus 3/- a day lodgings allowance: see above Table 1.4.

[158] WL, RAMC 830, letters home: 27 Sept. and 28 Oct. 1813; 28 Apr. 1814. Fenwick had been released on parole from the French army and therefore had no more need of the horse. As a staff surgeon, Murray revealed, he received free rations for two or three servants.

[159] Brown did not record where he initially took the army entrance exam. He qualified as a full surgeon in London in January 1808.

[160] TWA, Acc. No. 1132/5: letter 24 Feb. 1806. Interestingly, Lesassier, bound for Gibraltar in the same year, was given three month's pay in advance, plus travel money, an indication perhaps of the influence of his family: see Rosner, 41.

incurred, as Brown and others found, were usually hard to repay immediately. Two years later, now in Jersey, the debt to Beaumont was still outstanding and would remain unpaid until 1812, when Brown was stationed in Lisbon.

I am still grievously assailed by my old enemy poverty. I have what supports me, but I have not a farthing to spare. If I remain here long being away from the mess, I expect to save a little money; and send Jno. Beaumont £5, which I am ashamed to say circumstances have not yet enabled me to do.[161]

Indeed, the whole system of pay was likely to mire the incautious in permanent debt. Each officer had an account with the regimental banker in London to whom his pay was transferred. The banker then extended him credit, paid his bills and annual standing orders, and transferred sums on request to and from his family living in the British Isles. For most of the time, an officer had very little ready money. When he needed cash or wished to pay off a large debt, either at home or abroad, he drew up a bill of exchange on his bank, which a local merchant or retailer accepted on expectation it would be duly honoured a few months later. But living on credit was expensive. The officer had to pay the bank for looking after his pay, and raising cash and settling accounts by bills of exchange meant he was continually paying a premium on any service: such bills were only accepted at discount. Admittedly, sensible army agents looked to their own solvency, so seem not to have extended credit too far. When an officer fell too deeply into the red, his bills of exchange were not met, as John Murray's father discovered on one occasion when he tried to redeem a £9 note from his son.[162] But some army agents were greedy. There was the added danger, then, that an army agent might go bankrupt, as essentially happened to Window in 1827, and the prudent officer would suffer in the collapse as much as the profligate.[163]

As a result, the average surgeon had to make a herculean effort to save. How difficult this could be is demonstrated by the case of William Lindsay, assistant surgeon of the 36th, then surgeon of the 18th. Lindsay was a small landowner who had got into debt through borrowing and had had his family property expropriated in late 1817 to repay two bonds. To add to his problems, he was a disadvantaged only son who had to support his decrepit mother and two sisters, one sick and unmarried, another a widow with two children.[164] Presumably, they were cared for in part by the interest on the capital acquired from the sale of the land, provided it was not all consumed by repurchasing the outstanding bonds. But Lindsay also steadfastly contributed to their upkeep from his army salary, forwarding in the 1820s £4 10s. per month while he was an assistant, then £6 10s. when he was promoted to regimental surgeon.[165] Understandably as this

---

[161] TWA, Acc. No. 1132/6, 8: letters home 10 May 1808 and 4 Feb. 1812.
[162] WL, RAMC 830: Murray to his mother, 2 May 1811, apologizing.
[163] Ibid., RAMC MS 206, Officers Benevolent Fund, minute book, 71–2: 4 Oct. 1827. Window had been the Fund's original treasurer.　　　[164] He came from Lochmaben, Dumfriesshire.
[165] WL, RAMC 262/7/4: account with Greenwood and Cox.

was a third of his basic pay (9*s*., then 14*s*. per day), he had difficulty in maintaining the payments, all the more that his bankers, Greenwood and Cox, were unwilling to extend him limitless credit. The bankers expected any debt in their favour to be wiped out when they received his army arrears. If this did not happen, the hapless surgeon received a warning letter in which the bank made clear its displeasure, as in March 1825.

We beg leave to transmit herewith an abstract of your account showing an over payment of £26 4/3 which we will thank you to liquidate by leaving your accruing pay from 25 January. We must also request you will be so good as to provide in future for the monthly payments to Miss Ross [his niece] of £6 10/- should you wish the same to continue.[166]

Throughout his army career, Lindsay responded to his shortage of funds in the time-honoured tradition of the financially embarrassed: he borrowed from army friends and deferred paying his creditors or paid them only partially.[167] Mostly, he got by, but on one occasion, at the very moment his landed property was in administration, he got into serious trouble. In the course of the 1810s, he had run up the substantial bill of £62 10*s*. with the firm of John Cameron of Henrietta Street, Covent Garden (probably an outfitters). Initially, Lindsay had promised to pay Cameron with the prize-money he had forthcoming, but he had failed to do so, and in March 1816 the retailer threatened to take him to court.[168] Lindsay seems to have avoided this by giving Cameron a bill of exchange for the full amount, due to fall in on 18 March 1818. Cameron accepted the bill only to discover in June 1817 that the bill was not drawn on any house in any town. As Lindsay, then at Portsmouth, was on the point of embarking for Malta, Cameron demanded a bill drawn on a London house not an IOU. Lindsay did as requested and sent a new bill to be redeemed by the firm of Carsdale (?) the following spring. When spring came with Lindsay safe abroad, the bill of exchange was unsurprisingly refused. An irate Cameron played his last card and threatened to end Lindsay's career.

I cannot help feeling myself very cheated in this business for you must have known all along that it would not be paid . . . but as I cannot go on any longer and I am determined to bring this affair to a settlement—I have to inform you that if you do not remit me home immediately on receipt of this something satisfactory, I shall most certainly address your commanding officer on the subject previous to applying to His Royal Highness the commander-in-chief, for I will not let the business rest as it is at present.[169]

---

[166] WL, RAMC 262/7/4: account with Greenwood and Cox, letter of 5 Mar. 1825.

[167] His papers are full of letters from creditors: e.g. ibid., 262/7/7: letters from Currie of Regent Str. 2 Aug. 1825 and 11 July 1826, asking him to pay his account; 262/7/10: letter from a lieutenant late of 36th fallen on bad times, 31 Mar. 1824, calling in a long-standing debt.

[168] When enemy ships were captured by a British vessel, they became prizes. The vessels and their cargoes were sold and the proceeds divided among the crew on a sliding scale determined by rank. A similar system pertained in the army, where enemy booty was treated as a prize. In the army, however, the rewards were generally much less.

[169] WL, RAMC 262/7/8: Cameron to Lindsay, letters 30 Mar. 1816, 11 June 1817, 2 Apr. 1818.

How Lindsay wriggled out of the dangling noose remains unknown, but such ungentlemanly behaviour (if all too common among some sections of the officer corps) cannot have endeared him to the Army Medical Board. If they never ultimately knew about his account with Cameron, they must have been aware he did not repay loans from fellow officers. In his case, doing right by his family in Lochmaben—the most charitable interpretation of his conduct—cannot have helped speed his promotion.[170]

MAKING FRIENDS

Clearly, for Lindsay and many other medical officers, the army was not a path to riches. Most did not rise high enough in the service or stay for a long enough time to reap significant financial reward. They may have found themselves a comfortable billet for a number of years—apart from the time spent on campaign, of course—but few with the rank of regimental surgeon or below can have left with a large fortune. Joseph Brown must have displayed true Quaker restraint to have accumulated even a couple of hundred pounds by the end of the Peninsular campaign. What all medical officers, even juniors, acquired from their sojourn in the forces, on the other hand, were contacts.

Earlier in this chapter, we saw how important it was for a young surgeon to forge positive links with his commanding officer, if he were to progress relatively speedily through the service. But the colonel or his deputy was only one of many military officers in his own and other regiments with whom the socially adept would strike up a close acquaintance over the years. Like any other club, the mess would have been subdivided into smaller circles of sociability and most surgeons would have quickly become intimate with two or three officers who remained their friends for life. The sober Gibney may have found his first night in the mess 'monotonous', but he soon found congenial company. After supper he took coffee, then spent the rest of the evening playing the flute with one of his mess-mates, Captain Carpenter, who was a linguist, a man of learning and uninterested in hunting, gambling, drinking, and horse flesh. 'Carpenter and I became great friends continuing so for many years.'[171]

A surgeon's set was most likely to comprise officers of his own age and interests, such as the four devil-may-care companions with whom John Murray investigated the volcanoes of the Lipari islands in 1809.[172] On the other hand, it might comprise officers of all ranks, and, given the fact, that senior officers often had their wives

---

[170] It must be said, he never sent the family enough: e.g. ibid., 262/10/10: Eliza (his sister) to Lindsay, 12 Nov. 1825, begging he send her a sovereign so she can buy a pair of blankets for the winter.

[171] Gibney, 101–3.

[172] WL, RAMC MS 830, letter home 24 Sept. 1809. The friends had a serious interest in natural history, but they were young men enjoying a summer ramble and terrified their guides by summoning the devil that the locals thought lived in the volcanoes.

and children with them, be of mixed sex. When William Lindsay—who needed friends more than most—was stationed on Corfu with the 36th, he was intimate with his CO, Lieutenant Colonel Cross, his CO's wife and daughter, 'sweet Ellen', the CO's son William, a subaltern officer in the regiment, a Major Browne, a Lieutenant Macleod, also married, and an Ensign? Gilbert, not to mention his fellow medical officer Webster, another married man.[173] Much of Lindsay's friendship with Cross and his family can be put down to their ill-health and his success in convincing them he could treat their complaints.[174] But his other friendships seem to have been based on mutual affection. Cross took sick leave in 1821—his first long period of absence from his regiment in twenty years—and Browne replaced him as acting CO. The major and the assistant surgeon were so close that they shared a cottage together and when Lindsay fell ill with malaria the following year, Browne looked after him. As Lindsay informed his lieutenant colonel, still languishing in Italy, Browne was 'one in a thousand'.[175]

For an army surgeon, as for any other army officer, these tightly-knit webs of friendship were of great value. On a day-to-day basis, they helped to make a tedious spell of duty enjoyable or calm nerves on the eve of battle. Shortly before Waterloo, Gibney and his friends were treated to a bacon-and-egg dinner by another of his set in the regiment, Lieutenant Buckley, where they indulged in banter about the forthcoming engagement.

It was wonderful with what indifference we spoke or rather joked with each other on coming events. To one tall and big, the information was vouchsafed that his chances of being hit were good, so huge an individual forming a target not to be missed. To another, with an unusually prominent nasal organ, its liability to attract the enemy's attention to him was pointed out; and so everlastingly. The jokes were more personal than polite, and fell hard on such as rode badly, or rather, who were not thoroughly at home in the saddle.[176]

This was Gibney's first real taste of action and he must desperately have needed reassurance. A few days later half the regiment would be dead or wounded and Buckley would die of his wounds, his friend unable to save him.

Once formed, an army friendship could survive long bouts of leave and even a change of regiment. The fact that friendship circles were continually being split up and new ones created by the impermanence of army life was part of their utility. By the end of his career, any army officer would have friends dotted around the globe. Those back in Britain could be the most immediately useful. When a friend went on leave, he would take letters for the families of his set and perhaps

---

[173] WL, RAMC 262/8: collection of letters to and from Lindsay and his close friends, 1815–27. Webster was one of those from whom Lindsay borrowed money: see nos. 32, 32a, 33: Webster to Lindsay, 1 and 6 Mar. 1826; Lindsay to Webster, 2 Mar.

[174] Ibid., 262/8/3: Cross to Lindsay, 2 Apr. 1821, extolling his virtues as a doctor and asking him to send details of the medicines he gave Mrs Cross.

[175] Ibid., 262/8/4: Lindsay to Cross, 28 Aug. 1822. The letter expresses his condolences, if, as he fears, Ellen is dead.   [176] Gibney, 174.

even visit them to ensure their son was in good health, while, if based in London for any length of time, he would become the postbox through which mail to and from home would thereafter pass.[177] And a friend's assistance could be called upon when an officer got into a scrape. In early 1824, shortly before his promotion, Lindsay, back in the capital for the first time since 1817, received an urgent letter from Major Browne at Portsmouth with whom he had probably returned. Browne was being threatened with court-martial for having taken charge of the transport ship from a Lieutenant Hewitt during the voyage. His situation looked bleak because Sir Frederick Adam (the new Lord High Commissioner of the Ionian Islands) had informed Horse Guards that the 36th was lacking in discipline under Browne's temporary command. Lindsay was requested to approach McGrigor, who would have already received the surgeon's positive account of the state of the regiment, and ask the director-general to lobby on Browne's behalf. Lindsay was also to call at Horse Guards. 'You have such a manner with you and you would be so earnest and interested for me that you might avail on the Judge advocate general himself.'[178]

For junior army surgeons, in particular, especially those from relatively humble backgrounds, such friendships had a wider social utility. Their friendship circles introduced them into a far more elevated milieu and a much more English world than the one from which most had emerged. Browne's confidence in Assistant Surgeon Lindsay was not just flattering but a sign that the poverty-stricken son of a bonnet laird had socially arrived. Admittedly, surgeons were continually thrust into the affluent world of the urban and rural elite in the course of their army career, for wherever a regiment was temporarily stationed in the British Isles its officer corps was likely to be entertained by the local gentry or their urban counterparts and given balls in their honour. Gibney, for instance, remembered with affection the local Irish hospitality he had enjoyed while based in the barracks at Feathard and Cappoquin in 1814–15.[179] But such encounters were necessarily transitory and seldom led to any permanent connection with the local community. When the dashing Lesassier was stationed in Ireland six years before and tried to win the hand of an heiress of County Armagh, one Alicia Urwin, her father quickly stepped in to stop her contracting with a penniless surgeon.[180] Army friendships, in contrast, were more likely to reap social dividends.

Put simply, while cultivating the colonel might assist a surgeon up the army career ladder, it was forming lasting friendships with a wider group of officers which would ease his passage back to civilian life, especially if he were a relatively young officer placed on half-pay. A career in the army medical service provided a tyro surgeon with limited prospects the chance to enjoy a relatively high standard of living in an upper-class environment. The friendships he made in the officer mess could be his passport to a good marriage and a respectable practice once

---

[177] This seems to have been more reliable than passing them through the regiment's army agent.
[178] WL, RAMC 262/8/6: letter 11 Feb. 1824. Also later letters.
[179] Gibney, 133–41. Cappoquin's barracks were particularly appalling.   [180] Rosner, 60–8.

he came out. In the next two chapters, we explore how successfully army surgeons capitalized on these advantages. First, we reconstruct their later civilian career, where they had one, in order to discover if army service launched them into the ranks of the medical great and good. Second, we consider the social and economic position of their families when they died, to judge to what extent service in the army medical corps could be seen as a serious agent of social mobility.

5

Professional Life outside the Service

LEAVING THE ARMY

By the time of the battle of Leipzig in October 1813 the rank and file of the British army totalled over a quarter of a million men.[1] With the coming of peace in the following year the government was anxious to demobilize the armed services as rapidly as possible to save money. The majority of officers were put on half-pay.[2] As we saw in the previous chapter, medical officers were culled just as mercilessly as their combatant peers in the mess. Over the next few years two-thirds of the service would be placed on half-pay, many permanently.[3] As a result, young or old, the discharged medical officers had to settle back into civilian life, sometimes after twenty years or more following the colours. How they fared in Civvy Street is the subject of the present chapter.

Most of those discharged in the aftermath of the war had several years of retire-ment to look forward to (see Figure 5.1). Charles Brereton, who joined the army in 1813 and left in 1816, enjoyed half-pay for an astonishing fifty-six years while in practice in Beverley in Yorkshire. Out of the 315 who are known not to have died in service, twenty-five were on half-pay for over forty years. Strikingly eighteen of these had more than eleven years of service and in the case of John Grant, who was recalled briefly to the colours for the Waterloo campaign, twenty-three years. Such long retirements are partly explained by the unusual longevity of members of the cohort. Of the 204 who died in the United Kingdom, whose birth and death dates are recorded, eighty-eight lived to be over 70.[4] Thirty-seven died in their eighties and eight in their nineties. The longest lived was Francis Sievewright, who was born in Edinburgh in 1773, joined the army in 1813, retired as a staff surgeon in 1856, resided for a while in Dunoon in Argyllshire, and died in his native city in 1872 at the age of 99.

Some of the cohort, whenever they were released, were able to retire to a life of leisure. For whatever reason—age, amassed wealth, inheritance, connections—they

---

[1] J. E. Cookson, *The British Armed Nation 1793–1815*, (Oxford, 1997), 260, citing WO25/3225, which gives a total of 260,797 on 15 Oct. 1813.

[2] On leaving the army officers could either sell their commissions or more commonly go on half-pay. Registers of half-pay officers are to be found in TNA, WO23: see Simon Fowler, *Army Records for Family Historians*, Public Record Office Readers' Guide No. 2 (London, 1992), 15.

[3] See Ch. 4, pp. 194–7.   [4] The average age was 68.

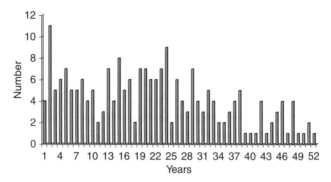

Figure 5.1. Length of Retirement

Note: This has been calculated from the last year placed on half-pay and does not include previous periods of half-pay.
Source: Doctors' Database, Tables: Doctors; Half-Pay.

enjoyed a large enough income to live as gentlemen. Henry Tytler, who prior to joining up in his mid-forties had gained a name as a translator of Latin and Greek, left the army at the age of 54 in 1806 and died in Edinburgh two years later, apparently no longer in practice.[5] Archibald Arnott from Dumfriesshire, who attended Napoleon on St Helena and retired as surgeon to the East Devonshire (20th) regiment in 1826, set himself up as a minor laird in the family home at Ecclefechan. When the *Medical Directory* was first published in 1845, he stressed his gentlemanly status by advertising the fact he had quit the profession.[6]

John Davy, the younger brother of Sir Humphry, had planned for his retirement for some time. In 1830 he married Margaret, the daughter of Archibald and Eliza Fletcher. Archibald was an Edinburgh advocate, friendly with prominent Whigs, such as the Broughams and Francis Jeffrey, and major literary figures, such as Dr Thomas Arnold and his wife and William Wordsworth and his sister. In 1843 John Davy and his wife decided to settle in the Lake District and built a house, Lesketh-how, near Ambleside in Westmorland.[7] In the following year he was posted to the West Indies and did not finally retire to the Lakes until 1848. Well before he decided to settle there, he had become medical adviser to Worsdworth and his family. Wordsworth's first surviving letter to him in the autumn of 1835 sought advice about the medical condition of both his daugher and his sister.[8] Although he continued to treat Wordsworth and his circle in retirement, he devoted most of his time during the last twenty years of his life to angling

---

    [5] See Ch. 7 for Tytler's literary activities.
    [6] *Medical Directory for Scotland* (London, 1845), 15.
    [7] www.spaceless.com/fletcher/flet11.htm (Oct. 2005); and Eliza Dawson Fletcher, Autobiography of Mrs. Fletcher of Edinburgh; With Letters and Other Family Memorials, ed. Lady Mary Fletcher Richardson (Carlisle, 1875), available at www.spaceless.com/fletcher/flet11.htm (Oct. 2005).
    [8] Alan G. Hill, *The Letters of William and Dorothy Wordsworth*, vi: *The Later Years: Part III, 1835–1839* (Oxford, 1967), 89.

and literary and scientific pursuits.[9] Already an established author and a fellow
of the Royal Society, he published a number of new works in the autumn of his
life including *Discourses on Agriculture, with Introductions on the Present State of
the West Indies, and on the Agricultural Societies of Barbados,* [10] *The Angler and his
Friend, or, Piscatory Colloquies and Fishing Excursions,*[11] and *On some of the More
Important Diseases of the Army, with Contributions to Pathology.*[12] Mrs Gaskell met
him in 1859 and described him as 'a gentleman of a stiff, precise, over-gentlemanly
manner', which she found rather frightening.[13]

Others retired to a more active civic life. William Byrtt, who was born and
died in Belfast, described himself, after leaving the army with twenty-three years
of service, as a 'gentleman' living at 40 Upper Queen Street in the Belfast directory
of 1843–4.[14] His father and grandfather and even his great-grandfather, who
seem to have been prosperous boot shoe makers in the city, had been 'connected
with the Corporation and Institution of Belfast', and Byrtt devoted his seven years
of retirement 'to the public good—the cause of the poor, the aged, the young, the
fatherless and the widow, was cherished by him'.[15] This catalogue suggests that he
drew on his medical knowledge in the conduct of his voluntary work. Some army
surgeons with the immediate means to retire, however, chose to hide their previous career when they were discharged. Richard Humfrey, who had been born in
Gosport, presumably to a family with naval connections, seems to have retired
in 1814 to a fashionable part of Bristol, where he lived until his death in 1843: in
1830 he simply listed himself in the local directory as a gentleman.[16]

A few of the cohort had been so badly wounded that they could never work
professionally again, or at least for any length of time. Peter Macarthur was retired
on full pay in 1816, 'being unfit for further service on account of a wound
received at the storming of Seringapatum, 1799'.[17] This did not prevent him from
emigrating to South Australia in 1834 to begin a new life as a pastoralist at
Arthurton in Victoria.[18] Edward Johnston was permanently disabled after volun-
teering in 1811 to carry dispatches from Tarifa to the 28th Regiment, then nearly
surrounded by the enemy at Medina Sidonia. He fell into the hands of guerrillas
and received thirty-two wounds—his skull was fractured and his left arm was left
semi-paralysed. He was placed on half-pay in 1816 and went to work as a physician
in Weymouth, but was forced to retire five years later.[19] It may have been through
the good offices of the king's son, the duke of Cambridge, to whom he was physician,
that he was granted an army pension. Michael Carmac, who was retired on full

---

[9] 'John Davy', *Proceedings of the Royal Society*, 16 (1867–8), lxxix–lxxxi. He did look after the
dying Wordsworth, who lived close by.   [10] (London, 1849).
[11] (London, 1855).   [12] (London, 1862).
[13] www.spaceless.com/fletcher/flet11.htm (Oct. 2005).
[14] *Belfast Directory* (1843–4), 279.   [15] *Belfast Newsletter*, 14 Oct. 1845.
[16] *White's Directory of Bristol*, 1830.   [17] TNA, WO25/3910, fo. 101.
[18] www.medicalpioneers.com/cgi-bin/index.cgi?detail=1&id=1559 (Sept. 2005).
[19] TNA, WO25/3910, fo. 80.

pay in 1807, and Andrew Ligertwood in 1816, seem to have been similarly disabled, while Andrew Broadfoot, who had had a distinguished army career, ended up deranged in the lunatic asylum at Chatham, and died aged 57 in 1837.

Many demobbed medical officers, on the other hand, would immediately have had to think about establishing themselves in civilian medical practice. In the absence of consistent series of local directories and of a medical directory until 1845 (by which time almost half the cohort was dead), it is impossible to say with certainty how many put up their plate. But it must be presumed most did unless they had other sources of income or career preferences. Half-pay, which for a full surgeon amounted to at least £120 a year, only provided a cushion for the provident against the exigencies of civilian life.[20] Although such pensions were larger than the stipends of many clergymen, the sum was not sufficient to maintain a family in real comfort. In consequence, even some of the cohort with long years of army service and senior positions sought to make civilian careers for themselves, such as Deputy Inspectors Charles Fergusson Forbes and Stewart Crawford who set up in London and Bath. McGrigor in 1814 would have been one of them, had he not been quickly offered the appointment of director-general, as he recalled in his memoirs:

I now began to look about me and to see what future prospects I had. Numbers of my friends, military, particularly, urged my entering on the practice of my profession as a physician in the metropolis. It then appeared I could do this with every prospect of success, known as I was to the whole body of officers who had then been in the Peninsula and through them to their relatives in London, many of them of the aristocracy, or most opulent individuals.[21]

Only a handful of the cohort, however, had forged such influential connections and could hope to put up their plate in London, at least initially. As we will see in the following sections, discharged medical officers spread themselves round the world in search of a comfortable civilian billet and could move several times in the course of their civilian career. Many, too, found establishing a successful practice, especially in the early years, difficult. Over the eight years 1816–23, 238 of the cohort were discharged either permanently or semi-permanently, suggesting altogether a total of about 700 army surgeons in search of employment.[22] At the same time 400 surgeons were retired from the navy.[23] The first reliable statistics for the number of physicians, surgeons, apothecaries, and medical students practising in Great Britain (excluding Ireland) were published in the analysis of the 1841 census, which recorded a total of 20,000. [24] If this was the approximate figure twenty years earlier, and it was in all probability lower, practitioners discharged

---

[20] See Table 1.4.   [21] McGrigor, 246.

[22] See Table 4.20. The cohort comprise every third surgeon in service in 1815: see Introd., In the years 1816–23 a total of 268 surgeons were released but this figure includes some thirty who were placed on half-pay, re-entered the army almost immediately, then were released again before the end of 1823. A few surgeons were placed on half-pay three times over the eight years, having re-entered on two occasions.   [23] TNA, ADM 105/1076.

[24] See Irvine Loudon, *Medical Care and the General Practitioner 1750–1850* (Oxford, 1986), table 19, 216.

from the army and navy would have represented an increase of some 5–6 per cent in the ranks of the civilian profession. This was a serious addition to the number of medical practitioners in a few years and can only have exacerbated the overcrowding of which many contemporaries complained.[25] The competition was guaranteed to be fierce.

In 1823 Thomas Speer, who was discharged himself on half-pay from the 5th Dragoons in 1817 and worked briefly at the Dublin Dispensary, prophesied a life of struggle for his erstwhile colleagues in the service now Europe was at peace:

These changes must mark a new era in our profession; the redundancy of practitioners is increased and increasing every day, whilst their necessity is diminishing every day. Whilst war raged, the stock though rapidly growing in one source, was rapidly diminishing in another, but now there scarcely seems any vent for the overstock which our laid-up fleets and armies have diffused over society…we see our medical men diffused over the Continent, practising in the cities and towns; and as to the numbers remaining at home, if each were to confine his attention and practice to one organ or one disease alone of the system, there would seem more than enough, according to the present rate and that which now appears established.[26]

Speer's analysis was greatly exaggerated, but did contain some grains of truth in that a sizeable number of discharged medical officers failed to make a go of civilian practice at first attempt. A number found their way back into the army when offered the chance. Over 40 per cent of those who left between 1816 and 1823 rejoined during those years, albeit sometimes only for a few years.[27] Thomas Montgomery Perrot, an assistant surgeon from Petworth in Sussex, was placed on half-pay in 1817 and settled in Stepney in London where he attended classes on surgery, chemistry, and midwifery, suggesting he was bent on a civilian career. His East End practice, however, cannot have been a great success for he accepted the summons to go back in again for a brief period the following year and again in 1819. Placed on half-pay for a third time in 1821, he returned into service once more in 1822, when he was appointed assistant surgeon to the 41st Regiment of Foot. He finally left the army in 1831 and settled in New South Wales, where he was a registered practitioner from 1839 to 1851.[28]

[25] The overcrowding of the profession is discussed ibid., ch. 10, 208–26.

[26] T. C. Speer, *Thoughts on the Present Character and Constitution of the Medical Profession by T. C. Speer, M. D., M. R. I. A. Late Physician to the Dublin General Dispensary &c.* (Cambridge, 1823), 39–40.

[27] One hundred and four of the 238 individuals placed on half-pay in these years returned to the colours. A small number of others would return at a later date. Thirty-six of the 104 would serve for less than five years and eleven for less than two. Twenty-five of the 104 would die in service, including a handful who had only been back in the army a few years. Over a quarter of the 104 returnees would remain in the service for at least ten years. These presumably formed a hard core of veterans of the French wars who decided from choice or circumstance to make the army their life. Among this group, James William Macaulay served for a further forty-one years: he was placed briefly on half-pay in 1816, returned the following year, then stayed in the army until 1858, when he retired on a handsome pension. His unusual career is discussed below, pp. 231–2.

[28] Information supplied by Stephen Due, editor of the Australian medical pioneers database, available at **www.medicalpioneers.com** (July 2005).

Alexander Lesassier, we have seen, was definitely forced back into the army through financial exigency in 1830. He had been trying desperately to be re-employed through-out the second half of the 1820s. His private life in turmoil and heavily in debt, he had no alternative but to return to the colours, describing it as his 'safest & most honourable asylum'.[29] So too was Andrew Anderson of Selkirk, son of a Lowlands surgeon and the brother-in-law of the late Mungo Park. Anderson joined the army as a hospital mate in 1805 and became surgeon of the 61st Foot in 1812. He was placed on half-pay on 25 December 1814 and returned home to the Scottish Borders, where he acquired a wife, Anne Cairns, daughter of a Peebles lawyer. On 1 January 1818, after three years on half-pay and presumably assisting in the family practice, he was placed on active service for a second time and transferred to the 92nd. After a short stay in Ireland, the regiment was posted to the West Indies, a tour of duty which Anderson would have given much to forgo. As his young wife made clear in a letter to Mungo Park's widow (her sister-in-law), her husband had no choice but to comply, since he could not afford to refuse. 'The doctor bids me tell you that he has no great relish for going to Jamaica. If he had £300, to build stable and barn at Shawwood [a small property in his possession near Selkirk], he would rather have gone on half-pay than gone out.'[30] Doubtless, there was not enough business in the Selkirk area for both himself and his younger brother, Thomas, who had taken over the family medical, practice in 1808. As it was, Anderson would remain in the army until 1833, only finally retiring at the age of 49 after completing twenty-four years in the service.[31]

Others too did not feel so comfortably off that they were ready to forgo their regular half-pay when the army became less accommodating in the late 1820s. William Milligan from County Cavan, who had for the previous seven years lec-tured to good audiences in Great Pultney Street in London on the theory and practice of medicine and materia medica, did not accept commutation but obeyed an order in 1829 to proceed to the penal colony in New South Wales with the West Suffolk regiment, where he seems to have hoped to settle. He founded a hospital that was later to become the Royal Perth, and had the distinction of having a street named after him. However, when his regiment was again posted to Madras in 1834, he went with them. After distinguished service there, he was invalided home and once again practised in Regent's Park until his death in 1846.[32]

For many surgeons, the decision to go back was lethal. Anderson survived, but his wife Anne died in the West Indies of yellow fever. James Rowland Morgan, who returned to the army in 1822, 'not expecting to be called again into active service',

[29] See Ch. 4. Rosner, 196.

[30] Sheila Scott, 'My Dear Cath…The Story of an Army Doctor's Wife' (1976): published transcription of Ann Cairn's letters home in WL, RAMC 1227.

[31] For Anderson's family: see Ch. 2, pp. 69, 88.

[32] John Brine, et al., *Looking for Milligan: The Fascinating Search for William Milligan a Pioneering Doctor of the Swan River Colony c.1795–1851* (Perth, 1991); www.medicalpioneers.com/cgi-bin/index.cgi?detail=1&id=3461 (Sept. 2005); and *Medical Directory* (1852), 641.

did his duty with disastrous consequences for himself and his family. He was posted to Columbo in Ceylon. On arrival 'by the upsetting of the Boat in which his family was going from the Ship towards the Shore, his Wife, youngest child, and Maidservant were drowned, and a great part of his Baggage was lost'. As a result he had to send his two other daughters home to be cared for by his elder brother, Rowland, at 'ruinous expense'. Within two years their father was dead, and Rowland petitioned the War Office for help.[33]

According to Lesassier, the quick-tempered John Hamilton, his uncle and professor of midwifery at Edinburgh, considered the discharged medical officer at fault if he failed to succeed in civilian practice. 'Medical gentlemen who had been in the army were totally uncalculated for private practice. Their manners he always thought far too unaccommodating & unpracticable for such a *difficult task*.' In addition, Lesassier noted, his uncle criticized them for drawing a salary whether they saw a patient or not.[34] In Lesassier's own case there may have been some truth in the gibe, for he admitted to being used to ordering patients about and found the patient-practitioner ethics of civilian practice uncongenial. 'It was a sorry fate to be forced to grovelling by suiting oneself to every one's caprice, in order to earn a petty livelihood.'[35]

His experience is echoed by that of Dr John Mackenzie of Kenellan near Dingwall, not one of the cohort, who equally found it impossible to transfer to civilian life, as he recalled in 1841. Mackenzie had joined the army in 1826 after studying in Edinburgh, London, and Paris, but his sojourn with the medical corps was soon curtailed by a change in his domestic circumstances.

I then married, and finding that a married man has no business in the army, I resolved to embark in private practice, expecting that, with the excellent opportunities of becoming acquainted with disease in every form which I had possessed in the army, and aided by numerous friends, I might rise easily in my profession. I settled in Edinburgh, and became a fellow of the College of Physicians.

However, Mackenzie found the transfer to civilian practice 'out of the frying pan into the fire'.[36] Instead, he turned to farming on the family's extensive estates in the north of Scotland, no doubt putting his scientific knowledge to good use.

In other instances, on the other hand, there is no reason to doubt an individual's commitment. It appears much more likely that initial failure in civilian life reflected inadequate forethought about where to put up one's plate. Andrew Anderson's decision to go home after nine years in the service is perfectly understandable, especially if he already had an eye on marrying a local girl. He ought, though, to have thought through the limited possibility of establishing himself successfully in a predominantly rural area.

[33] TNA, WO25/797, no fo.: return of service, 61–6 Foot, 1829. Information supplied by Morgan's brother. For the high death rate among returnees, see above pp. 196–7.   [34] Rosner, 130.
[35] Ibid.
[36] Quoted in Samuel Dickson, *The Principles of the Chrono-Thermal System of Medicine, with the Fallacies of the Faculty* (London, 1845), 184. Drew, no. 4141: Mackenzie's short army career.

Many, probably most, ex-medical officers, however, did not find it so difficult to make a success of civilian practice. The medical profession in the years following the end of the war may have been overstocked and highly competitive, but army surgeons were often well placed to come out on top. Besides their contacts and experience, which set them apart from their civilian peers, they were also, as a group, peculiarly well-qualified, as a reviewer in the *Edinburgh Medical Journal* acknowledged in 1816. 'Our brave troops had the advantage of being succoured by surgeons of first-rate talents and acquirements.'[37] At the time of their discharge, 70 of the 238 who went on half-pay in the years 1816–23, nearly a third, held MDs, whereas in a survey of 2,000 general practitioners in 1847 by Loudon only 13.5 per cent held such a qualification.[38] Moreover, a further 11 per cent of the army cohort took their MDs within four years of leaving the service.

Admittedly, not everyone agreed that this was a sensible investment. The former director-general of the medical service, John Weir, told Thomas Rolston, who had lost a leg at Tarragona in 1813, 'not to spend so much money in so unnecessary a manner'.[39] Yet, that said, there can be no doubt that an MD was perceived as giving the practitioner an edge in the medical marketplace. Thomas Speer believed that the degree was becoming highly sought after in the post-war era, thus eroding, as he pointed out, the old distinction between physicians and surgeons:

It is the appendage of M.D. that has become the character and decoration of the day, and that has made such extraordinary changes with us; it seems to hang as fluently on our names as crosses on French button-holes. Indeed, it is in the nominal physicians that the great redundancy of the profession now becomes manifest and it is the appendage which seems to have chiefly levelled its distinctions and barriers. Previous to this passion for letters, the line separating each branch had at least something clear and definite about it, although even then too much weakened; divisions of the profession then seemed to belong to the divisions of the human body ... Now however matters seem altered, there seems a general mixture, and M. D. seem to be the cabalistic letters that have charmed and united all parties together both in town and country; all branches of the profession are beginning to feel the influence of these magical letters; dentists are beginning to be bitten and we may naturally expect that chiropodists and bone-setters will soon follow.[40]

Speer, the pessimist, evidently thought there were now so many MDs in the country that the qualification had become devalued. But he clearly, as in his analysis of his army colleagues' prospects, was being unnecessarily alarmist. Army surgeons were ahead of the game. Moreover fifty-one of the 238 either were already or were to become licentiates, members, or fellows of one of the London, Irish, or Scottish colleges of physicians and surgeons, giving them direct access to the senior echelons of the profession in those countries and the accompanying patronage. These included John Robert Hume, a Fellow of the Royal Colleges of Physicians of

---

[37] *EMJ*, 16 (1816), 220–1.   [38] Loudon, *Medical Care*, 220.
[39] TNA, WO25/3904, fo. 144.   [40] Speer, *Thoughts on the Medical Profession*, 95.

Table 5.1. Place of Death of Those who had left the Service

Place of death	Born in England	Born in Ireland	Born in Scotland	Born in Wales	Born abroad	Unknown	All deaths	MDs
Africa	1	1	0	0	0	0	2	0
Australasia	0	1	1	1	0	0	3	0
Canada	2	0	3	0	0	0	5	3
Channel Island	3	1	3	0	0	0	7	4
England	61	18	20	1	3	6	109	60
Europe	3	6	2	0	1	2	14	7
India	0	1	1	0	0	0	2	0
Ireland	3	35	0	0	0	2	40	22
Isle of Man	0	2	0	0	0	0	2	2
Scotland	5	1	39	0	2	0	47	19
St Helena	0	1	0	0	0	0	1	0
At sea	0	1	1	0	1	0	3	0
Unknown	13	17	18	0	2	4	54	18
Wales	0	1	0	3	0	0	4	0
Total	91	86	88	4	9	14	293	138

Source: Doctors' Database: Table: Doctors 1.

Edinburgh and London, John Howell, a Fellow of the Royal College of Surgeons of London, Robert Shekelton, Fellow of the Royal College of Surgeons in Dublin, and Alexander Dunlop Anderson, a Fellow of the Faculty of Physicians and Surgeons of Glasgow.[41] In fact, as a group these experienced well-qualified army doctors, who were on the whole young and with their half-pay cushioned to an important extent against the vagaries of the market, must have represented a serious challenge to the cosy world of medical practice with its tight network of patronage and family connections. The threat they posed was magnified by their own close connections with the duke of Wellington and his senior officers, the heroes of the age.

In consequence, as we will see, a significant proportion of the cohort who went into private practice ended up as pillars of their local medical community.[42] Typical was John Howell, who was in the army for seventeen years and became one of the leading practitioners in Bristol in the thirty years after 1818. Some ultimately made enough money to retire and establish themselves as local worthies. The Yorkshire clergyman's son, Charles Boutflower, who described himself as a gentleman in the 1841 Liverpool directory, had previously been in practice in the 1820s in Colchester, a garrison town. In Liverpool he served as a town councillor and drainage commissioner and contracted typhoid in pursuit of his civic duties.[43]

[41] Although called a faculty, it had the same status as the royal colleges in licensing medical practitioners.   [42] See pp. 253–4.

[43] John B. Penfold, 'Charles Boutflower, FRCS: Surgeon in Wellington's Army and Hon. Surgeon to the Essex and Colchester Hospital', *History of Medicine*, 7/1 and 2 (1975).

Likewise Charles Waite who listed himself as an MD amongst the gentry in Woodford in Essex in 1832, had previously practised in Dublin.[44]

In the following sections, we look more closely at the fate of our cohort in civilian life. Altogether 293 of the cohort may be presumed to have died after they had left the service, and of these the place of birth is either recorded or can be assumed with certainty from other evidence of 279 (see Table 5.1). Of the 86 born in Ireland, the country of death of 17 is not known and 35 are known to have died there; of the 88 born in Scotland, the country of death of 18 is not known and 39 are known to have died there, and of the 91 born in England the country of death of 13 is not known and 61 are known to have died there. [45]

LIVING AND WORKING ABROAD

Speer was correct in claiming that a number of his contemporaries had decided to make their careers on the continent in preference to other parts of the world. At the time he was writing nine of the cohort on half-pay were in practice in France, one in Paris, and five in resorts popular with British gentry, Abbeville, Boulogne, Caen, and Saint-Servan (near Saint-Malo). Four also found their way to Italy, three residing in Florence, which was another favourite destination for British travellers. Of the fourteen who died in Europe, eight died in France, three in Italy, one in Gibraltar, one in Malta, and one in Belgium. Two of those who died in Europe would seem to have been born there. Romaine Amiel died in Gibraltar but came from Reiz near Toulon in France. He had trained at Montpelier and had been retired for fifteen years after thirty-eight years in the army when he died. Although the origin and precise place of death of Pasquale Bocca is unknown except that he died in Europe, he was educated at Palermo in Sicily. Two of the three, who died in Italy, had Italian wives. Their places of birth go unrecorded, though they both had British names. John Williams was married to Paola Nunciata Maria Roni and Edward Porteus to Domenica Schivoni. Six out of the fourteen who died in Europe came from Ireland, including Eugene McSwyny of Cork, who was buried in Paris in 1840, but little can be read into such small numbers. Some of those who died on the continent had either retired there or were on holiday. John Howell, who expired in Italy, had previously been in practice in Bristol and had presumably gone there for the sake of his health, while William Morrison, who died in Malta, was at the time of his death surgeon to the Perthshire volunteers. Sir James Brown Gibson, who died in Rome in 1868 and came from County Londonderry, was an honorary physician to the queen and body surgeon to the duke of Cambridge, commander-in-chief of Her Majesty's armies.

[44] *Piggot's Commercial Directory*, 1832–4.
[45] Since 93 of the cohort died in service (see Table 4.19), this leaves 68 of the 454 surgeons whose date of death or precise status (military or civilian) at the moment they died has not been determined.

It has not been possible to discover a great deal about the practices of those in Europe, but their place of residence suggests that they cared largely for the ex-patriot British community. A few held official posts. Thomas Walker was physician to the British Embassy in Russia, while Adam Neale, who died in France in 1832, had been medical officer to the British Embassy in Constantinople and was physician extraordinary to the duke of York. Edward Walsh from County Waterford was president of the medical board in Ostend, and James Dillon Tully from County Galway was president of the board of health and inspector of quarantine in the Ionian Islands before going back to the service as a deputy inspector in the West Indies, where he eventually died. These appear to have been British government appointments under the Privy Council Medical Department for which no doubt army medical officers were well qualified.[46]

It is striking, given the perception of the fortunes to be made in India, how relatively few chose to join the ranks of the East India Company as an alternative to remaining in the United Kingdom. Just two of those who had retired are recorded as dying there, far fewer than in Europe; probably the climate and the known risk to the health of medical officers was a deterrent. It is possible more of the cohort worked in India, but few others are listed as being resident there after they left the army, possibly because service with the East India Company disqualified them from half-pay.[47] Two died in Africa in the hospitable climate of the Cape. William Parrot, who had been serving in South Africa when he was discharged in 1841, was still living at Fort Beaufort when he died nine years later. On the other hand, Henry Collis Carter, who died at the Cape in 1848, had been retired for thirty years in Carlow in Ireland and appears to have emigrated. At least one other doctor retired to Africa, probably to take up a government appointment. This was Andrew Foulis, who went to the Gambia in the 1850s, but his place of death is unrecorded.

Although none of the cohort not on active service died in South America, one surgeon spent considerable time there. Robert Dundas in 1817 was appointed physician superintendent of the British hospital at Bahia in Brazil where he worked for twenty-three years. For the first thirteen he was on half-pay but in 1830 he was granted a pension. In final retirement in Liverpool he recalled the horror of practising in the country, no doubt echoing the experience of medical men in other tropical climates. He graphically described his visits to the aptly named Mizericordia hospital of the Escola de Medicina da Bahia:

My heart sank within me as I daily approached the gates of the hospital; and, even now, I can scarcely repress a shudder, as I recall to remembrance the human misery. Happily, my professional brethren in England are beyond the reach of scenes like these.[48]

[46] The records of the department do not survive but details of its activities can be gleaned from annual reports presented to Parliament, *Nineteenth Century Public Health and Epidemics: Some PRO Sources—Domestic Records Information 73*, available at **http://catalogue.pro.gov.uk/**.

[47] One who did spend time in India was William Dunlop: see below, n. 51.

[48] Robert Dundas, *Sketches of Brazil: Including New Views on Tropical and European Fever, with Remarks on a Premature Decay of the System Incident to Europeans on their Return from Hot Climates* (London, 1852), 395.

It was almost certainly such experiences that led only one of the cohort to retire in the West Indies, even though several had seen service there and practised amongst the civilian ex-patriot community. Joseph Gogill Leath from Norfolk was the exception. His final period of service abroad had been in Jamaica and Honduras from 1827 to 1830. On retirement, he then went back to Honduras as principal medical officer in the mid-1830s, but died in London in 1859. The Irishman Daniel Hagartye equally must have liked his last appointment. He had a most varied army career including a tour of duty in Ceylon, but was posted to St Helena in 1821 and remained there after he left the army later that year until his death in 1825.

Although there were obvious attractions in making a new life in Canada and Australia in the decades after Waterloo, not least in land grants for long-serving officers, it is difficult to be certain how many army surgeons chose to take advant-age of these opportunities.[49] Six retired medical officers in the cohort died in Canada and three in Australia, but at least ten had a civilian practice 'down under', albeit only a for a few years.[50] William 'Tiger' Dunlop was the most remarkable member of the cohort to die in Canada. After he returned to civilian life, he travelled round the world and tried his hand at journalism in London before being appointed the Canada Company's warden of woods and forests by John Galt, the novelist, who like Dunlop came from Greenock. Dunlop wrote enthusiastically about the country, doing much to promote Upper Canada as an emigrant destina-tion. After he left the Canada Company following a dispute over supplies to his 'Bloody Useless' militia unit, he entered the Canadian parliament where he was better known for his wit than his sagacity.[51] Among the Australian immigrants the most interesting was the Dubliner, John Arthur, who was posted to the colony in 1835. While still in the army, he became physician to the asylum at New Norfolk, Tasmania, and then on his retirement in 1839, the government's colonial surgeon on the island. He appears, though, to have become involved in a professional quarrel and was unable to settle in Australia permanently. Within a few years, he was forced to leave for Britain and died in London in 1853.[52]

The relative lack of attraction of making a career overseas was probably a reflec-tion of the confidence of most army surgeons that their qualifications, experience, and connections would give them an entrée to civilian positions in the United Kingdom. The common perception was that most medical students on complet-ing their training returned home to put up their plate. In his evidence to the select committee on medical education in 1834, George James Guthrie, who had risen to the rank of deputy general inspector of hospitals, claimed 'A Gentleman, after

[49] It seems likely that medical and regular officers in the army and navy could exchange their rights to half-pay and a pension for a grant of land.

[50] www.medicalpioneers.com/cgi-bin/index.cgi?detail=1&id=3461 (Sept. 2005).

[51] *Canadian Dictionary of National Biography*, vii. 261–3. Dunlop had gone to India immediately on retiring in 1817. He was called 'Tiger' because of his attempt to exterminate tigers from the Ganges island of Sagar.

[52] www.medicalpioneers.com/cgi-bin/index.cgi?detail=1&id=3461 (Sept. 2005).

having been educated . . . goes back to establish himself . . . in his native town.'[53]
Not surprisingly, given the place of birth of many of the cohort, only a handful of
army surgeons took this path on being stood down. There had been few attractions in returning to rural Scotland or Ireland, or even England, when they had
finished their initial training, where they would have had to compete with established practitioners. There was even less once they were established medical men
with qualifications and connections.

RETURNING TO IRELAND

Only 41 of the 142 members of the cohort who can be identified as being born
in Ireland are known to have died in their country of birth, and of these 35 had
definitely left the service, of whom 15 died in the same county in which they were
born (See Table 5.2). There were almost certainly more as the place of death is
unknown of 17 of the 86 members of the cohort who were born in Ireland and
died no longer on active service. Moreover, the destruction of testamentary
records in Ireland in 1922 makes it difficult to trace place of death unless recorded
in the half-pay or pension records.[54]

One of the obstacles to returning to rural Ireland was the restriction of the
Dublin Corporation of Apothecaries, which used its charter to limit the 'practice
of pharmacy strictly to its own members'. As an editorial in the *Edinburgh
Medical Journal* commented in 1818, 'it has at this moment a most injurious
operation in preventing the many excellent practitioners who have been released
from the service of the army and navy from settling in the country parts of Ireland,
where there is a grievous want of good general practitioners, and where these
valuable men would be of the highest benefit to the country'.[55] David Linn, who
unusually was a member of the corporation, was able to practise as both a surgeon
and an apothecary in Larne after he left the army, while Thomas Atkinson got
round the charter by going into partnership with his brother, an apothecary, in his
home town of Ballina in County Mayo.[56] Other returnees presumably advertised
their services as simple surgeons and/or physicians, if they had degrees. For those
who chose to settle in rural towns, there was a decided preference for county or
diocesan towns of the Church of Ireland, such as Armagh, Clogher, Monaghan,
and Tuam, where they could ply their trade amongst the Protestant clergy and
members of the ascendancy. The Edinburgh MD, Thomas Dillon, who seems to
have come from a gentry family, went home to Galway where he cut quite a figure
in the county, serving as a magistrate, surgeon to the Galway infirmary and the
dispensaries at Westport, County Mayo, and Tuam in County Galway, physician

[53] *Report from the Select Committee on Medical Education*, 1834, part II, Q. 4902, quoted in
Loudon, *Medical Care.*, 44. Cf. what was said above, pp. 95–6.
[54] John Grenham, *Tracing your Irish Ancestors*, (Dublin, 1992), 48.
[55] *EMJ*, 14 (1818), 19.   [56] *Piggot's Directory of Ireland*, 1824.

Table 5.2. County of Death in Ireland of Those
who had left the Service

County	Number	Born in Ireland
County Antrim	3	3
County Armagh	1	1
County Cork	1	1
County Donegal	2	2
County Down	1	1
County Dublin	13	10
County Galway	3	3
County Limerick	1	0
County Londonderry	3	3
County Mayo	1	1
County Monaghan	2	2
County Sligo	1	1
County Tipperary	1	1
County Tyrone	1	1
County Wexford	3	2
County Wicklow	3	3
	40	35

Source: Doctors' Database: Table: Doctors.

to the county gaol, and the local medical referee for the Britannia and Minerva Assurance Companies.[57]

It is perhaps not coincidental that some of those who died in rural Ireland had property, even though owning land during this troubled period could be as much a liability as an asset. Charles Farrell was born in County Longford and retired as inspector-general of hospitals in 1833 to a family property Dalyston at Loughrea, in County Galway. He was a wealthy man, reputedly having made a fortune while serving in Ceylon between 1815 and 1826, probably through dealing in opium.[58] Shortly after settling in Galway he paid the Encumbered Estates Commissioners £14,800 for an additional 1,040 acres for his estate.[59] It was property which took John Frederick Clarke, who was born in Dublin and equally rose to the rank of inspector-general of hospitals, to Mount Kennedy in County Wicklow, when he left the army in 1846. He died within a year.[60] Gideon Gorrequer Dolmage almost certainly went back to Tipperary because his brother Julius owned estates there.[61] Gabriel Rice Redmond tried his luck in Caen and then in County Wicklow, before inheriting an estate in Wexford from an uncle he claimed to be

[57] *Medical Directory* (1853), 830.

[58] Dietmar Rothermund, *An Economic History of India from Pre-Colonial Times to 1991* (London, 1993), 26.

[59] Entry in *Burke's Landed Gentry of Ireland* (London, 1912), 453, and Pádraig Glave, 'The Encumbered Estates Court and Galway Land', in Gerard Moran (ed.), *Galway History and Society: Interdisciplinary Essays on the History of an Irish County* (Dublin, 1996), 410.

[60] TNA, Prob 11/2086.   [61] Entry in *Burke's Landed Gentry of Ireland*, 144.

his father.[62] Others also clearly had property, such as Martin Cathcart, who died at Gartnannovagh House in County Londonderry, Denis Murray who died at Enniscorthy Lodge County Wexford, or John Dick, who died at Bellefield, County Wicklow, and was a JP.

Atkinson and Dillon were elected fellows of the Royal College of Surgeons in Dublin late in their careers in 1844 and 1845, while Farrell and Murray became Fellows of the London Royal College of Surgeons in 1843 and 1844. It is a matter of conjecture as to why four doctors working or just residing in the west of Ireland should have wanted such recognition.

The disadvantages of practising in rural Ireland are, perhaps, best confirmed by the fact that thirteen of the forty who settled in Ireland after they left the army died in Dublin. Five of these came from the city. Although Dublin, by far the largest city in Ireland, had ceased to be a political capital after the union of 1801, it remained an important cultural, administrative, economic, and social centre. The viceroy kept court at Dublin castle, Trinity College Dublin continued to have a vibrant medical school, and many Protestant landed families, whose sons had served in the war, still maintained town houses, providing ample opportunity for civilian practice.

Robert Shekelton, who died there in 1867, came from Dundalk in County Louth, and lived at 59 Upper Leeson Street, the same street as his fellow army surgeon James William Macauley at No. 58. These were fashionable residences and reflected their success in Dublin medical circles. Shekelton was well connected with one brother already in practice in the city.[63] Robert became a fellow of the Royal College of Surgeons in Dublin in 1816, the year he left the army. He quickly established himself as an obstetrician. He was appointed assistant master of the Rotunda Lying-in Hospital in Rutland Square in 1817 and became master thirty years later. He was among the first vice-presidents of the Dublin Obstetrical Society, which was established in 1838, and lecturer in midwifery and the diseases of women and children at Trinity College, and was the first in Ireland to use chloroform in deliveries.

Macauley, a native of Dublin, whose brother-in-law William McAuley was a leading apothecary in the city, was on leaving active service appointed assistant surgeon to the Royal Military School for Soldiers' Children in Phoenix Park and to the Royal Hibernian School, making him technically still a full pay officer.[64] In 1829 he became physician to Kilmainham gaol and the following year assistant surgeon and apothecary to the neighbouring Royal Kilmainham Hospital, which

[62] See p. 91.

[63] The younger brother John was appointed curator of the Royal College of Surgeons in 1820, where he was responsible for anatomical demonstrations. He was considered to be one of the most promising surgeons in Dublin, but died prematurely of septicaemia in 1824. Eoin O'Brien, Anne Crookshank, and Gordon Wolstenholme, *A Portrait of Irish Medicine: An Illustrated History of Medicine in Ireland* (Dublin, 1984), 105, and J. D. H. Widdess, *The Royal College of Surgeons in Ireland and its Medical School 1784–1984*, 3rd edn. (Dublin, 1984), 68–9.

[64] Kirkpatrick archive, Royal College of Surgeons, Dublin.

had been established by the duke of Ormond in 1680 as Ireland's equivalent of Chelsea Hospital. He was appointed surgeon and physician to the hospital in 1853. Despite the prestige of these positions, he was never elected to the Dublin colleges possibly because of his Catholic connections, having to make do with a membership of the London Royal College of Surgeons in 1828.[65]

Oliver Dease, who had been apprenticed to Charles Hawkes Todd, a distinguished Dublin surgeon, retired in 1816 to become surgeon to the Dublin Westmoreland Lock hospital, presumably with the aid of his Dease relatives.[66] His career was cut short by his early death just five years later. Nothing is known of the civilian careers of the other three army doctors, who were born and died in Dublin, and only about one other of the further five, who died there and were born elsewhere in Ireland. Edward Walsh, who was born in County Wexford, retired to fashionable Glasniven in Dublin from his position as president of the medical board at Ostend. There he devoted himself to his literary pursuits, which are discussed in a later chapter.[67]

Of the forty members of the cohort who died in Ireland after they had left the service, up to five may not have been born there. Three definitely came from England but the place of birth of the other two cannot be traced. At least one, judging by his name, John Bickerson Flanagan, who was born in Stoke Damarel in Devon, was of Irish origin. Flanagan had only just left the army when he died at Dublin in 1845. His motivation for settling in Ireland was probably because he had served there, and two of his children had been born in the country. Although a few of the thirty-five Irishmen married locally in the county they came from, such as Michael Devitt in County Sligo, in only one or two cases was marriage a deciding factor in choice of residence. Robert Constable went to live at his wife's family property Prior Park near Clonmel in Tipperary when he left the army in 1805, and Robert Dudgeon from Dublin settled in his wife's home town of Warrenpoint when he finally retired in 1825.

GOING HOME TO SCOTLAND

A slightly higher proportion of Scots than Irish who had left the service died in their native land: 39 out of 88 (some 44 against 40 per cent) (See Table 5.3). However, a much higher proportion (21 of the total) died in their county of birth than in Ireland. At least 4 of the 39 had practised elsewhere before going home, including Henry Muir, who had been inspector of health in the Ionian Islands and Cephalonia before retiring to his native Strathaven in Lanarkshire, William Forrester Bow from Edinburgh who initially practised at Alnwick, and John Easton who had first set up his plate at Bootham in Yorkshire.

---

[65] For his background, see Ch. 2 under 'Religion'.   [66] See p. 54, n. 122.   [67] See Ch. 7.

Table 5.3. County of Death in Scotland of Those who had left the Service

County	Number	Born in Scotland
Aberdeenshire	3	3
Angusshire	1	0
Ayrshire	3	3
Banff	2	2
Dumfriesshire	2	1
East Lothian	1	1
Fife	2	2
Kirkcudbrightshire	1	1
Lanarkshire	5	5
Midlothian	16	13
Morayshire	2	1
Perthshire	3	3
Roxburghshire	1	1
Stirlingshire	2	1
Sutherlandshire	1	0
West Lothian	1	1
Wigtownshire	1	1
Total	47	39

Source: Doctors' Database: Table: Doctors.

The attraction of returning to the family hearth was frequently linked to property and family connection in the medical establishment. Alexander Dunlop Anderson, who came from an established medical dynasty in Glasgow, set up in practice there when he left the army in 1820. Although his father was a Greenock merchant, his uncle, Alexander Anderson, had been one of the original managers of the Glasgow Royal Infirmary and held the prestigious position of dean of the faculties at the University of Glasgow from 1778–1780. He died in 1815. A cousin William Dunlop, who died in 1811, had, also, been a lecturer in clinical surgery in Glasgow Royal Infirmary.[68] No doubt it was family influence that gained him an appointment as a surgeon to the infirmary in 1823. He confirmed his position in local society by marrying in 1829 Sarah, the daughter of Thomas McCall, a wealthy merchant from Blantyre. He became physician to the infirmary in 1838.[69] William Richardson Gibb, whose father Gavin was professor of oriental languages at Glasgow University, similarly settled in Glasgow when he left the army in 1819. Like Anderson, he made an advantageous marriage into the mercantile community and became surgeon to the Royal Infirmary in 1821.[70]

Medical connections and filial loyalty took several back home to other parts of Scotland. Andrew Ligertwood returned to practice with his father John, who was

[68] W. Innes Addison, *The Matriculation Albums of the University of Glasgow from 1728 to 1858* (Glasgow, 1913), entries 1527 and 4948. [69] Ibid., entry 7471.
[70] Ibid., entries 3692 and 6155.

a physician and surgeon at Foveran in Aberdeenshire. Shortly after his return from North America in 1816 John Douglas joined his father Robert and his elder brother, another Robert, in practice in Hawick, a fast-expanding Borders mill town. His brother Robert had also been an army surgeon, serving throughout the Peninsular war, but not part of the cohort. John Douglas became a respected member of the local community and after the death of his father and brother 'The Doctor' in the town. Under the terms of the Cotton Mills Act of 1819, which prohibited the employment of children under the age of 9, he examined the 'piecer children'.

When a little one came in he would say: 'What is your name, and where do you live?' 'Please sir, I am Annie Morrison and we live in Needle Street,' might be the reply. 'Oh, aye, I ken your mother,' the Doctor would say. 'And what age are you,' was the next question. 'Twelve past in March, sir.' 'Aye, did your mother tell you to say that?' 'Yes, sir.' Soliloquising, he would say, half aloud: 'Yes, yes, a little kind; that will do, my dear: you can go,' and the child was passed, much to its relief.

During an outbreak of cholera in 1849 he worked tirelessly, and when he died in 1861 an impressive memorial was erected to him by townspeople in the Wellgate cemetery.[71]

The other motive for setting up in practice near home in Scotland was family reputation in the community. John Grant, whose father had been factor on the duke of Gordon's massive Strathspey estate in north-east Scotland, set up his plate in Forres after Waterloo. No doubt taking advantage of his father's position, he became a leading figure in the community, serving as dean of guild in 1824 and provost in 1830 and founding the medical hall and library.[72] John Riach went back to Perth where his father had been a teacher in the influential Perth academy, one of the leading schools in provincial Scotland. After rejoining the colours in 1813 after six years on half-pay and again in 1826 after another five years of half-pay, suggesting he failed to establish himself in civilian practice, he finally retired to his home town in 1841. An added attraction might have been that his brother William, a major in the 79th Regiment—the Cameron Highlanders—had also retired there. When John died in 1864 the *Perth Courant* made no reference to his medical career and simply commented: 'Thus another of the now few remaining "Waterloo men" has passed away. He was a good though humble soldier of Christ.'[73] John Poyntz Munro almost certainly set up his plate in Inverness because he had family connections there. Similarly his namesake William Munro (not in the cohort), who retired as an inspector-general of hospitals, settled at Bellgrove, a small estate near Campbeltown because his son was in practice as a lawyer there. He became so respected in the community that when he died the whole town went into mourning.[74]

[71] Charles John Wilson, 'Hawick and its People', *Transactions of the Hawick Archaeological Society* (Hawick, 1902), 28.

[72] Robert Douglas with Sir James Robert Brown and Dr Muir, *The Annals of Forres* (Forres, 1934), 212.   [73] *Perth Courant* (17 May 1864), 3, col. 2.

[74] TNA, Prob 11/2085, and NAS, SC51/32/11.

Property appears to have been a deciding factor in persuading at least ten of the cohort to return to their homeland. Alexander Browne had been born in 1798 at Langlands, a substantial farm at Twynholm, north of Kirkcudbright, which the family owned. His father died in 1812 and his only brother in 1824, leaving his widowed mother and two sisters living at the farm. His mother died in 1836, but it was not until 1850 that Alexander retired from the Royal Hampshire Regiment after twenty-five years' service to join them. A classical scholar, he devoted the remaining twenty years of his life to antiquarian pursuits. He became a close friend of Dr John Carlyle, the historian's brother, who retired from London to Dumfries. Carlyle described him as 'one of the best men I ever knew'.[75] Archibald Arnott after he came out of the army in 1826 purchased the interests of his surviving brother and sisters in the family home of Kirkconnel Hall, near Sanqhuar in Dumfriesshire. He rebuilt the house and lived there with his elder sister and his brother John and his wife and children. Unmarried, he died in 1855.[76] Alexander Thomson, whose father had been a factor in Wigtownshire and had purchased the Torhousemuir estate in 1799, retired on half-pay in 1810.[77] He practised at first in London and then, possibly because he was unwell, went to live with his brother on his substantial property at Machremore Castle outside Newton Stewart in Kirkcudbrightshire. Richard William Batty, who came from Kirk Andrews upon Esk in Cumberland, made preparations for his retirement well in advance. On his return from the West Indies in 1802 he purchased the modest estate of Broats, just across the border on the road from Kirkpatrick Fleming to Annan in Dumfriesshire.[78] He eventually took up permanent residence there when he finally left the army in 1806. Although John Easton died in Edinburgh after practising in civilian life in England, he presumably had retired in the interim to the estate he owned at Constance Hill in Dumfriesshire which produced an annual income of over £200.[79]

John Robb, who was an inspector-general of hospitals, retired from the army following the death in 1821 of an elder brother William, who left the whole of his substantial fortune to him. As the youngest brother, his inheritance was fortuitous, a result of the financial embarrassment of another brother, Charles. He not only inherited Blackburn, his brother's estate in the Carrick Hills to the south of Ayr, but also a partnership in the Ayrshire Banking Company.[80] Rich and prosperous, he married Jessie (Janet) Campbell, the daughter of Richard Campbell of Craigie, a large nabob estate near Ayr. In 1814 William Paton of Castlebeg retired to his family seat at Durham House in Torryglen in Fife to live the life of a gentleman near his wealthy bachelor brothers James and Alexander,

[75] Alison Mitchell (ed.), *Pre-1855 Gravestone Inscriptions and Index for the Stewarty of Kirkcudbright*, vol. v (1996), no. 25a, p. 175, and P. H. MacKerlie, *History of the Lands and Their Owners in Galloway with Historical Sketches of the District*, vol. v (Edinburgh, 1879), 275–7.

[76] James Arnott, *The House of Arnott* (Edinburgh, 1918), 120–1.

[77] MacKerlie, *Lands and their Owners in Galloway*, vol. ii (Edinburgh, 1877), 334.

[78] NAS, Dumfriesshire sasines, 1781–1820, no. 1929, 14 July 1802.

[79] NAS, SC70/1/141, fo. 724.   [80] NAS, RD5/205, 118–25.

both of whom had been surgeons in the East India Company. When James died in 1834 William inherited his property at Middleton of Pitgobar in Muckhart along with over £2,000.[81]

When Alexander George Home joined the army in 1826 (one of the small number of surgeons in the cohort who did not serve during the French wars)[82] he was ostensibly already a rich man, having come of age and inherited Whitefield, the family estate near Edinburgh, and the residue of the Manderston estate near Berwickshire.[83] His forebear George Home had been a Jacobite and his Whitefield estate in Berwickshire had been forfeited after the 1745 rebellion. However, through his wife, George inherited Manderston from Alexander Cairncross, bishop of Raphoe. George was succeeded by his brother Alexander, who married a fortune and purchased property between Edinburgh and Leith that he renamed Whitefield to keep the title in the family. But Alexander was extravagant and much of the Manderston property was sold before the birth of his grandson, our Alexander George, was born in Demerara in 1805. Alexander George's father, Alexander's son, was a naval officer, variously described as a lieutenant and a captain. He was member of the colony's governing council, but died within a year of his son's birth, and his mother brought him up. It is difficult to know what Alexander George's motives were in joining the army. When he retired after a long career in 1852, he lived at Whitefield, and played a part in the civic life of Edinburgh.[84]

Others inherited more modest fortunes. George Brown, who finally retired as surgeon major of the Grenadier Guards in 1858, returned to live in Aberdeen where his father had left him property.[85] Francis Sievewright returned to Edinburgh as he and his brother had property in the city that they had inherited as children from their father David, a successful London merchant.[86] Alexander Cuningham inherited Canonmills house in Edinburgh and retired there in 1834.[87]

In at least three instances marriage was the deciding factor that brought the eight members of the cohort born elsewhere to Scotland. Alexander Melville, who had been born in St Vincent's and had started his civilian career in London, retired to Montrose, his wife's hometown, suffering from a disease of the spine. He died in 1855 in the aftermath of learning he had lost everything in the Panamanian bubble.[88] Marriage to Elizabeth Gibb took William Galliers, who came from Shropshire, to Stirling where he was in practice from the time he was discharged in 1816 until his death in 1861.[89] George Adams from Dublin almost certainly settled in Forres because he had married Jane Roy from Ardersier in Inverness-shire

[81] NAS, Fife sasines 1836, no. 2589, and 1843, no. 1203, and SC20/50/9, 660.
[82] See p. 18.
[83] NAS, Berwickshire sasines 1823, no. 441, and Edinburgh sasines 1823, no. 3533.
[84] *Burke's Landed Gentry* (London, 1871), see under Hume of Ninewells.
[85] NAS, Aberdeenshire sasines 1859, no. 2356.
[86] NAS, Edinburgh sasines 1805, no. 11085. The family home Greenlaw at Glencorse to the south of Edinburgh had been sold to become a barracks after the Napoleonic wars.
[87] NAS, SC70/1/127, 459.
[88] Information supplied by Nigel Dalziel of Montrose Museum.   [89] NAS, SC67/36/44.

four years before leaving the army in 1818. They must have met when he was serving with the Royal North British Fusiliers at Fort George. In civilian practice in Forres he numbered amongst his patients Sir William Cumming, the Brodie of Brodie and Colonel Fraser Drummond.[90]

Even among native Scots marriage seems to have influenced choice of residence. Ebenezer Black from Kelso in Roxburghshire probably put up his plate in 1821 at Haddington in neighbouring East Lothian because his wife Elizabeth Grieve, whom he married in 1821, came from there. When his father William died in 1827 neither he nor his brother, an Ottawa merchant retired in Jedburgh, had any interest in running the family's woollen mill in Kelso. Instead Ebenezer's eldest son, also William, took over with the help of an advance of £2,000 from his father.[91] George Gordon Maclean when he left the army settled at Cruden, north of Aberdeen, where he married Frances Angus from nearby Udny in 1820. He took his MD in 1819 from Marischal College where he had been an arts student from 1808 and graduated MA in 1812 before he joined the army. Although his military service had never taken him out of Europe, his interests were in oriental languages and theology. In 1826 he was elected Murray lecturer at King's College for the winter session, charged with inculcating 'just and liberal notions of pure and undefiled religion and virtue without descending to party distinctions and controversy'.[92] Nine years later he was appointed professor of oriental languages at Marischal College, a position he held until 1860.

As in Ireland, the capital was overwhelmingly the destination of choice of those who settled in Scotland. Out of the sixteen of the cohort who died there, six were natives of the city. However, unlike army surgeons from other parts of Scotland none seems to have returned to join his father in practice. Nor, unlike either Glasgow or Dublin, did any of the six have connections with the medical establishment. Nevertheless two of them were able to break into the tight knit Edinburgh medical community. David Maclagan, whose military colleagues held him in high regard, decided to return home to Edinburgh in 1816 and set up in practice in the heart of the New Town. Five years earlier he had married into an Ayr medical family, the Whitesides, who hailed from the Isle of Man and had been involved in smuggling. He was immediately elected a fellow of the Edinburgh Royal College of Surgeons. Unusually amongst his peers, he was an Episcopalian but prudentially switched to the Church of Scotland. He was also a Whig and a supporter of reform, who was not afraid to voice his opinions in public alongside Henry Cockburn and Francis Jefferey. The 1820s was an important juncture in Scottish politics with the Whigs in alliance with the radicals gradually winning the struggle for reform, not just of local and national government but of a whole raft of institutions long dominated by Tories.[93]

[90] NAS, SC26/39/4, 489.   [91] NAS, Haddington sasines 1827, no. 1399.
[92] Peter John Anderson, *Officers and Graduates of University & King's College Aberdeen MVD–MDCCCLX* (Aberdeen, 1893), 77–8.
[93] William Ferguson, *Scotland 1689 to the Present* (Edinburgh, 1987), Ch. 9.

In 1822 the Whig John Thomson resigned as professor of military surgery at Edinburgh, which was in the gift of the Crown.[94] At the time tension between the two political factions was running high following the acquittal in June of the Whig James Stuart of Dunearn for the murder in a duel of the Tory Sir Alexander Boswell.[95] Maclagan's name was put forward by the Whigs as a well-qualified candidate since he had already lectured on the subject the winter before.[96] George Ballingall, who had seen service in the Far East, India, and at Waterloo, challenged Maclagan. There was a third candidate, a Dr George Augustus Borthwick, the brother-in-law of the lord provost, George Kinnear, a leading Tory banker.[97] Maclagan submitted testimonials from four of his colleagues in the army medical service, McGrigor, Guthrie, William Fergusson, and Theodore Gordon (not the member of the cohort), all of whom praised his surgical skills in the field.[98] Guthrie wrote: 'I do hope that the ability and talent displayed by you on many occassions during the Peninsular War; under circumstances of unexampled difficulty and danger will not on this occasion be overlooked.' Ballinghall only submitted one testimonial from an army medical officer, McGrigor himself. The rest were from army officers under whom he had served.[99] In October Sir Robert Peel, the home secretary, wrote to the 2nd Viscount Melville, then rector of the University, affirming that the best-qualified candidate 'irrespective of any other considerations' must be appointed.[100] Although Maclagan was undoubtedly the best qualified, Ballingall, whose political and religious opinions were more acceptable, was nominated by Melville and duly received the royal commission.[101] Nevertheless, Maclagan did succeed in gaining the presidency of the College of Surgeons in 1826 and after the triumph of reform had the unique distinction of also being elected a fellow of the Royal College of Physicians in 1855.[102] He was appointed physician in ordinary to the young Queen Victoria in 1838. He was a man of varied interests, becoming a fellow of the Royal Society of Edinburgh and a member of the Society of Antiquaries, the Royal Scottish Society of Arts, and the Society of Nature and Chemistry. When he died in 1866 the *Scotsman* newspaper, admittedly of Whig and Liberal sympathies, showered him with praise: 'This good old man—who never made an enemy and never lost a friend—the valued family

[94] For a discussion of Thomson's Whig opinions see L. S. Jacyna, *Philosophic Whigs: Medicine, Science and Citizenship in Edinburgh, 1789–1848* (London 1994).

[95] *The Trial of James Stuart Esq., Younger of Dunearn* (Edinburgh, 1822).

[96] Inferred from the testimonial of Professor John W. Turner, EUL Special Collections, ref. SD 6234, and quoted in Matthew H. Kaufman, *The Regius Chair of Military Surgery in the University of Edinburgh, 1806–55* (Amsterdam, 2003), 119.

[97] Ibid. 114, and EUL, Special Collections, notes on alumni and staff.

[98] Kaufman, *Regius Chair*, quoted *in extenso*, 117–20; of these Fergusson is the only one who is not a member of the cohort.   [99] Ibid. 115–16.

[100] BL, Add MSS 40317, fo. 5, cited in Kaufman, *Regius Chair*, 114.

[101] Ibid. 114 and 120–3.

[102] Clarendon H. Creswell, *The Royal College of Surgeons of Edinburgh: Historical Notes from 1505–1905* (Edinburgh, 1926), 245.

doctor and friend—the public-hearted citizen—the genial companion of our best men for fifty years.'[103]

James Buchan, who retired as deputy inspector of hospitals in 1819, let no such political sensibilities stand in his way. He was elected president of the Royal College of Physicians in that December and later served as physician to Edinburgh Royal Infirmary, governor of the Orphan's hospital and physician to Heriot's Hospital.[104] John Kinnis, another deputy inspector, who came from Dunfermline, retired to Edinburgh in 1851 after thirty-six years' service. He set up home in Rutland Square in the fashionable New Town of Edinburgh with the help of a loan of £855 from his wealthy elder brother, who had been provost of Dunfermline.[105] He was elected a Fellow of the Royal Society of Edinburgh for his work in improving health in Ceylon. Although he seems to have intended to enter civilian practice, he was dead within a year.

Little is known of the others who settled in Edinburgh. At least two only had modest general practices: Andrew Anderson and William Wallace.[106] Anderson, who finally left the service in 1833, settled at 40, Minto Street, one of the meaner parts of the New Town, where his neighbours were merchants rather than professional men.[107] Two failed to establish themselves permanently in the Scottish capital. One was Lesassier, whose lacklustre civilian career has been referred to on several occasions. The other was James William Watson, a native of the city and MD of the university in 1812. He seems to have tried to break into the Edinburgh medical fraternity when he left the army in 1814 to take up the post as lecturer in chemistry as substitute for the distinguished and well-connected Professor Thomas Hope at Edinburgh University. Such appointments were often the route to preferment, but in 1819 he re-enlisted, eventually retiring to Bath as a deputy inspector of hospitals in 1850.[108]

ENGLAND: THE LAND OF PROMISE

Altogether 109 of the cohort died in England after they had left the service, 37 per cent of the number known to have died in civilian life (see Table 5.4). But as might be expected, they came from all over the British Isles. The origin of six is unknown, 61 were born in England, 18 in Ireland, 20 in Scotland, and 1 in Wales (see Table 5.1). Strikingly 55 per cent held or were to take MDs, overwhelmingly from Scottish universities. Even though thirteen came from medical

[103] *Scotsman* obituary reprinted in *EMJ*, 10/11 (1865–66), 94.
[104] W. S. Craig, *History of the Royal College of Physicians of Edinburgh* (Oxford, 1976), 499 and 503.
[105] Peter Chalmers, *Historical and Statistical Account of Dunfermline*, vol. ii (Edinburgh 1859), 335, and NAS, SC20/50/26, 347–51, inventory of the estate of William Kinnis, died 7 Feb. 1851.
[106] NAS, SC70/1/106, fo. 240; SC70/1/121, p. 121: wealth on death, £378 and £154 respectively. Cf. with the average value of the estates of cohort members dying in Midlothian: see Table 6.6.
[107] *Edinburgh Post Office Directory* (1849–50), 201.
[108] EUL Special Collections, notes on alumni and staff.

Table 5.4. County of Death in England of Those
who had left the Service

County	Number	Born in England
Berkshire	3	3
Cheshire	1	0
County Durham	2	2
Devon	7	3
Dorset	2	1
Essex	2	2
Gloucestershire	5	3
Hampshire	3	0
Herefordshire	1	1
Kent	3	2
Lancashire	2	1
London	49	26
Shropshire	1	1
Somerset	11	3
Suffolk	1	1
Surrey	3	3
Sussex	3	0
Warwickshire	3	2
Westmorland	1	1
Wiltshire	1	1
Worcestershire	2	2
Yorkshire	2	2
Unknown	1	1
Total	109	61

Source: Doctors' Database: Table: Doctors.

families, only two, Christopher Alderson and William Maurice, can with certainty
be identified as joining their fathers in practice.

Alderson's father, Dr John Alderson, had first moved to Hull in the 1780s to
serve with the West Norfolk Militia, which was stationed there. Setting up his
plate, he established a large practice covering the East Riding and across the
Humber in north Lincolnshire and became physician to the General Infirmary in
Hull. The eldest son of the family, Christopher was appointed physician to Hull
Royal Dispensary in 1817, the year after he was placed on half-pay, and was
elected president of the Hull Medical Society in 1821. Like John Schetky, he was a
competent water colourist, particularly of botanical subjects. It was perhaps for
this skill that he re-enlisted in May 1821 to take part in what seems to have been
a scientific expedition to America and to serve as surgeon to the 62nd regiment in
Nova Scotia. In October 1823 he returned with a mass of specimens including a
collection of insects and seeds and specimen plants for Hull Botanic Gardens.
He was appointed physician to the Hull General Infirmary in 1824 and became
joint proprietor of the Sculcoates Refuge for the Insane which had been founded

by his father. In 1828, the year before his untimely death, Christopher served as chairman of the Hull Botanic Gardens Committee.[109] His father Dr John Alderson died in September 1829, seven months after Christopher, and the practice was inherited by his fourth son James (1794–1882), another physician, who was, probably, at that date, established in London.[110]

William Maurice's civilian career was much more prosaic. Born in Bristol, the son of Joseph Maurice, a Welsh Unitarian surgeon apothecary, he had served as assistant surgeon with the elite Queen's Own Dragoon Guards. He had been discharged in August 1814 but recalled for the Waterloo campaign. Finally retiring in 1818, he had returned to Bristol to assist his father. Despite being an apprentice of the distinguished Bristol surgeon William Hettling and known to Richard Smith, a leading medical figure in the city, he never sought preferment. His father left Bristol shortly after his return to retire to his native Wales and William continued in practice as a surgeon in Upper Maudlin Street.[111]

Although John Mort Bunny returned eventually to Berkshire where his father, Joseph, had been in practice in Newbury, it was to live the life of a gentleman and not to be a doctor. By the time his father died in 1810, Bunny senior described himself in his will as a gentleman and the family practice was in the sole hands of his eldest son, Joseph Blandy.[112] When John Mort Bunny left the army in 1818, he clearly felt that there was not enough business in his home town for him to set up his plate alongside his brother, all the more that Joseph Blandy, who would die in 1834, had started to train his own son, another Joseph (1798–1865), to follow in his footsteps.[113] Understandably, therefore, John Mort practised first in London and then in Norfolk, Some time before he died, however, in 1848, he had retired back to his native town, still a bachelor, and was probably living with one of his two surviving brothers or nephews. It is most likely he was taken in by his youngest brother Edward Brice Bunny, who lived at Church Speen outside Newbury. Edward married in to the gentry and became a deputy lieutenant and a JP. His own son changed his name to St John on inheriting Sinfold Lodge, near Horsham in Sussex.[114]

Yet, if only two Englishmen returned home to join their father in practice, there were many more Bunnys. Twenty-six of the sixty-one Englishman who died in their native country after quitting the army eventually went back to their place of origin, eleven to London. George Paulet Morris, an inspector of hospitals who had joined the service in 1778, set up his plate in the West End of London when he retired in 1802, just as his father had done after leaving the army as a physician many years before. James Anthony Topham, an assistant surgeon, retired to his

[109] J. A. R. Bickford and M. E. Bickford, *The Medical Profession in Hull, 1400–1900* (Kingston upon Hull, 1983), 1–4; R. L. Luffingham, *John Alderson and his Family*, Centenary Monograph no. 21 (Hull, 1995); id., *The Manuscript of Sir James Alderson*, Centenary Monograph no. 22 (Hull, 1995); and information supplied by Mr Susan Sharp of Harpenden, a descendant.
[110] See p. 86.　　[111] BRO, Richard Smith papers 35983/36h, fos. 349–51.
[112] TNA, Prob 11/1509.　　[113] Joseph junior took his doctorate at Edinburgh in 1823.
[114] *Burke's Landed Gentry* (London, 1952), entry for St John of Sinfold.

home town of Darlington in 1838 after thirteen years' service, only to die within three years. William Roberts, who had served as surgeon to the West Kent Militia before joining the army in 1805, returned to practise with his brother Edwin in Lewisham when he was discharged in 1816.[115] James Williams, after twenty-one years' service, retired in 1817 to his home county of Worcestershire to live at Martin Hussingtree where his brother George was vicar and his sister Mary kept house.[116] Stephen Panting eventually went back to Wellington in Shropshire where his father had been vicar. Admittedly, this was probably out of necessity rather than choice. He may well have preferred to settle in Lichfield where he had been in practice prior to joining up and where one brother was a canon of the cathedral and the other a lawyer in the city. However the accusations of fraud made by Mrs Docksey, the sister of his former partner Peter Garrick, made that impossible.[117]

These surgeons went back to their place of origin either to go into practice or live in retirement among family and friends. Unlike a number of Scots and Irish surgeons who returned home, none inherited a family property. In 1805, shortly after the death of his first wife, Assistant Inspector William Greaves, born at Burton-on-Trent, 'beged leave to retire' from the service after twelve years. Thereafter until his death in 1848, he lived at Mayfield Hall in Staffordshire, eventually becoming deputy lieutenant of the county and a justice of the peace.[118] He never owned the hall, however. The property had been owned by his family since his great great grandfather's day and in the early nineteenth century was owned by his elder uncle, the Reverend George Greaves. William did not even own the moveables in the hall until 1823 for these were the property of his other uncle, the land agent, Robert Charles Greaves, who bequeathed them to the army surgeon on his death. In other words, William was simply the tenant.[119]

Only one or two of the surgeons born in England seem to have settled in the county where their wives were born.[120] George Peach, who came from Leicester, left the army as a surgeon in 1815 and the following year married Elizabeth (whose maiden name is unknown) at her home in Mapperton in Dorset. They went to live at Childe Okeford in the east of the county, buying two small farms of about 170 acres.[121] Similarly very few of those born outside England seem to have been influenced by marriage in their choice of residence, with the exception of John Kidston and Stewart Crawford. Kidston, who came from Midlothian

[115] Colonel H. Bonhote, *Historical Records of the West Kent Militia* (London, 1909), 415, and *Bagshaw's Kent Directory*, 1846.   [116] TNA, Prob 11/1934, 1966 and 2168.
[117] See Ch. 2.   [118] TNA, WO25/3910, fo. 59.
[119] www.gravesfa.org/gen228.htm (Sept. 2005); TNA, Prob 11/1675 and Prob 11/1743: wills of William's two uncles. When George died in 1828, there is no mention of Mayfield in his will. The Hall may already have been sold to Joseph Tunnicliffe who owned it in 1851: see www.ashbourne-town.com/villages/mayfield (Oct. 2005).
[120] William Greaves's two wives were close relatives but neither came from Staffordshire, although one was brought up at Ingleby Hall, just across the border into Derbyshire, see Ch. 6.
[121] Deduced from John Hutchison, *History and Antiquities of the County of Dorset*, vol. iv (London, 1870), 82, where his daughters are described as the owners of the property.

and had married over twenty years earlier, no doubt retired to Bath in 1816 to be near his wife's family. Crawford, a physician to the forces from County Tyrone, married in the same city in 1799 and settled there when he left the army six years later, setting up his plate in the fashionable Circus. He was appointed physician to the Bath United Hospital in 1808 and was one of the founding proprietors of the Bath Royal Literary and Scientific Institution in 1824, serving on the short-lived laboratory subcommittee in 1829.[122] Some of the surgeons who settled in England outside their place of origin may have been encouraged to do so by the presence of other relatives. Thus, on leaving the army in 1814 John Barr, who came from Glasgow, joined his uncle Alexander in practice as a surgeon and apothecary at Fletching in Sussex, inheriting his house and property when he died in 1827.[123]

The majority of those who settled in England outside their place of origin selected their new residence either out of choice or because of the prospects of employment. Most opted for somewhere within striking distance of home but potentially more lucrative. Pennel Cole, who came from Ludlow in Herefordshire, could not return there as his brother Thomas Caesar Cole had already put up his plate in the small town. Instead when he returned from Canada in 1783 after almost twenty years of service he was appointed surgeon to Worcester Infirmary in the next-door county. He soon began to take lucrative apprentices at the hospital, each paying between 200 and 250 guineas.[124] On retiring from the hospital in 1815 after thirty-one years of service when he was succeeded by his son Herbert, astonishingly he re-enlisted at the age of 65 for the Waterloo campaign.[125] Although on half-pay and living in France, he was promoted deputy inspector of hospitals in 1821. He died in Worcester in 1833.

Charles Brereton from humble Bawtry in the south of Yorkshire, who left the army in 1816 after less than two and half years' service, similarly could not go home where his brother, if perhaps no longer his father, was in practice. Instead, he purchased the practice of a Mr Dixon in the minster town of Beverley, 60–70 miles away.[126] He built up a large practice in the East Riding and became a prominent figure in the town. In 1823 he married Caroline, the daughter of Alderman William Osbourne, a wealthy Hull timber merchant and sawmiller, who also owned a shipyard at Kingston-on-Spey in the north-east of Scotland. A man of literary tastes with a valuable library and a cabinet collection of geological specimens, he chaired the meeting which led to the foundation of a mechanics' institute and became a frequent lecturer. He was elected mayor in 1832 and chief magistrate in 1845. He was committed to the dispensary movement and gave

[122] Information supplied by the archivist of the Bath Royal Literary and Scientific Institution, 15 Feb. 2003.   [123] TNA, Prob 11/1733.

[124] Joan Lane, *Worcester Infirmary in the Eighteenth Century*, Worcester Historical Society Occasional Publications no. 6 (Worcester, 1992), 35.   [125] Ibid. 157–8.

[126] Beverley of course was in the same county but Yorkshire was a vast size and he could hardly be said to have gone home.

freely of his services to the poor. He died a respected local figure on Christmas Day 1872.[127]

Joseph Brown, of Quaker stock from North Shields in Northumberland, married a Scot while stationed in Kent in 1818 and the following year left the army after ten years' service. He settled in Sunderland in neighbouring County Durham and became a local celebrity. Not only did he occupy 'the highest position in this town, but in all the north of England his name was well known, and his consultations frequently led him to Darlington, York, Barnard Castle, Shields and Newcastle at a time when railways were not and when journeys like these serious undertakings'. Despite his exertions, moreover, he 'never wearied of doing good to the poor; his advice and assistance were freely given'. He served as medical officer to the infirmary in Sunderland from 1822, shortly after its foundation, until his death in 1868. A Liberal in politics, he was one of the town's first magistrates and served as mayor in 1840. He presided over the subscription library and as chairman of the sanitary committee led a campaign to improve the homes of the poor. So respected was his service to the community that the townspeople presented him with a testimonial of £1,000 in 1858.[128]

John Jeremiah Bigsby from Nottingham, who settled in Newark in the same county when he left the army in 1826 after eleven years' service, had an almost identical civilian career although he was by no stretch of the imagination a liberal. He was senior physician to the town's dispensary, president of the local mechanics institute, and a committee member of the Stock library. He served as mayor, as an alderman, and a magistrate. He was noted for his 'unostentatious charity, and for the unceasing interest he took in the education of the poor children in his immediate neighbourhood'.[129] While serving in Canada from 1818, he became interested in geology and was assigned to the British/American Survey, for whom he seems to have worked until retirement. By the time he set up his plate in Newark he had contributed to a number of learned periodicals, including the *American Journal of Science*, and he continued to write up his scientific discoveries while in civilian practice. In the late 1840s, having never been back to Canada, he penned what was in effect a guide for tourists and would-be immigrants.[130] After his second wife came into money he retired from practice about 1850, moving to London's fashionable west end where he could indulge his lifelong interest in geology. His *Thesaurus siluricus* (an account of North American fossils) earned him a fellowship of the Royal Society in 1869, and the Murchison medal

---

[127] Manuscript history of the Brereton family by Mrs Marjorie Salkeld, available in the Beverley Reference & Local Studies Library.

[128] 'Death of Dr. Brown', *Sunderland Telegraph*, 20 Nov. 1868, and W. Robinson, *The Story of the Royal Infirmary, Sunderland* (Sunderland, 1934), 115.

[129] 'Dr John Jeremiah Bigsby', *Proceedings of the Royal Society*, 33 (1881–2),pp. xvi–xvii.

[130] *The Shoe and Canoe, or, Pictures of Travel in the Canadas, Illustrative of their Scenery and of Colonial Life with Facts and Operations on Emigration, State Policy, and other Points of Public Interest* (London, 1850).

of the Geological Society in 1874.[131] Unlike his colleagues cited above, Bigsby had had no prima-facie reason not to go back to his home town when he went on half-pay for a second time in 1826, for Nottingham was a big town and his father at the beginning of the century had been surgeon to the hospital. It seems likely, though, that Bigsby senior had been retired for several years and had gone to live in the countryside.[132] Perhaps there were too many well-established practitioners in the city by the 1820s, and John Jeremiah thought Newark a better bet.

A few Englishmen, on the other hand, set themselves up a long way from home. John Howell from Cambridge, whose wife came from Devon, settled in Bristol when he retired in 1816 as a staff surgeon. Although still nominally on active service, he had spent much of the previous two years studying at Edinburgh where he gained his MD. An evangelical member of the Church of England, he chose to live in the select residential district of Clifton, a parish with churchmanship to his taste. He soon involved himself with the recently established Clifton Dispensary, becoming senior physician.[133] He plunged himself into Bristol society, engaging in scientific, literary, philanthropic, educational, and evangelical societies. In 1828 he stood as a candidate in the election for surgeon to Bristol Royal Infirmary against Dr Wallis. Howell's supporters were 'the Evangelical or pious people', while 'all those who were not straight-laced joined the ranks of Dr Wallis'. The two sides quickly divided into 'Saints' and 'Sinners' and scandal mongers put it about that Dr Wallis often drove out unaccompanied with ladies. It was a neck-to-neck race and when Wallis emerged victorious the crowd roared 'Huzzah for Wallis and the Sinners, Down with the Saints'. Nevertheless, Howell was elected physician to the infirmary the following year.[134] In 1830 he was visited by Sir James McGrigor, who was keen to see over the Bristol Royal Infirmary. Possibly in an attempt to get him back into the army, McGrigor promoted him deputy inspector of hospitals.[135] During the cholera outbreak of 1832 Howell served as secretary to the board of health in Bristol, issuing a stream of instructions to contain the spread of the disease. During the 1830s as a committee member of the Bristol Institute for the Advancement of Science, Literature and the Arts, he applied himself to the development of its library and museum. He donated books and curios himself.[136] He contributed to the Friends of the Established Church in

[131] *A Brief Account of the Thesaurus Siluricus with a Few Facts and Inferences* (London, 1867), and www.geolsoc.org.uk/template.cfm?name=medallistsfrom1831_(July, 2005).

[132] Bigsby had been apprenticed to his father in the second half of the 1800s, so Bigsby Snr must have been in practice until at least 1810.

[133] C. Munro Smith MD, *A History of Bristol Royal Infirmary* (Bristol, 1917), 302.

[134] Ibid. 441–4.   [135] BRO, Richard Smith papers 35893/36m, fo. 155.

[136] Ibid., fo. 232, which contains a report of the 10th annual meeting, recording that he had presented fourteen Roman Egyptian coins and rare scientific books including *A Statistical, Commercial, and Political Description of Venezuela, Trinidad, Margarita, and Tobago: Containing Various Anecdotes and Observations, Illustrative of the Past and Present State of these Interesting Countries; from the French of M. Lavaysse: with an Introduction and Explanatory Notes, by the editor* [Edward Blaquière] (London, 1820).

Ireland, the Gloucester and Bristol Diocesan Church Building Society for new churches and chapels, and the city's Magdalene House, Blind Asylum, and School of Industry.[137] He retired from Bristol to Datchet in Buckinghamshire in the mid-1850s, before moving to Palermo in Sicily, where he died in 1856.

Surgeons who were born outside England and wanted to establish themselves in the English provinces frequently had to supplement their civilian practice with less glamorous work. Thus, George Russell Dartnell, who came from County Limerick, set himself up as a private asylum keeper at Henley-in-Arden in Warwickshire, when he left the army in 1857 with the rank of deputy inspector after thirty-seven years of service. He seems to have run Arden House as an asylum for twenty-one years, proudly promoting himself in the *Medical Directory* as the inventor of the improved military truss and the author of a paper in the *British Medical Journal* on branding for desertion.[138]

The other sensible option was to go into practice in one of the flourishing English spa towns, where there were many old army and naval officers taking cures. Edward Johnston from County Monaghan, who left the army in 1816 became physician to the Weymouth Infirmary.[139] William Gibney from County Meath, who retired on half-pay in 1818, set up his plate at 9, Rodney Terrace in Cheltenham, where he practised with great aplomb for forty years. For most of this time he was also physician to the Cheltenham dispensary and to the female orphan asylum. He also wrote a pamphlet extolling the virtues of the local waters.[140] Even in retirement he could not escape the allure of the spa, for he moved to Totnes in 1865, noted for its Leech Wells. Other outsiders tried their luck at Bath, the largest spa of them all.[141] The Irishman, Stewart Crawford, as we saw above, was an army surgeon who lived and died in the town and became a figure of real consequence. Others stayed for a short while, including the Irishman Frederick Albert Loinsworth, who was there for a year between postings. Two outsiders who lived in the town wrote about the curative effects of mineral waters, the Irishman Thomas Charlton Speer in his Edinburgh MD thesis in 1812 *De natura aquae*, and William Lempriere, a native of the Channel Islands, who published a work on the alumnious chalybeate waters of the Isle of Wight in the same year.[142]

Surprisingly few surgeons set themselves up in garrison towns such as Canterbury, Colchester, the Isle of Wight, Walmer, and Windsor, probably because there was

---

[137] BRO, Richard Smith papers 35893/36m, fos. 184, 190, 202, and 205.

[138] www.ancestry.com: census 1861, 1871; *Medical Directory* (1873), 391.

[139] *Medical Directory* (1846).

[140] *Seaside Manual of Invalids and Bathers* (London, 1841), and *A Medical Guide to the Cheltenham Waters, Containing Observations on their Nature and Properties; the Diseases in which they are Beneficial or Hurtful; the Rules to be Observed During their Use* (Cheltenham, 1821).

[141] Only one Englishman practised in Bath. This was James Muttlebury from Wells, who will be encountered in Ch. 6. Gibney, fittingly, died in Bath.

[142] *A Report on the Medicinal Effects of an Alumnious Chalybeate Water, Lately Discovered at Sandrocks, in the Isle of Wight; Pointing out its Efficacy in the Walcheren and other Diseases incident to Soldiers who have been Abroad, and more Particularly the Advantages to be Derived from its Introduction into Private Practice* (London, 1812).

too much competition from serving medical officers. Those who did so, apart from Charles Boutflower who settled in Colchester, again came from outside England. The Scot John Lorimer established himself at Canterbury, while his fellow countryman John Lightbody practised at Walmer, where the duke of Wellington spent much of the summer. The Irishman George Frederick Albert ended up at Windsor, having started his civilian career in the Isle of Wight, which was garrisoned to protect the naval base at Portsmouth. Two other surgeons, too, went to live briefly in the Isle of Wight before going into practice elsewhere: the Scot, George Robertson Baillie, and William Lempriere, mentioned above.

METROPOLITAN PRACTICE

An analysis of the county of death in England confirms an even greater concentration in the capital, London, than in either Scotland or Ireland. Of the cohort forty-nine died in London or Middlesex and of these eight were born in Ireland, nine in Scotland, two abroad, and one in Wales.[143] The attraction of London was even greater than Dublin or Edinburgh, not simply because after the union of the Irish and British parliaments in 1801 it was the only seat of government, but also because the guards regiments were permanently garrisoned there. As McGrigor himself pointed out, an army medical officer would have ready access to the aristocracy when developing his practice.[144] It was probably no coincidence that nineteen of those who died in London and Middlesex had reached the rank of deputy inspector-general of hospitals or above, representing a third of all those who achieved this rank in the cohort. Strikingly only three of these high-ranking army doctors had been born in the city.[145] Nobody of this rank died in Dublin, only three in Edinburgh, and, tellingly, five in Bath.

The most glittering career in the cohort was undoubtedly that of George James Guthrie, who left the army as a deputy inspector of hospitals in 1814 to practise in London. Although he refused McGrigor's instruction to re-enlist for the Waterloo Campaign, he did attend the military hospitals at Brussels and Antwerp after the battle to treat the wounded and to pursue his medical research.[146] In 1815 he published his acclaimed study of gunshot wounds and on his return to London began lecturing on surgery.[147] He was the driving force behind the foundation of the Westminster Ophthalmic Hospital in 1816 and its first surgeon with his army friend and member of the cohort Charles Fergusson Forbes as physician. He persuaded the duke of Wellington to be its president, and in 1823 he dedicated his treatise on the operative surgery of the eye to him

---

[143] The place of birth of three is unknown.   [144] See n. 21, above.
[145] The place of birth of only one is unknown.   [146] See above, pp. 197–8.
[147] G. J. Guthrie, *A Treatise on Gun-Shot Wounds, on Inflammation, Erysipelas, and Mortification, on Injuries of Nerves, and on Wounds of the Extremities Requiring the Different Operations of Amputation* (London, 1815).

and his vice-presidents.[148] His surviving correspondence suggests he milked his connections with the aristocratic patrons for all it was worth, dropping names and writing sickeningly sycophantic letters. On 21 September 1840, he wrote, for example, to the duke of Gordon, with whom he had served in the Peninsula:

Your Grace was so good as to direct a box of grouse to be sent to me in August but I was unfortunately out of town, having allowed myself this year 3 weeks with my Lord Panmure at Brechin [Angus], which is the reason I did not return my many thanks for your Grace's kindness in thinking of me.[149]

A furious row broke out between Guthrie and Forbes in 1828 over the treatment of the eye following the publication of an article in the *Lancet*. Guthrie commenced legal proceedings and when Forbes was *subpoenaed* by the defendants he resigned. Hale Thomson, a young surgeon and supporter of Guthrie, challenged Forbes to a duel which was fought in broad daylight on Clapham common. Both assailants fired three shots in the air before the seconds intervened. Forbes refused a similar challenge from Guthrie on the grounds that he had withdrawn his suit. Forbes remained in private practice with a large number of patients amongst the nobility and wealthy. He was knighted in 1844, an honour that eluded Guthrie.[150]

Guthrie was elected assistant surgeon of the Westminster Hospital in 1826 and full surgeon in 1827 when he was also elected a fellow of the Royal Society. At the hospital he gave lectures free of charge and spectators flocked to watch him operate wearing an enormous checked apron which covered him completely. His staff included William Bewicke Lynn, a fellow army surgeon and Londoner with whom he had served in the Peninsula, and the young Joseph Lister, but largely because of his popularity with the public and his notoriously impolite directness he was distrusted by his colleagues.[151] In 1828 he was appointed the Hunterian professor of anatomy, physiology, and surgery of the Royal College of Surgeons and served as the college president for three terms in 1833, 1842, and 1854. Publications flowed from his pen throughout his life. An obituarist remarked: 'his influence on the progress of medical science in his own time was that of an earnest advocate and an attractive teacher of whatever appeared simple and straightforward in practice, and of all surgical doctrines that professed to be based on correct anatomy'.[152]

Robert Keate, who had risen to the rank of inspector-general of hospitals without ever leaving London, pursued an equally brilliant civilian career. As a young man

---

[148] G. J. Guthrie, *Lectures on the Operative Surgery of the Eye: Being the Substance of that Part of the Author's Course of Lectures on the Principles and Practice of Surgery which Relates to the Diseases of that Organ: Published to the Purpose of Assisting in Bringing the Management of these Complaints within the Principles which Regulate the Practice of Surgery in General* (London, 1823).

[149] West Sussex County RO, Chichester, Goodwood Collection, MS 1611, fo. 705.

[150] *Medical Directory* (1853), 998, and *DNB*, *sub* Guthrie.

[151] John Langdon-Davies, *Westminster Hospital: Two Centuries of Voluntary Service* (London, 1952), 109 and 278.

[152] 'George James Guthrie', *Proceedings of the Royal Society*, 8 (1856–7), 272–4.

he enjoyed the patronage of his influential uncle Thomas Keate, who in 1792 had defeated John Hunter's favoured candidate, Everard Home, to become surgeon at St George's hospital. An outstanding surgeon, Thomas had succeeded Hunter as surgeon-general to the army, a position he had held until 1810.[153] His nephew, Robert, joined the army at Chelsea barracks in 1793 as a hospital mate and at the same time enrolled as a student at St George's. While still in the army he was appointed his uncle's assistant at St George's, carrying out all his operations for him, and finally in 1813 became full surgeon. He was remembered as 'an excellent colleague, but inclined to be irritable'.[154] Like Guthrie, he published his surgical findings, for example in 1819 a 'History of a Case of Bony Tumour containing Hydatids successfully removed from the Head of a Femur'.[155] In private practice he was surgeon to George III, George IV, William IV, Queen Caroline, Queen Adelaide, and Queen Victoria. He recalled towards the end of his life: 'I have attended four sovereigns and have been badly paid for my services. One of them now deceased owed me nine thousand guineas.' Perhaps by way of recompense, he was twice offered a baronetcy and twice declined.[156] John Phillips, another inspector of hospitals with a similar lack of overseas service and a practice in fashionable Pall Mall, also served as surgeon to George IV both as regent and king.[157] Such royal appointments may not necessarily have been lucrative, but they brought prestige and opportunity to extend practice amongst the aristocratic court circles.[158] George Paulet Morris, yet another inspector of hospitals but who had at least served in America, France, and the West Indies, had such an extensive practice amongst courtiers in St James that he had to resign as a physician to the Westminster Hospital.[159] Similarly sought after were Samuel Hadaway from Edinburgh, who put up his plate in Dean Street, off Park Lane, when he retired as an inspector-general of hospitals in 1870,[160] and the well-connected Michael Lambton Este. Este practised in the Albany when he left the services, catering for the enthusiasm amongst members of the royal family and the well-to-do for sea bathing and various forms of hydrotherapy which had interested him for over twenty years. He numbered amongst his patients and patrons the royal dukes of Kent and Sussex, Sir George Sinclair MP, and Joseph Hume MP.[161]

Caring for the medical wants of those in public life could bring unwanted calls for attendance. John Robert Hume, a Scot who retired as an inspector of hospitals in 1821, set up in Mayfair and was recruited by the duke of

[153] See Ch. 1.
[154] Terry Gould and David Uttley, *A Short History of St. George's Hospital and the Origins of its Ward Names* (London, 1996), 121–2.   [155] *Medical-Chirurgical Transactions*, 10 (1819), 278.
[156] Gould and Uttley, *St George's*, 123.   [157] TNA, WO25/771, fo. 32.
[158] W. F. Bynum, 'Medicine at the English Court', in Vivian Nutton (ed.), *Medicine at the Courts of Europe 1500–1837* (London, 1990), 262–89.
[159] Venn, iv. 471, and J. G. Humble and P. Hansell, *Westminster Hospital 1716–1966* (London, 1966), 40.   [160] NAS, SC70/4/215.
[161] *Remarks on Baths, Water, Swimming, Shampooing, Heat, Hot, Cold and Vapor Baths*, reprinted from the edn. of 1812 (London, 1845), 79–85.

Wellington as his personal physician. On the evening of 20 March 1829 he was summoned to be at Colonel Sir Henry Hardinge's house at seven o'clock the following morning. On arrival he discovered that Hardinge, who had lost a hand at Waterloo, had agreed to act as a second in a duel. He refused to name the parties, only saying 'they were persons of rank' and 'begged of me particularly to keep near him on the ground that I might witness everything that took place'. John Hume set off by coach with the pistols to Battersea Fields. On alighting he was disturbed to see Hardinge and the duke of Wellington, then prime minister, riding towards him. Before he could say anything, the duke greeted him 'in a laughing manner, "Well, I dare say you little expected it was I who wanted you to be here".' Shortly thereafter to Hume's horror the earl of Winchilsea and Viscount Falmouth appeared on the ground, their coachman having taken them to the wrong place. Just days before, as the whole of London knew, Winchilsea had publicly taunted Wellington in the House of Lords over his government's proposals for Catholic emancipation. Waving a large white handkerchief, he accused him of 'an insidious design for the infringement of our liberties and the introduction of Popery into every department of the State'. Although he disapproved of duelling, Wellington considered for the honour of the government he had no alternative but to respond to the challenge. After some discussion, Hume handed the pistols to Wellington and Winchilsea. Wellington, who was a poor shot with pistols, fired first and deliberately wide and then Winchilsea fired in the air. The affair was not yet over as Wellington insisted on a formal apology.[162] Hume was much relieved when the matter was settled and Wellington and Hardinge had ridden off. He later reported to the duchess: 'In meetings of this nature the principals are supposed to commit themselves entirely to the guidance of the seconds and thus become in their hands almost passive agents. On this occasion the Duke conformed himself strictly to the rule and I could not help admiring how meekly and submissively he conducted himself through the whole of this affair.'[163]

There were others in the cohort who achieved prominence in London medical circles. John Constantine Carpue, a well-travelled Londoner, left the army in 1811 as staff surgeon to the York Hospital in Chelsea, 'being apprehensive of being ordered on foreign service' to become consulting surgeon to the National Vaccine Institution at St Pancras. For ten years, he had already been lecturing in anatomy at the York and offering classes to private pupils. When he retired, he concentrated on his private anatomical teaching, in which he 'far exceeded his most sanguine expectations: and his original mode, and impressive style of instruction soon procured him overflowing audiences'.[164]

---

[162] Richard Holmes, *Wellington: The Iron Duke* (London, 2003), 274–5.

[163] University of Southampton Library, Wellington papers, WP1/1004/16: report by Dr J. R. Hume to the duchess of Wellington, of the duel between the duke of Wellington and Lord Winchilsea, 21 Mar. 1829.   [164] See p. 120.

He obtained his cadavers from resurrectionists and was lampooned by Thomas Hood in his poem on the subject, *Mary's Ghost*:

> 'Twas in the middle of the night,
> To sleep young William tried,
> When Mary's ghost came steeling in,
> And stood at his bed-side.
>
> O William dear! O William dear!
> My rest eternal ceases:
> Alas! my everlasting peace
> Is broken into pieces....
>
> The body-snatchers they have come,
> And made a snatch at me;
> It's very hard them kind of men
> Won't let a body be!...
>
> The arm that used to take your arm
> Is took to Dr. Vyse:
> And both my legs are gone to walk
> The hospital at Guy's....
>
> I can't tell where my head is gone,
> But Doctor Carpue can:
> As for my trunk, it's all pack'd up
> To go by Pickford's van.
>
> The cock it crows—I must begone!
> My William we must part!
> But I'll be yours in death, altho'
> Sir Astley has my heart.[165]

For thirty-four years Carpue lectured winter and summer three days a week in the morning on anatomy and twice in the evening on surgery, earning the sobriquet 'the chalk lecturer' for his readiness to resort to the blackboard. Charging his pupils twenty guineas a course, he reputedly undercut the medical schools.[166] As well as being a gifted teacher, Carpue was also a skilled surgeon publishing papers on the reconstruction of the nose and the removal of gallstones.[167] He was invited by the prince regent, personally, to operate on the nose of Captain Latham. In recognition of his surgical achievements, he was elected a fellow of the Royal Society in 1816.

[165] Walter Jerrold (ed.), *The Complete Poetical Works of Thomas Hood*, (London, 1906), 70 and 76: first published in *Wims and Oddities*, 2nd series, 1827. The reference to Sir Astley is to Sir Astley Cooper. Dr Vyse cannot be identified.

[166] 'John Constantine Carpue', *Proceedings of the Royal Society*, 66 (1846), 638–9; *Lancet* (10 Aug. 1846), 617–21, and DNB, *sub* Carpue.

[167] *Account of Two Successful Operations for Restoring a Lost Nose from the Integument of the Forehead in the Cases of Two Officers of his Majesty's Army* (London, 1816), and *History of the High Operation for the Stone, by Incision above the Pubis* (London, 1819).

Henry Davies, another Londoner who left the army in 1818 as a surgeon, set up in practice as an obstetrician in Saville Row. He served from 1821 as physician-accoucheur at St Marylebone Hospital and later as lecturer on midwifery and the diseases of women and children at St George's hospital. George Gregory, who was born in Canterbury, left the army in 1816 to become physician to St George's and St James's Dispensary in London. A regular contributor to medical journals, he was appointed a lecturer in medicine at the Windmill Street School of Medicine and from 1842 a lecturer at St Thomas's. Samuel Dickson, who returned from Madras in about 1830, set up in practice in Piccadilly where over the next thirty years he waged a campaign against the practice of bloodletting. Although he was right, much of his writing was eccentrically paranoid and at times verged on the libellous.

By the present medical management, the greatest fool in London may make ten thousand a year with ease, while the ablest medical talent may not find bread. There are men now making that income who know no more of rational medicine than the people who consult them.[168]

Nevertheless, he had his admirers, including Dr Hume, principal medical officer at Fort Pitt (not a member of the cohort) and George Russell Dartnell, the deputy inspector-general of hospitals mentioned earlier.[169] John Gordon Smith, who left the army as an assistant surgeon in 1815, joined Guthrie at the Westminster Ophthalmic Hospital. He found it hard, however, to establish a civilian practice, but instead accepted the appointment of physician to the fabulously rich duke of Sutherland, whom he accompanied on his travels. This gave him the leisure to write and during the 1820s he published four books on forensic medicine and edited the *London Medical Repository*.[170] As a result he was appointed lecturer in medical jurisprudence at the Royal Institution in 1825 and professor of the same subject at University College in 1829. However, he failed to attract pupils and turned to writing more popular books as a means of making a living such as *The English Army at Waterloo and in France*.[171] He died a broken man in the Newgate debtors' prison in 1833.

Given that a very few of the cohort who settled in London listed themselves in directories, it is difficult to know if they all entered civilian practice. It must be assumed that some from their seniority and length of service retired. Joseph Skey from Gloucestershire retired in 1842 as an inspector-general of hospitals after thirty-six years in the army to live in London where his cousin the distinguished surgeon Frederick Carpenter Skey was both in practice and professor of anatomy at the Royal College of Surgeons. Although his cousin was listed in the London

[168] Samuel Dickson, *The 'Destructive Art of Healing' or Facts for Families* (London, 1853), 65.
[169] Id., *Fallacies of the Faculty, with the principles of Chrono-Thermal Medicine* (London, 1865), 75.
[170] DNB, *sub nomine*. The four works were: *The Principles of Forensic Medicine* (London, 1821), *An Analysis of Medical Evidence* (London, 1825), *The Claims of Forensic Medicine* (London, 1829), and *Hints for the Examination of Medical Witnesses* (London, 1829).
[171] (London, 1830). Another title was *Santarem; or, Sketches of Society and Manners in the Interior of Portugal* (London, 1832).

directory and later the Medical Directory, Joseph Skey was not. Little, however, can be inferred from such omissions without some corroborating evidence.

MOBILITY, SUCCESS, AND ENGAGEMENT

This chapter has explored the lives of the cohort outside the army. Once placed temporarily or permanently on half-pay, a lucky few—either because they were only finally demobbed in late middle age, or because they had inherited a private income—were able to retire. The large majority, however, had to earn a living through private practice. Only army doctors at the top of the career ladder received enough from their half-pay or pension to live comfortably without plying their profession.[172] Hardly any of the cohort set themselves up in their home county and only a minority from Scotland and Ireland in their native land. Most army surgeons, once they had left the service, gravitated towards England and, to a lesser extent and sometimes only after settling for a time in the British Isles, to the colonies and the continent of Europe. What is striking is their mobility. They not only did not return home in most cases, but they frequently practised in more than one place. Although probably more than half came from rural backgrounds, often in remote parts of the United Kingdom, their careers after the army were essentially urban, building on the middling milieu of merchants and manufacturers that had dominated British towns and cities for centuries.

We know very little about the professional *cursus* of the wider medical profession, but it seems highly unlikely that many medical practitioners, apart from those drawn to London, set up their plates far from their birthplace.[173] In this respect, the cohort's service as army surgeons had stood them in good stead. Having joined the army in many cases because they had limited prospects in their native locality, the service had given them the experience and contacts they needed to set up in a more congenial environment. It was not simply that the army had turned fledgling doctors into old lags and introduced them to the right sort of people. In addition, through their mixing for several, and often many, years with, for the most part, social superiors in the officers' mess, the army had steadily divorced them from their various regional backgrounds and given them a gentlemanly, British patina which allowed them to settle in virtually any town in the empire.

It is clear, too, that many made a great success of their civilian practice. Undoubtedly, some were unable to adapt to Civvy Street and scuttled back to the army as fast as they could. Most, though, became pillars of their local medical community. Although given the lack of sources, it is difficult to trace all their careers, there is sufficient evidence to suggest many not only prospered but also continued to contribute to practice and medical knowledge particularly as teachers and hospital doctors. More important than the handful who became royal doctors

[172] See Table 1.4.   [173] See Ch. 2.

or consultants to the great and good were the surgeons who received civic medical appointments. At least 63, some 20 per cent of those who returned to the United Kingdom, secured hospital appointments (in infirmaries or dispensaries), usually by breaking into close-knit medical societies where outsiders were not often welcome. This is testimony to their ability, to the value of their commitment to training and development, and to the high status enjoyed by the army medical service under McGrigor. Just as it is improbable that the wider medical profession was so well educated, so it is unlikely that such a large proportion of medical practitioners scaled the heights of the civilian profession.

Furthermore, many of the cohort, irrespective of their social origin or place of birth, were fully engaged in their host community. They were frequently much more than highly thought of medical practitioners. The active role several played in civic life and voluntary organizations confirms both their standing and their wider cultural and political interests, even if only the exceptional, such as Bigsby and Joseph Brown, were local councillors. The avowed Whig or Liberal politics of a minority at first sight sits oddly with their military service. But it was perfect positioning for those who had settled in Edinburgh and the north-east of England and sought professional and civic success in the new reform world of the 1830s and beyond.

Taken together, then, the experience of these army medical officers, wherever they chose to settle and from wherever they came, either socially or geographically, only serves to corroborate their singularity within the greater profession. At their most successful, they were the Lydgates of the late Hanoverian and early to mid-Victorian world, although George Eliot's creation had never been in the armed forces. In their commitment and engagement with their host communities, they encapsulate the wide-ranging interests of the best-educated professional men from the time of the Renaissance. At the same time they collectively presage the professionalization of medicine later in the nineteenth century. Moreover, for many, as we will see in the following chapter, the reward of a successful civilian practice was wealth as well as status.

6

Fortunes and Families

MEDICAL WEALTH

While there is no disagreement amongst historians about the growth of the professions in the first half of the nineteenth century, there is much that remains to be explained. Penny Corfield claims that the professions 'advanced into and consolidated their position in the broad embrace of Britain's respectable middle class', 'circles within which professional men moved easily'.[1] Such a statement begs as many questions as it answers. What were the parameters of the middle class and who qualified to belong to it? How dynamic was it and was it possible to rise above it or drop out of it? At the beginning of her study, Corfield demonstrates convincingly that the elite or upper class was accessible to those with sufficient talent and wealth to gain admission.[2] As Habakkuk showed in his Ford Lectures, it was easy enough for the improvident amongst the gentry and the aristocracy to face ruin, particularly as more children survived into adult life and needed to be provided for.[3] The long depression after the Napoleonic wars released large tracts of land on to the market in distressed sales making it possible for the ambitious *nouveaux riches* to set themselves up as country gentlemen. Popular novels are peopled with wealthy merchants and manufacturers aping the gentry, such as Mr Jorrocks, R. S. Surtees's foxhunting London grocer. Men from the professions feature infrequently and more ambiguously. Surtees's Dr Roger Swizzle and Dr Sebastian Melo are unashamedly on the make in the fast-expanding spa town of Handley Cross, but Walter Scott's Dr Gray in *The Surgeon's Daughter* enjoyed a modest income of £200 a year and did not aspire to joining the ranks of the landed gentry—'He was a plain, blunt man, who did not love restraint, and was unwilling to subject himself to that which was exacted in polite society'.[4] The political economist, Patrick Colquhoun estimated in 1815 that an annual income

[1] P. J. Corfield, *Power and the Professions in Britain, 1700–1850* (London, 1995), 237, and P. J. Corfield, 'Concepts of the Urban Middle Class in Theory and Practice: England, 1750–1850', in B. Meier and H. Schultz (eds.), *Die Wiederkehr des Stadtbürgers: Stadtreformen im europäischen Vergleich, 1750–1850* (Berlin, 1994), 114–35. [2] Ibid. 11–13.
[3] John Habakkuk, *Marriage, Debt, and the Estates System: English Landownership 1650–1950* (Oxford, 1994).
[4] R. S. Surtees, *Handley Cross* (London, 1854), and Sir Walter Scott, *The Surgeon's Daughter* (Edinburgh, 1827).

of £300 was average for the profession, while lawyers could expect to earn £400.[5] Loudon in his study of the income of general practice concluded from several case studies that by the early nineteenth century 'it was probably the rule that rank-and-file practitioners were men of property and substance in the country. In the cities, while it was probably true that the poor practitioners were sometimes very poor, the richest could be very rich indeed.' The evidence on which he based this conclusion is remarkably slim and contains no examples of investment in land which would qualify for the title 'men of property'.[6]

The only time that individual wealth becomes visible is at death when the probate value of a proved estate, if it has a value, is a matter of public record. There are problems with the use of such probate valuations as an accurate reflection of total wealth just because landed property, houses and buildings, and funds held in trust under marriage settlements were excluded.[7] If Loudon is correct in his assumption that doctors had indeed become 'men of property' then probate valuations will seriously understate their wealth. This is very evident in the case of William Paton, a member of the cohort, who died on his estate of Durham at Torryburn in Fife in 1844. The family had lived and farmed in the area for generations, but his father John had become a doctor and his three sons, James, William, and Alexander had followed him into the profession. James and Alexander joined the East India Company while William joined the army. James died unmarried in 1836, leaving his land and property including Castlebeg House, along with moveable assets valued at £2,332 to his two brothers and two sisters.[8] William, who had left the army in 1814, died in 1844, also unmarried, and left everything including assets valued at £8,222 to his brother Alexander.[9] He in turn died in 1852 and left the whole of his estate to Edinburgh Royal Infirmary, including assets valued at £7,991. The Infirmary managers sold the whole of his estates which realized £37,556, more than four times the probate valuation.[10] There are other less well-documented instances of members of the cohort who owned substantial agricultural estates, which would not have featured in their probate valuations. George Peach, who died in 1852 at Millbrook House at Child Okeford in Dorset where he had extensive farming interests, left £8,000.[11] Archibald Arnott, who died in 1855 at Kirkconnell Hall in Ecclefechan in Dumfriesshire with an estimated rental income of some £300 a year, left over £10,000.[12] Alexander Brown, who died on his estate at Langlands near Twynholm in Dumfriesshire in 1872, left

[5] Patrick Colquhoun, *A Treatise on the Wealth, Power and Resources of the British Empire* (London, 1815), 124. The figures quoted in Anne Digby, *Making a Medical Living: Doctors and Patients in the English Market for Medicine, 1720–1911* (Cambridge, 1994), 164, of £200 and £300 are incorrect.

[6] Irvine Loudon, *Medical Care and the General Practitioner 1750–1850* (Oxford, 1986), 100–25.

[7] See for example Nicholas J. Morgan and Michael S. Moss, 'Listing the Wealthy in Scotland', *Bulletin of the Institute of Historical Research*, 59/140 (Nov. 1986), 189–95.

[8] NAS, SC20/50/23, fo. 745.   [9] NAS, SC20/50/15.

[10] EUL, Special Collections department, minutes of the managers of Edinburgh Royal Infirmary, minute of Mar. 1854, 132–3.   [11] TNA, Prob 11/2237, fo. 648.

[12] NAS, SC15/41/10, fo. 760.

£16,515.[13] Charles Farrell, who had spent almost £15,000 on extending his Dalyston estate in Galway, died in 1855 leaving £10,000.[14] Alexander Home, who had inherited Whiteside, the family property between Edinburgh and Leith, left £3,468, which included his outstanding rental income but not the value of the property.[15]

It could be argued that such under-representation of wealth might affect only estates with larger probate valuations. There are, however, examples in the cohort of those who are known to have had substantial property investment, leaving relatively small sums. Richard Batty, who seems to have farmed on a large scale at Broats near Gretna Green, left just £742 and Alexander Robertson, who owned Hallylands farm near Perth, left only £300.[16] Such instances, though, were uncommon. In fact, it would seem that, contrary to Loudon's claim, property ownership was the exception rather than the rule among the cohort and was usually a consequence of inheritance rather than a deliberate investment strategy. This can be easily proven in the case of surgeons retiring to Scotland, where all property transactions have been registered since 1617: Paton, Brown, Arnott and Hume, for instance, all inherited land. Furthermore, testamentary evidence suggests that this was more generally true. Army surgeons frequently owned a house or tenement, but those who owned landed property had usually come into it: Farrell was left his estate by a relative, while Constable and Peach acquired theirs through marriage. It can be safely concluded, then, that probate valuations can provide at least some guide to social status and professional success or failure and complement the handful of individual case studies used by Loudon and others.[17] Although these exclude the value of the property, they do include outstanding rents, and wills also often refer to the ownership of house property, either as a dwelling or an investment.

It is difficult to know how pervasive marriage settlements were amongst the cohort. They are only referred to in two wills and in both cases the value of the estate is considerably under-represented. George Robertson Baillie left £1,000 and his marriage settlement was worth £5,000, while John Gogil Leath left £6,000 and his settlement was worth the same amount. The fact, though, that there is virtually no reference to marriage settlements in the surgeons' wills would suggest that they can be safely discounted in the use of probate valuations in the large majority of cases. They probably only affect the larger fortunes.

Until very recently, individual case studies were the only approach that was practical, except for the study of the super-rich whose enormous probate valuations were relatively easy to identify from the Inland Revenue registers in the National Archives.[18] It is only with the advent of civil registration in 1858 that annual probate registers were published summarizing details of all estates proved

[13] NAS, SC16/41/30, fos. 45–53.   [14] NAI, IR4/237/19.
[15] NAS, SC71/1/75, fo. 282.   [16] NAS, SC15/41/4, and NAS, SC 49/31/17, fos. 150–60.
[17] Loudon, *Medical Care*, loc. cit., n. 6 above.
[18] W. D. Rubinstein, *Men of Property: The Very Wealthy in Britain since the Industrial Revolution* (London, 1981).

in England and Wales. However, since 2002 the National Archives of the United Kingdom at Kew and of Scotland in Edinburgh have begun to make available on-line the registers of the Prerogative Court of Canterbury and all wills proved in Scotland.[19] The coverage of the two sources is not identical, as not all wills and estates proved in England and Wales were registered with the Prerogative Court of Canterbury, but this is an important development. Moreover, some local record offices, for example Cheshire and Gloucestershire, have also begun to publish indexes to diocesan registers on the web.[20] Information, too, about estates in Ireland is more readily available than is often believed. Although the originals did not survive the fire in the Public Record Office in 1922, an index of Irish wills proved in the ecclesiastical courts has been recently published.[21] Such resources are also increasingly available in countries that were formally part of the British empire. The South African National Archives boasts a remarkably complete on-line catalogue that includes testamentary references. Coverage in Canada varies from province to province. These new on-line resources make it possible to search precisely for individuals and identify death dates not available from other sources. In the United Kingdom outside Scotland, dates of death can also be used to search the probate registers in the Public Record Office for valuations of estates.[22] Similarly, although Irish probate valuations have also been lost, the Inland Revenue indexes held in the Public Record Office in Dublin are annotated with valuations and can be used providing the date of death is known.

Altogether probate valuations have been located for 181 individuals or 40 per cent of the cohort. Apart from fourteen who died abroad or in the Channel Islands and the Isle of Man, the rest died in the United Kingdom of Britain and Ireland, representing the large majority of those who died there after they left the service. Of the remainder, it can be presumed that the fact that no probate valuations can be traced suggests they left less than £100. For example William Roberts of Lewisham's will is registered in the Prerogative Court of Canterbury but no probate valuations can be traced.[23] By far the largest number of recorded estates, some 60 per cent, were in England, followed by 22 per cent in Scotland, some 4.5 per cent in Europe and 10 per cent in Ireland (see Table 6.1). The average value of estates in England is larger by a factor of between four and seven than that found by Digby in her analysis of probates of professional men in 1858 that she placed in the range one to two thousand.[24] The wealth amongst the cohort was concentrated in London and the home counties with over 60 per cent of the wealth left by the cohort (see Table 6.2). The average wealth in London was over £10,000, which was £3,500 more than its nearest rivals Gloucestershire with

---

[19] These can be found at Documents Online in the National Archives Website, www.documents-online.pro.gov.uk/, and at Scotland's People, www.scotlandspeople.gov.uk.

[20] www.cheshire.gov.uk/Recoff/eshop/Wills/home.htm and www.york.ac.uk/inst/bihr/probate-%20.htm.

[21] *Index of Irish Wills 1484–1858*, Irish Record Index vol. i (Dublin, 2003).

[22] Scotland is excluded because estate valuations have always been a matter of public record.

[23] TNA, Prob 11/2105.   [24] Digby, *Making a Medical Living*, 138.

Table 6.1. Distribution of Estates of Army Surgeons by Country

Country of death	Total value (£s)	Number of estates	Percentage of number	Average per country(£s)	Percentage of total value
Channel Islands	900	2	1.1	450	0.08
England	737,620	107	59.11	7,093	61.47
Europe	54,150	8	4.41	6,769	4.59
India	2,000	1	0.55	2,000	0.17
Ireland	58,606	18	9.94	2,930	4.96
Isle of Man	2,000	1	0.55	2,000	0.17
Scotland	311,570	41	22.65	7,989	27.41
W. Indies	2,450	2	1.1	1,225	0.21
Wales	300	1	0.55	300	0.03
Total	1,180,479	181			

Source: Doctors' Database: Tables: Doctors, Wealth1.

Table 6.2. Distribution of Estates of Army Surgeons by County in England

Place of death	Total value of estates (in £s)	Number of estates	Average per county (£s)	Percentage of total value
Berkshire	8,000	3	2,667	1.1
Cheshire	4,800	1	4,800	0.65
Devon	28,950	7	4,136	3.92
Durham	2,300	2	1,150	0.31
Dorset	17,000	3	5,667	2.30
Essex	3,950	3	1,317	0.54
Gloucestershire	46,000	7	6,571	6.24
Hampshire	7,500	4	1,875	1.02
Herefordshire	2,500	1	2,500	0.34
Kent	15,022	5	3,004	2.04
Lancashire	8,000	3	2,667	1.08
London[a]	447,998	43	10,407	60.67
Shropshire	20,000	1	20,000	2.71
Somerset	56,000	9	6,222	7.54
Suffolk	1,000	1	1,000	0.14
Surrey	4,500	2	2,250	0.61
Sussex	15,000	3	5,000	2.03
Warwickshire	2,750	3	917	0.37
Westmorland	14,000	1	14,000	1.90
Wiltshire	9,550	2	4,775	1.29
Worcestershire	16,000	1	16,000	2.17
Yorkshire	5,300	2	2,650	0.72
Total		107		100

[a] Includes Middlesex.

Source: Doctors' Database: Tables: Doctors, Wealth 1.

£6,500 and Somerset with £6,200. This finding coincides with Anne Digby's conclusion that 'London surgeon-princes might command very high annual incomes at the peak of their careers'.[25]

Concentration of wealth generally in the south-east of England was well known to contemporaries. Writing in 1816 Simon Gray, a civil servant in the War Office, used the returns for the income tax, introduced to help fund the war against Revolutionary France, to calculate the rise in incomes between 1801 and 1811 and their distribution. From these data he was able to show the overwhelming dominance of London. One in thirteen taxpayers earned more than £60 in Middlesex and one in forty-two over £200 a year, whom he defined as rich, and of these the average income was £1,090. He calculated that the 'metropolitan county possesses, in income of £60 and upwards, £91,084 per square mile'. No other county approached this scale of riches. Although in Kent one in twenty earned more than £60, just one in 116 could be classified as rich. In Essex one in twenty-one earned more than £60 and only one in 137 were rich. The popularity of Bath amongst the well to do was evident from the figures for Somerset, which ranked second amongst the rich with one in eighty-seven earning more than £200 a year with an average of £640. Counties remote from London, particularly those in the west, dependent for the large part on animal husbandry, were poor and those in Wales very poor. Analysing the growth in incomes during the war, Gray detected some significant changes in counties with mineral resources and burgeoning industries. Incomes had grown most rapidly in Staffordshire, Lancaster, Kent, Surrey, and the East Riding of Yorkshire.[26] These conclusions have been confirmed by William Rubinstein in a recent analysis of the wealth holders leaving more than £100,000. Between 1809 and 1839 some 70 per cent of such fortunes were left in the metropolis, declining thereafter as the increased prosperity observed by Gray began to show up in probate valuations.[27]

Neither Gray nor Rubinstein disaggregated their findings by occupation. An investigation of all those describing themselves as medical practitioners in the 1865 probate calendar for England suggests that members of the cohort were on average much wealthier than the profession as a whole. If the enormous fortune of £250,000 left by William Silver in Bristol in 1865 is discounted, they were richer by some 63 per cent, £6,880, compared with £4,221 (see Tables 6.2 and 6.3).[28] Interestingly the pattern of wealth holding in the profession in 1865 was much less concentrated in the metropolis. Almost certainly the number of medical fortunes is understated as some practitioners preferred to describe themselves

[25] Digby, *Making a Medical Living*, 164–5, fig. 5.1.

[26] Simon Gray, *The Happiness of States: or, an Inquiry Concerning Population, the Modes of Subsisting and Employing it, and the Effects of All on Human Happiness* (London, 1815), 455–59.

[27] W. D. Rubinstein, 'The Role of London in Britain's Wealth Structure, 1809–99: Further Evidence', in John Stobart and Alistair Owens (eds.), *Urban Fortunes, Property and Inheritance in the Town, 1700–1900* (Aldershot, 2000), 136.

[28] William Silver has proved hard to trace. He does not appear in Dr Richard Price's index of west country doctors held in the BRO nor in the local trade directory. The authors are grateful to Anne Bradley of BRO for this information.

Table 6.3. Distribution of Estates of Medical Practitioners Recorded in 1865

County	Number of estates	Total value of estate (in £s)	Average per county (in £s)	Percentage of total value
Berkshire	2	13,000	6,500	1.22
Berwick-upon-Tweed	2	2,600	1,300	0.24
Buckinghamshire	3	24,000	8,000	2.25
Cambridgeshire	1	2,000	2,000	0.19
Cheshire	3	3,500	1,167	0.33
Cornwall	3	1,220	407	0.11
Cumberland	3	3,600	1,200	0.34
Derbyshire	2	3,600	1,800	0.33
Devon	8	80,950	10,119	6.58
Dorset	5	2,600	520	0.24
Durham	4	21,500	5,375	2.01
Essex	4	8,300	2,075	0.78
Gloucestershire	11	26,950	2,450	2.52
Hampshire	10	28,600	2,860	2.68
Hertfordshire	2	9,000	4,500	0.84
Huntingdon	1	200	200	0.02
Isle of Wight	2	7,000	3,500	0.65
Kent	13	33,250	2,558	3.11
Lancashire	31	101,670	3,280	9.52
Leicestershire	3	11,250	3,750	1.05
Lincolnshire	4	4,350	1,088	0.41
London[a]	51	264,870	5,194	24.81
Norfolk	6	27,750	4,625	2.56
Northamptonshire	2	1,050	525	0.10
Northumberland	3	7,200	2,400	0.67
Nottingham	1	450	450	0.04
Oxfordshire	1	9,000	9,000	0.84
Shropshire	3	6,100	2,033	0.57
Somerset	10	56,200	5,620	5.26
Staffordshire	5	8,700	1,740	0.81
Suffolk	4	5,100	1,275	0.47
Surrey	6	28,800	4,800	2.7
Sussex	11	41,500	3,772	3.89
Warwickshire	5	5,200	1,040	0.48
Westmorland	1	600	600	0.06
Wiltshire	3	54,000	18,000	5.05
Worcestershire	2	2,600	1,300	0.24
Yorkshire	22	159,600	7,255	14.94
Total	253	1,067,860	4,221	100

[a] Includes Middlesex.
Source: Probate calendar 1865, First Avenue House, London.

as gentlemen in their wills and their families or executors respected this wish in probate valuations. Amongst members of the cohort, this was common throughout the United Kingdom and therefore cannot explain the significantly lower proportion of fortunes in the metropolis among all those who admitted to being medical men. As Rubinstein has shown, those leaving over £100,000 in London declined to around 50 per cent of the total by the mid-1860s but not to less than 25 per cent which is the case of medical practitioners in the 1865 calendar. More interestingly is the higher averages than for the cohort in several counties (singly or collectively), such as Buckinghamshire, Devon, Durham, and Yorkshire. In the case of Devon and Yorkshire this can be attributed to two substantial fortunes left by Jacob Bickford Bartlett of Teignmouth (£60,000) and Henry Blegborough of Richmond (£90,000), but in Buckinghamshire and Durham six of the seven recorded left more than £5,000.

Although there needs to be much more investigation of professional fortunes, these marked differences confirm that after the war there were much greater opportunities for former army medical officers in London than their civilian counterparts. Interestingly the same does not seem to be true of Bath, where they would have faced aggressive competition from the many Dr Swizzles of this world. It may also be due to the shift of royal patronage, critical for metropolitan success, away from Bath during and after the regency. However the second largest medical fortune left in Bath in 1865 of £12,000 was that of Thomas Anderson, an army surgeon on half-pay not in the cohort, who had served with the 3rd Regiment of Foot or the Buffs. In neighbouring Gloucestershire where Cheltenham and Bristol were almost as fashionable as Somerset's Bath, members of the cohort were considerably more prosperous than their peers when Silver's enormous fortune is discounted. The same is true for both Devon and Dorset if Bartlett's large estate is discounted, but seems to be less so for Kent, Surrey, Lancashire, Warwickshire, and Yorkshire and not the case in Essex. The fact that few of the cohort died in rural and industrializing counties perhaps emphasizes the difficulty of gaining a foothold in a tight knit medical community where work was hard to come by unless there was an existing family or professional connection.

The distinctive geographical pattern of the wealth holding of the cohort is clearly evident when compared with an equivalent cohort of 430 naval doctors, who served during the French wars (Table 6.4). The distribution of the wealth of the eighty-six who died in England whose estates can be traced conforms much more closely to that of the profession as a whole in 1865 (Table 6.3) than to that of army doctors (Table 6.2).[29] They were only some 8 per cent on average better off than the profession and their wealth was more geographically distributed. As might be expected from anecdotal evidence the south coast maritime counties of Kent, Hampshire, and Devon are strongly represented and only 30 per cent of the wealth was left in London. Interestingly the average value of wealth of metropolitan naval doctors was significantly higher than that of London medical practitioners who died in 1865, £6,578 as compared to £5,194. Elsewhere Bath had no attraction for retired naval surgeons, whereas Bristol with its busy

[29] The authors with the help of Dr John Cardwell have constructed a database of 430 doctors who served in the Royal Navy during the French wars, see Introduction.

Table 6.4. Distribution of Estates of Naval Surgeons by County in England

County	Number of estates	Total value of estate (in £s)	Average per county (in £s)	Percentage of total value
Berkshire	2	7,500	3,750	1.90
Cheshire	2	6,300	3,150	1.60
Cornwall	1	3,000	3,000	0.76
Devon	9	24,900	2,767	5.31
Dorset	2	8,000	4,000	2.03
Essex	1	16,000	16,000	4.05
Gloucestershire	5	35,000	7,000	8.87
Hampshire	9	44,800	4,978	11.35
Hertfordshire	1	0	0	0
Isle of Wight	1	4,000	4,000	1.01
Kent	15	32,200	2,147	8.16
Lincolnshire	2	3,200	1,600	0.81
London[a]	18	118,400	6,578	30
Norfolk	2	23,000	11,500	5.83
Northumberland	1	6,694	6,694	1.70
Suffolk	2	5,800	2,900	1.47
Surrey	6	28,600	4,767	6.24
Sussex	1	2,000	2,000	0.51
Unknown	4	5,260	1,315	1.33
Warwickshire	1	20,000	20,000	5.07
Yorkshire	1	100	100	0.02
Total	86	394,754	4,590	100

[a] Includes Middlesex.

Source: Naval Surgeons Database (see above, Introduction, p. 20): Tables: Doctors, Wealth1.

port and Cheltenham with its spa did with a higher average than even those from the army.

The metropolitan concentration of wealth is also evident to a lesser extent among the eighteen members of the army cohort who died in Ireland and whose probate valu-ations can be traced and the forty-one in Scotland (Tables 6.5 and 6.6). In Ireland 48 per cent of their total wealth was left in Dublin and of the remainder 18.5 per cent represents the estate of the wealthy Charles Farrell of Dalyston. These figures, however, must be treated with caution as, because of the loss of records, probate valuations have only been traced for 36 per cent of the fifty surgeons who are known to have died in Ireland, and eight of the eighteen are for those who died in Dublin. Nonetheless, despite the paucity of figures, the valuations for rural counties, even discounting Farrell's exceptional fortune, suggest that practice outside Dublin was not as unrewarding as contemporaries suggested.[30]

By contrast in Scotland it has been possible to locate probate valuations for forty-one of the fifty-five members of the cohort who died there, more than

[30] *Burke's Landed Gentry of Ireland* (London, 1958), *sub* Charles Farrell.

Table 6.5. Distribution of Estates of Army Surgeons by County in Ireland

Place of Death	Total value of estates (in £s)	Number of estates	Average per county (£s)	Percentage of total value
Armagh	20	1	20	0.04
Donegal	2,100	1	2,100	3.90
Dublin	25,898	8	3,237	48.12
Galway	10,000	1	10,000	18.58
Londonderry	2,169	1	2,169	4.03
Mayo	450	1	450	0.83
Meath	4,000	1	4,000	7.43
Tipperary	2,358	1	2,358	4.38
Wexford	450	1	450	0.83
Wicklow	6,200	2	3,100	11.19
Total		18		100

Source: Doctors Database: Tables: Doctors, Wealth1.

Table 6.6. Distribution of Estates of Army Surgeons by County in Scotland

Place of Death	Total value of estates (in £s)	Number of estates	Average per county (£s)	Percentage of total value
Aberdeenshire	7,184	3	2,395	2.31
Ayrshire	72,960	3	24,320	23.42
Banff	2,519	1	2,519	0.81
Dumfriesshire	10,976	2	5,488	3.47
East Lothian	3,839	1	3,839	1.23
Fife	8,222	1	8,222	2.64
Kirkcudbrightshire	16,515	1	16,515	5.3
Lanarkshire	43,106	5	8,621	13.84
Midlothian[a]	100,383	14	7,170	32.22
Morayshire	830	2	415	0.27
Perthshire	9,213	3	3,071	2.96
Roxburghshire	576	1	576	0.20
Stirlingshire	8,413	2	4,206	2.96
West Lothian	2,232	1	2,232	0.72
Wigtownshire	200	1	200	0.06
Total		41		100

[a] Includes Edinburgh.

Source: Doctors Database: Tables: Doctors, Wealth1.

80 per cent, the same figure as for England (107 out of 134).[31] Fourteen died in Midlothian, leaving some 32 per cent of the wealth, and five in Lanarkshire, leaving about 14 per cent. Although 25 per cent was left in Ayrshire, this can be

---

[31] Total death figures in the British Isles include those who died in retirement and on service and those whose status has not been determined: hence the discrepancy with the totals given in Tables 4.19 and 5.1.

Table 6.7. Distribution of Estates of Army Surgeons by Range by Country

Country	Less than £500	£500–1,000	£1,000–5,000	£5,000–10,000	£10,000 and above
England	22	7	35	20	23
Ireland	8	0	6	2	2
Scotland	9	4	14	5	9

Source: Doctors' Database: Tables: Doctors, Wealth1.

attributed to two very large estates, John Robb who left £36,795 in 1845 and John Ferguson who left £35,568 in 1856. Robb's fortune came to him largely by chance from the family's Ayr banking business and an advantageous marriage into a local Nabob family.[32] It has not been possible to trace the source of Ferguson's fortune. As he made his career in the army and never rose above the rank of surgeon, it either had similar mercantile origins or was the result, in part like Farrell's, of his five years of service in Ceylon between 1832 and 1836. If these two large Ayrshire fortunes are discounted, then the proportion left in Edinburgh rises to almost 50 per cent. The average wealth in Edinburgh of £7,170 is markedly higher than the £4,271 of the 117 describing themselves as doctors whose estates were proved in the Edinburgh commissary court between 1827 and 1845.[33]

Average wealth holding disguises huge variations from those who left next to nothing to the London society practitioner Michael Este, who left £60,000 (Table 6.7). Altogether a third left more than £5,000, which, although not a great fortune, was substantial. It would have taken Walter Scott's Dr Gray twenty years to earn such a sum which he could not conceivably have saved and it would have even taken a military inspector-general of hospitals on £2 a day almost eight years. The geographic distribution of these military estates must be treated with care. Moderate wealth resulting from professional practice and combined with half-pay reinforced the mobility experienced in military service. In Devon, two of those who left over £5,000 had practised in London after leaving the services, the Scotsmen William Henry Burrell, a deputy inspector-general, and William Robertson, a surgeon. John Davy, Sir Humphry Davy's brother, who left £14,000, had only retired to Westmorland late in life. The Irishman George Richard Melin, a staff surgeon who left £2,000, had practised in Dublin before retiring to Warwickshire. Charles Whyte, who made his career in the army and retired as a deputy inspector-general, had a home in Devon until he left the army and settled in Bristol, where he left £12,000 at the end of a long life. John Easton, who died in Edinburgh worth £2,814, had practised in Yorkshire before retiring to his native Scotland.

---

[32] See Ch. 4. Also, *Burke's Landed Gentry* (London, 1952), see entry for Plowden-Wardlaw family.
[33] Abstracted from the Edinburgh commissary court records in the NAS. Since *Calendars of Confirmation and Inventories* were not published in Ireland or Scotland until 1875, it has not been possible to make similar comparisons with the probate valuations of the whole profession as in England.

Eight of those who died in London had not spent all their retirement there and it must be presumed that some of their lifetime savings had been accumulated elsewhere. John Jeremiah Bigsby, who left £9,000, had only moved from Newark to London after his second wife came into money. John Gogil Leath, who left £6,000, had worked as principal medical officer in Honduras, and William Dawson, who left £12,000, had spent much of the time he was on half-pay practising in Jamaica. Nevertheless those who left the largest fortunes spent the whole of their retirement in London practice: Michael Lambton Este £60,000, Charles Collier £50,000, John Robert Hume £40,000, and Robert Keate £35,000. What emerges is a complex picture of mobility and wealth, which was probably novel.

Although 78 out of the 107 members of the cohort with estates in England left more than £1,000, military service did not necessarily guarantee financial rewards (see Table 6.8). Lack of wealth at death neither equates to military rank or place of death. George Frederick Albert and Joseph Thomas, both deputy inspectors of hospitals, left £200 and Alexander Robertson, an inspector of hospitals, £300. Eleven

Table 6.8. Distribution of Estates of Army Surgeons by Range by County in England

County	Less than £500	£500– £1,000	£1,000– £5,000	£5,000– £10,000	£10,000 and above
Berkshire	1	1		1	
Cambridgeshire					
Cheshire			1		
Devon	1		2	4	
Dorset			1	2	
Durham		1	1		
Essex	1		2		
Gloucestershire	3	1		1	2
Hampshire	1		3		
Herefordshire			1		
Kent	2	1	1		1
Lancashire			3		
London	9	2	10	8	14
Shropshire					1
Somerset	1		4		3
Staffordshire					
Suffolk			1		
Surrey			2		
Sussex			2		
Warwickshire	2		1		
Westmorland					1
Wiltshire		1			
Worcestershire					1
Yorkshire	1			1	
Total	22	7	35	20	23

Source: Doctors Database: Tables: Doctors, Wealth1.

of the forty-three with estates in London left less than £1,000. William Maurice, who practised apparently successfully for many years in Bristol, left £200, and William Roberts, who had a long civilian career in an established family practice in Lewisham, left next to nothing. It is possible that some of these low valuations can be explained by *inter vivos* gifts. These have been dismissed as unimportant by Rubinstein, but this opinion has not gone unchallenged.[34] The best-documented example in the cohort is that of George Guthrie, arguably the most distinguished surgeon of his generation. The probate valuation of his estate was only £450, but this is misleading as twelve years before his death in 1856 he had settled £12,000 on his daughter Anne Leonora. An insufferable snob, Guthrie was persuaded to lend this sum at 4 per cent to the wholly improvident 2nd duke of Buckingham. The duke assured Guthrie that as soon as his son the marquess of Chandos came of age in September 1844 the debt would be secured by a mortgage over part of his estates. Guthrie can have taken no advice before entering into this arrangement, as he would have discovered that the duke was head over heels in debt. On attaining his majority Chandos learned of his father's astonishing extravagance and witnessed the breath-taking expenditure for the visit in January 1845 of Queen Victoria to Stowe, his fabulous country seat in Buckinghamshire. He refused to become ensnared in his father's financial mismanagement and Buckingham fobbed Guthrie off with the promise to assign him three life policies. Matters reached a head in the spring of 1847 when Chandos and a cartel of leading creditors took action to force Buckingham to address his financial difficulties. As a result all the family property was made over to Chandos on the condition that a schedule of debts, which did not include the name of Anne Guthrie, was paid. Unaware of these manoeuvres, Guthrie, finding the half-year dividend had not been paid, had a meeting with Buckingham and his son in June. Buckingham pleaded that this was a 'debt of honour he could not forgo'. Chandos could make no promises and did not have the heart to tell Guthrie the true state of affairs. The gullible Guthrie left, believing that the 'Duke of Buckingham and Lord Chandos, father and son, were acting cordially together as their manner implied, for the preservation of honour of a family of even Royal descent, and had no idea of anything like reservation or deception'. Matters dragged on and it eventually dawned on Guthrie that he had been duped. The debt was still unpaid at the time of his death.[35] Equally large wealth holding can also be understated as a result of *inter vivos* gifts. Robert Keate, who left £35,000, had already made over £6,950 to his two daughters on their marriage.[36] Such evidence is scanty and can only serve to add a further note of caution in the use of probate valuations.

[34] W. D. Rubinstein, 'The Victorian Middle Class: Wealth, Occupation and Geography', *Economic History Review*, 2nd series, 30 (1977), 603–4, and Morgan and Moss, 'Listing the Wealthy in Scotland'.
[35] WL, RAMC 1759, George James Guthrie muniment collection, letters concerning £12,000 lent to the duke of Buckingham, 1844, and *Stowe Landscape Gardens* (National Trust, 1997), 80–2.
[36] TNA, IR 26/2105, fo. 858; Prob 11/2259, q. 762.

When the distribution of the estates by range of wealth of the cohort who died in England is compared with the estates of medical men recorded in the probate calendar for 1865 (Table 6.9), the most striking differences is the proportionately fewer estates of over £5,000 among the latter (some 15 per cent compared with

Table 6.9. Distribution of Estates by Range of Medical Practitioners Recorded in 1865

County	Less than £500	£500– £1,000	£1,000– £5,000	£5,000– £10,000	£10,000 and above
Berkshire	0	0	1	1	0
Berwick-upon-Tweed	0	1	1	0	0
Buckinghamshire	0	0	0	2	1
Cambridgeshire	0	0	1	0	0
Cheshire	1	1	1	0	0
Cornwall	2	1	0	0	0
Cumberland	0	1	2	0	0
Derbyshire	0	1	1	0	0
Devon	3	1	2	0	2
Dorset	2	3	0	0	0
Durham	0	0	2	2	0
Essex	1	1	1	1	0
Gloucestershire	3	1	7	0	0
Hampshire	1	1	6	2	0
Hertfordshire	0	0	2	0	0
Huntingdon	1	0	0	0	0
Isle of Wight	0	1	0	1	0
Kent	3	4	5	0	1
Lancashire	9	5	11	4	2
Leicestershire	1	1	0	1	0
Lincolnshire	2	1	1	0	0
London[a]	9	10	20	7	5
Norfolk	4	0	1	0	1
Northamptonshire	1	1	0	0	0
Northumberland	1	0	2	0	0
Nottingham	1	0	0	0	0
Oxfordshire	0	0	0	1	0
Shropshire	0	1	2	0	0
Somerset	2	0	4	2	2
Staffordshire	3	0	2	0	0
Suffolk	0	1	3	0	0
Surrey	0	1	4	0	1
Sussex	3	1	4	2	1
Warwickshire	2	0	3	0	0
Westmorland	0	1	0	0	0
Wiltshire	0	1	0	1	1
Worcestershire	0	1	1	0	0
Yorkshire	8	3	6	2	3
Total	63	45	96	29	20

[a] Includes Middlesex.

Source: Probate calendar 1865, First Avenue House.

almost 40 per cent). The proportion of those with estates of between £1,000 and £5,000 (36.94 compared with 32.71 per cent) is much the same but there is again quite a wide discrepancy between those leaving less than £1,000 (42.69 per cent compared with 27.1 per cent). There was also much less concentration of wealth in the metropolis with 24.49 per cent of medical practitioners who left more than £5,000 in 1865 resident there compared to 51.16 per cent in the army cohort. Moreover as well as the fabulously rich William Silver another four of the eight doctors recorded in 1865, who left £20,000 or more, died in the provinces,[37] whereas only two of the nine members of the cohort who left such a sum in England died outside London, Richard Humphrey in Gloucestershire who left £25,000 and Stephen Panting in Shropshire £20,000.

The concentration of the larger fortunes in the metropolis is less evident in Scotland, with only four of the nine of the cohort who left more than £10,000 living in the Scottish capital.[38] Since a much greater proportion of members of the cohort from Scotland came from landed backgrounds, this is perhaps not surprising. As larger estates were sometimes recorded in the Edinburgh commissary court, some comparison can be made between the estates of the 117 doctors recorded there between 1827 and 1845 and the forty-one members of the cohort with estates in Scotland. As in England the lower proportion of estates of more than £5,000 is striking with 17 per cent compared to 34 per cent in the army cohort. Like England, too, a much smaller proportion of the army cohort left less than a £1,000: some 32 per cent compared with 50 per cent of medics recorded in the commissary court. The proportion leaving between £1,000 and £5,000 is much the same, 34 per cent compared with 32 per cent. Although the richest of the cohort who died in Edinburgh were not as rich as five of their wealthiest peers included in the 117 estates, the wealth of at least three of those was not derived entirely from metropolitan medical practice. Richard Kellet (£37,502) and John Gilchrist (£17,461) had served with the East India Company and Thomas Charles Hope (£54,705) was a well-connected professor at the University of Edinburgh.[39]

In any study of larger fortunes, it is difficult to determine how far they reflect inheritance or are the product of lifetime providence. It would seem likely from their background that the majority of the cohort who left substantial sums accumulated their wealth during their professional life. Digby and Loudon have both shown from case studies that this was perfectly possible even in the first half of the eighteenth century.[40] The richest member of the cohort, Michael Lambton Este, was left nothing by his father Charles when he died in 1828 with an estate of

[37] These were Henry Blegborough of Richmond, who left £90,000, Jacob Bickford Bartlett of Teignmouth £60,000, William Frowd Seagram of Warminster £45,000, and Philip Harrison of Norwich with £25,000.
[38] These were David MacLagan, who left £25,523, John Murrary £22,068, James Buchan £20,032, and Alexander Cunningham £15,692.
[39] For a description of this source see Cecil Sinclair, *Tracing Your Scottish Ancestors: A Guide to Research in the Scottish Record Office* (Edinburgh, 1990), sect. 5.14–15. For Hope, see Ch. 3.
[40] Digby, *Making a Medical Living*, Ch. 5, and Loudon, *Medical Care*, 100–3.

£17,000 on the grounds that he was already comfortably off.[41] After he left military services, Michael Este pursued a career in the same sort of quackery as Dr Swizzle and Dr Melo and left £60,000 at his death.[42] Charles Collier, whose father William died when he was young and whose father-in-law was a Church of Scotland minister, must have made his £50,000 partly as principal medical officer of Mauritius and partly from his London practice. John Robert Hume, who retired as an inspector-general of hospitals, was the son of Joseph Hume, a surgeon to the forces and later in practice in Hamilton, who, although he educated his sons, did not leave them much money. John Robert Hume's £40,000 estate almost certainly derived from his extensive private practice in London. John Murray, whose friend and fellow surgeon Andrew Anderson described as 'surgeon to most of Britain', must have made his £22,000 with his 'skilful hand'.[43] Although Robert Keate was well connected, his father was only a minor canon at Wells Cathedral with several other children to be provided for, and it must be assumed his fortune of £35,000 was accumulated in the course of his professional life in London. It is known that the fathers of four members of the cohort, whose estates were valued at £10,000 or more, left nothing to speak of. These were Robert Maclagan, whose son David left £25,000, Hugh Buchan, whose son James left £20,000, the Reverend William Williams, whose son James left £16,000 and William Crawford, whose son Stewart left £12,000.

Apart from John Robb (£40,000), Alexander Browne (£16,515), and Archibald Arnott (£10,234) who are known to have inherited property, the only other member of the cohort who left more than £10,000 who can be definitely linked to dynastic wealth is Alexander Dunlop Anderson (£27,522). This connection, however, brought him an extensive share of what is called 'the best practice' from which no doubt the bulk of his wealth derived.[44] Moroever, there were several of the cohort who clearly received little benefit from having rich relations. Captain John Piper of Colyton House in Devon left £12,000 divided amongst his three sons and daughter, but his son Samuel Ayrault Piper, a member of the cohort, left only £3,000. Similarly Alexander Thomson, whose brother Charles rented Machermore Castle at Newton Stewart in Wigtownshire, left £200, John Mort Bunny, whose brothers were a well-to-do banker, lawyer, and surgeon in Newbury, left £800, and the long-lived Francis Sievewright, whose father was a rich London merchant, had an estate of £1,436.

It is more difficult to discover why some members of the cohort failed to make much from their careers. In a few cases this is obvious: Andrew Anderson (£378) had bad luck; Lesassier (£700) suffered from a mixture of improvidence and licentiousness; Alexander Broadfoot (£300) ended his days in the lunatic asylum at Chatham;[45] while Crawford Dick (£597) was discharged on grounds of ill

[41] Will of Este Snr.   [42] See Ch. 7 for Este's interest in balneology.
[43] EUL, Att 84.6.20 (2): dedication to Andrew Anderson's Edinburgh thesis 1816.
[44] V. G. Plarr, *Plarr's Lives of the Fellows of the Royal College of Surgeons of England*, 2 vols. (London, 1930), i. 22–3.   [45] TNA, WO25/3911, fo. 13.

health and was cared for by his brother on the family's tenant farm in Ayrshire. But for the most part the reason can only be guessed at. Many set up in unpromising parts of the country. Daniel Owen Davies (£300) probably paid the price of returning home to Llangrandog in Cardiganshire where incomes were notoriously low. Gray reckoned it to be the poorest county in the United Kingdom with only one in 164 of the population earning more than £60 a year.[46] Similarly, William Williams (£450) was ill-advised to return to Llanfair Dyffryn Clwyd in the more prosperous, but still relatively disadvantaged, Denbighshire. So too were Thomas Atkinson (£450), who worked in the wilds of County Mayo, and James Barlow, who spent his civilian career in unpromising Limerick and left nothing to speak of. Likewise, Backsall Lane Sandham, who similarly had no estate to leave, must have found it hard to eke out a living in remote Sutherland. In at least three cases it is possible to link civilian failure to a stained military record. John Gray Hibbert (£100) was found guilty at a court martial in 1817 and lost two years' seniority. Both David MacLoughlin (£200) and William Dowell Fry (£24) were also dismissed from the service, although Fry was subsequently reinstated. In another it can be linked to professional incompetence. Michael Fogerty (£450) was described as being 'perfectly useless' in his War Office record.[47] On the other hand John Price (£450) was commended for his 'eminent services in Egypt during the plague epidemic' and finished his career as a physician to the forces.[48]

It is possible to make a guess that some others passed on the bulk of their wealth before death not necessarily in gifts but by investing in the education and training of their children and if they had none their nephews and nieces. Jose Harris, commenting on the period 1870–1914, claimed that 'the aim of many a middle-class father was not to provide his sons with an inheritance after his death: it was to provide them with the education, deportment and business connections to establish their independence while he was still alive'.[49] Alexander Robertson (£300) stated in his will that he had provided his three eldest sons with a 'liberal education and procured situations in which they ought to be capable of doing for themselves'. They appear to have been in trade as his third son Duncan was a merchant in Kingston, Jamaica.[50] Robert Brown (£600) financed at least three of his six sons through medicine and it is unlikely that he did not provide a similar start in life for the others. Despite his lack of funds, Andrew Anderson (£378) had by the time of his death secured a captaincy for his eldest son in the 78th Highlanders, the Rosshire Buffs, and a position for his second son with a Hong Kong merchant.[51] Robert Shekleton (£300). a successful Dublin practitioner, put one son through medicine and went to the expense of establishing another as a barrister. George Guthrie (£450) sent both his sons to Westminster; one became a surgeon and the other went on to Cambridge to

[46] Gray, *Happiness of States*, 455. [47] TNA, WO25/3909, fo. 49.
[48] TNA, WO25/3909, fo. 133.
[49] Jose Harris, *Private Lives, Public Spirit: Britain, 1870–1914*, (Oxford, 1993), 70.
[50] NAS, SC 49/30/17, fos. 150–60. [51] NAS, Edinburgh sasines 1862, no. 5099.

become a clergyman. Lack of wealth at death did not necessarily imply an impoverished lifestyle. John Douglas (£576), a respected doctor in Hawick, had a well-appointed residence, a fine library, slept in an Elizabethan bed, and was waited on by servants.[52]

Comparison of the wealth left by the cohort with the rest of the medical profession provides little guide as to their position in society. Although the growth of the professions is viewed as integral to the rise of the middle class, there has been little research into their relative intra- or inter-professional staus or economic standing.[53] Corfield, in her study of the professions from 1700 to 1850, tellingly placed lawyers and the clergy before doctors in her analysis of their individual experience, although she admitted that 'this was a key period in which the status of "medicine" rose'.[54] Most commentators, such as Digby and Loudon, resort either to contemporary comment or to a small number of well-documented case studies. Before the recent improvements in access to testamentary records, such research was impossible and could only be conducted using the more manageable but bulky printed calendars of probates and confirmations of a later date. Evidence drawn from the Scottish calendars at the end of the end of the nineteenth century after a period of unparalleled prosperity north of the border suggests that for anyone to leave an estate of more than £10,000 was unusual, a little more than 5 per cent of all estates (Table 6.10).[55] This more than suggests that the thirty-four members of the cohort (about 21 per cent of the 181 whose valuations have been traced) who left such a fortune can be considered rich and to have moved in the upper echelons of middle-class society.

In the professions, which included accountants, architects, engineers, lawyers, ministers of religion, and teachers as well as doctors, the proportion of those leaving £10,000 or more in Scotland was significantly higher than for the population as a whole, confirming the contemporary perception of the professions as 'the head of the great English [*sic*] middle class' (Table 6.11).[56] There again professional estates only contributed a small proportion of the super-rich—less than 10 per cent. It is clear, too, as might be expected, that there were more wealthy lawyers than doctors and clergy. Thirty-two lawyers left more than £10,000, twenty-one doctors and fifteen ministers of religion. There seem to have been more wealthy clergy in England, where episcopal and deaconal stipends were high. Digby in her analysis of probate valuations of professional men in 1858 puts the law and the Church before medicine amongst higher wealth owners, but interestingly in the range £2,000 to £8,000 medicine is in second place, and between

---

[52] NAS, SC62/44/38, fo. 972.

[53] See for example K. Theodore Hoppen, *The Mid-Victorian Generation 1846–1886* (Oxford, 1998), 40–9.   [54] Corfield, *Power and the Professions*, 136.

[55] These data have been abstracted from the printed Scottish *Calendar of Confirmations and Inventories*, described in Sinclair, *Scottish Ancestors*, sect. 5. 24–5. The datasets from which these figures are drawn can be obtained from Glasgow University Archives.

[56] H. J. Perkin, *The Rise of Professional Society: England since 1880* (London, 1989), 84.

Table 6.10. Fortunes of over £10,000 left in Scotland in 1881, 1894, and 1901

Year	Number of estates	Number of estates of £10,000 or more	%
1881	5,330	270	5.07
1894	7,021	335	4.77
1901	7,263	449	5.18
Total	19,614	1,054	5.37

Source: Scottish probate calendars, 1881, 1894, 1901.

Table 6.11. Professional Fortunes of over £10,000 left in Scotland in 1881, 1894, and 1901

Year	Number of estates	Number of professional estates	%	Number of professional estates of £10,000 or more	%
1881	5,330	281	5.27	25	8.9
1894	7,021	314	4.47	25	6.96
1901	7,263	269	3.7	27	10.07
Total	19,614	864	4.41	77	8.91

Source: Scottish probate calendars, 1881, 1894, and 1901.

£100 and £600 medicine takes the lead.[57] This only emphasizes that the richest fifth of the army cohort were peculiarly affluent.

MARRIAGE

Unlike the conclusions of Leonore Davidoff and Catherine Hall in their study of family fortunes, the wives of members of the cohort played an important role in the disposal of their husband's estates.[58] This is perhaps only to be expected as wives of army officers had inevitably to live independently of their husbands during the French wars and often while they were abroad in peacetime. Whereas Davidoff and Hall found that only 28 per cent of wives acted as executors, of the 114 wills of members of the cohort which have been located, wives were named as executors in 41 (36 per cent) and 24 acted alone. Given that 27 of the wills were for unmarried men and at least six wives were dead, the proportion is over 50 per cent, which is nearer the 70 per cent identified by Peter Earle in his

[57] Digby, *Making a Medical Living*, 164–5, fig. 5.1.
[58] L. Davidoff and C. Hall, *Family Fortunes: Men and Women of the English Middle Class 1780–1850* (London, 1987), 211.

study of the London middle class a century earlier.[59] In a further eight instances a daughter was named in the absence of the wife, in another five sisters, in a further three nieces, and in one a mistress. However in the thirty-five estates of £10,000 or more only nine wives were named as executors and only in four did they act alone and in one instance with a daughter. In only one instance, that of David Maclagan, is a father-in-law named, but in his case there were twelve trustees including his wife and two of his sons.

Altogether 259 members of the cohort (57 per cent) are known to have been married and 63 (14 per cent) are thought never to have been married. Of those who were married, 19 were married twice and one, Samuel Ayrault Piper, three times. Of the 230 whose year of first marriage is known, 85 were married before or during the French wars and all but 27 married while their husbands were either in the service or would return to the colours in the future. Although it has only been possible to discover the place of birth of just 10 per cent of the wives, the place of first marriage is recorded for 224. The majority of the cohort married outside their county of birth, confirming that, as Earle observed in London between 1660 and 1730, marriage continued to be a matter of choice not of family pressure or connection.[60] Several were married a long way from home, often when stationed abroad. Henry Davies, who came from London, was married in Bermuda in 1814, Donald McNeil from Inverness-shire in Jamaica in 1805, and Edward Porteus in Florence in 1834 while inspector of health in the Ionian Isles.

Only forty-six of the husbands were married in the same county in which they were born. The place of death of thirty-five of these is known and just half died in the same county. At least three of their spouses were born elsewhere. Helen Dixon, who was born at Morpeth in Northumberland, married William Henry Burrell in Leith in 1827, presumably at the home of his parents, and then lived in Exmouth in Devon. Eliza Johnston from Hackney married Samuel Dickson in Edinburgh in 1832, again presumably at the home of his parents, and then lived in London. Given that only five of the birthplaces of these wives is known it is likely that far more came from other counties. All told, the place of birth of twenty-eight wives is known and of these only eighteen were married in the same place in which they were born. Frequently, then, neither bride nor groom had any long-standing connection with the place where they wed. William Gibney came from Westmeath and his wife Frances Dwarris from Warwick and belonged to a family with West Indian connections, but they married in a Northamptonshire church.

Through their wives a number of the cohort from nonconformist backgrounds became reconciled to the established Church, which would suggest that marriage could be a convenient way of burying a socially embarrassing background. Carpue had been brought up a Catholic but all of his five daughters were baptized at St Anne's Soho. Alderson was reared as a Presbyterian but similarly seems to have

---

[59] Peter Earle, *The Making of the English Middle Class: Business, Society and Family Life in London, 1160–1730* (London, 1989), 315.   [60] Ibid. 185–92.

accepted Anglicanism. He married Maria Hill at St George's Hanover Square on 2 November 1810 and all their children in the following decade were christened in the Church of England. A son, Richard, was even baptized in St Mary's Hull, an ancient parish church of his home town, a city where his father remained a prominent practising dissenter. Not all nonconformists, however, ended up as Anglicans. Maclagan had been raised in Edinburgh as an Episcopalian. On marriage to Jane Whiteside of Ayr, granddaughter of a moderator of the General Assembly, he must have begun to revise his spiritual options. On being released from the army and setting himself up in Edinburgh New Town, he became a staunch Presbyterian and worshipped first at St Andrew's and then St George's, Charlotte Square.[61]

Marriage was certainly a way of consolidating social status. Although the occupations of only thirty-one of the wives' fathers is known, the evidence suggests that in choosing their spouses many army doctors were seeking social advancement through establishing themselves in respectable professional families (see Table 6.12). Some married within their social milieu. Robert Keate, whose father was a prebend, married the daughter of Henry Ramus, a civil servant in the East India Company. Henry Tytler, whose father was a Church of Scotland minister, married the daughter of a merchant; while John Kinnis, whose father was a tablecloth manufacturer, married the daughter of a surgeon. A significant number, however, 'traded up'. George Guthrie, a persistent social climber whose father sold surgical goods, made a match with the daughter of the lieutenant-governor of Prince Edward's Island. Joseph Brown, whose father was a brewer, draper, and shipowner, married a colonel's daughter. Samuel Barwick Bruce, whose father was a doctor, married the daughter of the land agent of the earl of Ripon's Studley Royal estates in Yorkshire. John Davy married into the Fletcher family, well-to-do Edinburgh Whigs, that his brother's reputation and connection gave him access to: his father-in-law, already dead when he tied the knot, had been an advocate.[62] Only William Greaves is known to have married within his family. His first wife was his cousin, Anne Lydia Greaves, the daughter of his paternal uncle, the land agent, Robert Charles, while he shared a common great-grandfather with his second, Sarah, née Evans, the daughter of a clergyman.[63]

Much the same impression of 'trading up' is gained from the careers of the twenty-nine brothers-in-law, representing twenty-two families (see Table 6.12). The large majority had professional careers. Seven were in the medical profession, including Andrew Anderson's famous brother-in-law, the explorer Mungo Park. Three were in law, including William Gibney's distinguished brother-in-law, the judge and classical scholar Sir Fortunatus William Lilley Dwarris.[64] Two were clerics, one of whom held the prestigious living of Southwell Minster in Nottinghamshire. There were five army or naval officers, although three of

---

61 Norman L. Walker, *David Maclagan* (London, 1884), 32.

62 Eliza Dawson Fletcher, *Autobiography of Mrs. Fletcher of Edinburgh*, available at www.alexanderstreet4.com/cgi-bin/asp/bwld/getvolume.pl?S4649 (Oct. 2005).

63 www.gravesfa.org/gen228.htm (Sept. 2005).   64 DNB, *sub nomine*.

Table 6.12. Occupations of Sons, In-Laws, and Grandsons

Occupation	Sons	Fathers-in-law	Brothers-in-law	Sons-in-law	Nephews	Grandsons
Agriculture	4	3	2			
(Gent farmers)	(1)					
(Planters)		(1)				
(Tenants)	(1)					
(Land Agents)		(2)				
Business	10	5	5	2	2	3
(Artisan)			(1)	(1)		
(Finance)	(7)					(2)
(Manufactures)	(1)		(2)	(1)		
(Merchant)	(2)	(5)	(1)		(2)	(1)
Professions	124	23	22	17	41	33
(Administration)	(3)	(3)		(1)		(3)
(Armed Forces)	(44)	(8)	(9)	(3)	(7)	(6)
(*Lieut. Cols and above*)	*(9)*	*(1)*	*(1)*			
(Church)	(15)	(5)	(2)	(5)	(8)	(9)
(Education and Science)	(3)				(2)	(1)
(Engineering)	(4)					(1)
(Law)	(13)	(4)	(4)	(2)	(9)	(4)
(*Barristers*)	*(7)*	*(1)*		*(1)*		*(1)*
(*QCs*)	*(2)*					
(Medicine)	(42)	(3)	(7)	(6)	(15)	(9)
(*Medical professors*)	*(3)*					
(*Physicians*)	*(17)*	*(2)*	*(2)*	*(3)*	*(8)*	
(*Surgeons to the forces*)	*(12)*		*(3)*	*(1)*	*(3)*	
White Collar						1
Total	138	31	29	19	42	37
No. of families	88	30	22	17	23	17
Names Known	379	61	87	40	137	71
Possibly died young	120					
Putative adults	259					
Percentage identified	53.3	50.8	33.3	47.5	30.6	52.6

Source: Doctors' Database: Table: Relationships1.

these were McGrigor's brothers-in-law. The remainder, a quarter, were in either agriculture or trade.

The age at first marriage is known for 211 of the cohort. The average age was 34, which is five years older than that in Davidoff and Hall's study, but almost the same as the age they concluded upper middle-class men became heads of households.[65] There were, however, wide differences (Figure 6.1). George Henry Rutlege from County Sligo married Maria Tyrill in Dublin in 1810 and John Richard Elmore from London married Francis Holroyd in Cork in 1808, both at the age of 18. The oldest to marry for the first time was Alexander Stewart, who

[65] Davidoff and Hall, *Family Fortunes*, 222 and 233.

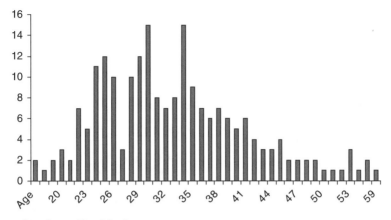

Figure 6.1. Age at First Marriage
Source: Doctors Database: Tables: Doctors, Relationship 2.

at the age of 60 took Frances Brown, eighteen years his junior, to be his wife in 1848. It has only been possible to discover the year of birth and marriage of forty-two of the first wives of members of the cohort, who had an average age of 26, a much wider age gap than Davidoff and Hall discovered.[66] Only two were older than their husbands, William Henry Burrell who at 32 was eight years his wife's junior, and John Davy who at 40 was seven years his. A few older doctors in the cohort married very young wives. James Moffitt was 46 when he married the 16-year-old Eliza Sweeny in 1835, and Alexander Melville was 39 when in 1822 he married the 21-year-old Elizabeth Sutherland, who nursed him through his long illness at her parent's home in Montrose.

The evidence supports Peter Earle's conclusion that those who married later in life left the largest fortunes.[67] Only three out of the twenty-five members of the cohort, who married before the age of 31 and whose probate valuation is known, left more than £10,000, while eleven out of seventy-one who married over the age of 30 did. The average value of the estates of those who married before the age of 31 was £3,950 and of those who married later was £6,142. This impression is further confirmed by the average value of the estates of the twenty-nine who did not marry and whose probates have been traced, which was almost £6,922.

Wives could expect a peripatetic existence after they married if as in the majority of cases their husbands were still in the army. The first three children of Thomas Fiddes and Anne Galland, who were married in Malta in 1827, were born on the island where Fiddes was stationed from 1828. Their last child was born in Ashton, Cheshire, in 1833 and he died on his way to a posting at Halifax in Canada with his family in 1835. James Steele Huston and Eliza Brown were married in Canada in 1822, their first two children were born in Amhertsburg in

---

[66] Ibid. 325.   [67] Earle, *English Middle Class*, 182.

Ontario in 1825 and 1827, their third in Quebec, their fourth in Chatham in Kent, their fifth in St John's, Newfoundland, and their last at Cove (Queenstown), County Cork, in 1836. He died in Dublin two years later. The seven children of George Johnston and Mary Anne Carter, who were married in 1815, were born in Canada, Edinburgh, Chester, Castlebar (Co. Mayo), Dublin, and Corfu.

Some wives seemed to have refused to accompany their husbands, such as Jane Kelsall, who married Tully Daly in 1815: all bar one of her six children were baptized at St Luke's in Chelsea, where she kept a succession of family homes. It is ironic that the first time she accompanied him, he was drowned trying to save the life of one of his children at the Cape of Good Hope.[68] All the six children of Clementina Dawkin and her husband William Williams were baptized at their home at Kidwelly in Carmarthenshire, between 1826 and 1835, while he was serving in Ireland and Gibraltar. There is little to suggest that wives put pressure on their husbands to seek civilian careers as only twenty-seven left the army for the last time within five years of marriage. There were thirty-four whose husbands served a further twenty years before retirement. The longest (45 years) was Francis Sievewright, who married Isabella Hill in 1798, fifteen years before he joined the army. During his military career he was constantly on the move, serving nearly all the years after the war in the West Indies, Ceylon, and India. He finally retired from Bengal in 1855. It is perhaps not surprising that only a daughter of their marriage is recorded. Another lengthy army marriage was William Henry Young to Maria Dent in 1815. She accompanied him to India in 1823 where they remained until 1854, Maria bearing five children.

One of the perils of a military marriage might be thought to be widowed early and left with a young family to educate. Sir James McGrigor was conscious of this possibility, establishing a benevolent society for widows of the hospital and regimental medical staff to provide annuities which could be purchased. Perhaps because virtually all the members of the cohort had survived the war or joined afterwards, the risk of early widowhood was relatively low. Of the 213 members of the cohort whose date of first marriage and date of death is known, only 38 (some 18 per cent) died within ten years of the ceremony and of these 15 were over the age of 40 at their wedding. There are 124 wives who were either certainly widowed or whose date of death is known. The average length of their marriages was of just under 20 years; 27 enjoyed 30 years or more. The longest was that of David Maclagan to Jane Whiteside, which lasted from 1811 until his death in 1865. McGrigor himself was married to Mary Grant for forty-eight years. Nevertheless 67 out of the 185 members of the cohort, who are known to have had families, died with children under 16 years of age. Eliza Bigg was widowed after seven years of marriage to Edward Smith Graham and left with three young sons to bring up on a widow's pension, the youngest of whom was less than a year old.[69] Joanne Hagartye was widowed in 1825 when her husband Daniel died

---

[68] TNA, WO42/12/020.   [69] TNA, WO42/19/201.

on St Helena, leaving her with a son and three daughters, one of whom was born two days after his death. There is no record of how she fared. A widow's pension was not a matter of right unless her husband had purchased an annuity from the benevolent fund and every case was considered on its merits by the board of the medical department.[70] Widows had not only to apply in writing to the War Office to prove their need, but also to send copies of their marriage licence and baptismal certificates for all their surviving children. After the death of her husband John in 1836, Eliza Murray wrote to the board to tell them that after sixteen years of marriage she was left with a family of four and the eldest had not yet reached his fourteenth birthday.[71] William Dyer Thomas instructed his executors to approach McGrigor to ensure his wife Rosa received any pension she might be entitled to.[72] Captain Irwin of the 63rd Regiment wrote from Cape Town on passage to Australia in 1829 to inform the War Office that Dr Tully Daly had drowned with his eldest son, aged 9, but that his widow intended to travel on to Swan River (Perth), where she hoped to maintain herself with the assistance of her fellow passengers.[73] She was awarded a pension. A widow whose husband had a blemished record could expect harsh treatment. John Williamson was found guilty at a court-martial in Jamaica in 1825, but died before sentence could be confirmed. His widow appealed in vain for a pension to support herself and her daughter.[74] Proven need was supposed to be the criteria for granting a pension, but this is not altogether clear. Jane Pinchney, the widow of John Fisher, and Caroline a Court, the widow of Stewart Crawford, both received pensions even though their husbands both left £12,000. At least fourteen widows whose husbands left more than £1,000 got pensions, compared with twenty-two who left less.

SONS

The average family size of the 185 members of the cohort who are known to have had children was 3.8, which compares with 2.8 in medical families in the 1880s and 1890s.[75] These figures have to be treated with caution, however, as they largely reflect children who had survived at least the first critical years of their life as they are mostly drawn from information supplied by widows to the War Office. There were sixty-two families of five children and more and sixty-seven of two or less. The largest family was that of John Phillips, whose wife Frances Crew bore thirteen children from 1783 to 1803 during his long military career that took him to the rank of inspector of hospitals. James Muttlebury and Alexander Robertson

[70] Simon Fowler and William Spencer, *Army Records for Family Historians* (London, 2000), 29–31.
[71] TNA, WO42/34/900.   [72] TNA, Prob 11/1877, q. 321.
[73] TNA, WO42/12/020.
[74] WL, RAMC MS 206, 68–70. The children did receive support from the Orphans Fund, see pp. 192–3.
[75] J. A. Banks, *Victorian Values: Secularism and the Size of Families* (London, 1981), 98–9.

both had eleven children and John Harper Sprague ten. There is no obvious correlation between wealth at death and family size. John Phillips left £16,000, James William Macauley (8 children) £14,000, Alexander Dunlop Anderson (8 children) £27,522, and Robert Keate (7 children) £35,000, whereas Alexander Robertson (9 children) left £300, Robert Brown (8 children) £600, and William Roberts (9 children) had no estate worth recording.

It is difficult to test Jose Harris's hypothesis that investment in the education and training of children was of more importance than inheritance, but such evidence as there is suggests a need for qualification. Much of what has been written about education in this period has tended to emphasize the increasing plurality of formal provision available to the middle class rather than investigating the more challenging subject of family experience and strategies.[76] Of the 379 sons of 159 members of the cohort that have been identified, it has only been possible to discover the schools that 23 attended and the place of higher education of 78, of whom 14 went to the Royal Military Academy at Sandhurst, one to Woolwich, and one to Addiscombe (the Indian Army's college). Since school rolls for leading public schools and matriculation records for all eight universities in the United Kingdom are readily accessible, this suggests contrary to the perception of many historians that the sons of these professional men were not being prepared for a career through public schools and universities. Moreover several of the sons who did matriculate at universities came from the few families where higher education was well established.[77] Andrew George Anderson and his brother Thomas McCall Anderson, who matriculated at Glasgow in 1850 and 1852 respectively, were surrounded by three generations of relatives with a university education. Their great uncle John Anderson had been professor of natural philosophy and by his will founded the Andersonian University.[78] Robert William Keate (Oxford 1814) and Edward Keate (Woolwich 1833) came from a family with a long tradition of university attendance. Their grandfather, great-grandfather, great-great-grandfather, and three of their father's brothers had been at Cambridge. Only in three cases did all the sons in a family receive higher education. Francis Leigh sent his three sons and Robert Shekleton his two to their *alma mater* Trinity College Dublin, while Charles St John's three sons went to Sandhurst. There is a correlation between father's wealth and higher education. Of the 52 sons who received higher education and whose father's wealth is known, the fathers of 41 (79 per cent) left almost £2,000 or more and 32 £8,000 or more. This was also true in Scotland, where entrance to university was supposed to have been more democratic and less expensive. Habakkuk argued that even for the aristocracy and gentry cost of education inhibited the entry of younger sons into the learned professions which required a degree.[79] There is no indication that there was any preference by order

[76] See for example Davidoff and Hall, *Family Fortunes*, 234–40.
[77] Cf. what was said in Ch. 2.
[78] W. Innes Addison, *The Matriculation Albums of the University of Glasgow from 1728 to 1858* (Glasgow, 1913), no. 872.   [79] Habakkuk, *Marriage, Debt and the Estates System*, 114.

of birth in deciding which sons should receive a higher education, even amongst the worse-off members of the cohort.

The occupations of 138 of the 379 sons have been identified, representing 88 families. Childhood mortality probably accounted for a third. John Davy's family may well have been typical. Of his five children, his two younger sons, Humphry and John Miles, died of scarlet fever as infants, and his eldest daughter, Elizabeth, of consumption in her early twenties. Only his eldest son, Archibald, and younger daughter, Grace, survived into adult life.[80] If this is the case, then it would leave only some 120 sons of the cohort whose careers have not been traced. Of these it can be assumed a good proportion settled outside the United Kingdom. One member of the cohort whose sons definitely did so was James Muttlebury. Muttlebury came from Wells in Somerset and when he left the army he spent the 1820s practising in Bath. In 1832, however, he left for Canada to take over land that he had acquired in York township (early Toronto) but was dead within a few months. His wife and children seem to have stayed in England but three at least of his sons—Rutherford, Frederick Creighton, and James William—eventually settled in the colony, where they practised as barristers.[81]

Although it may have been possible to discover the occupations of more sons through the time-consuming scrutiny of probate calendars and local directories, it was beyond the scope and resources of this study. The impression gained from the occupations of those who can be certainly identified is that members of the cohort, irrespective of their country of origin, understandably wanted their sons to consolidate or maintain the status that they had come to enjoy as army surgeons. For the most part, this meant that sons followed their fathers into the professions, even if only a handful attended the top public schools and less than a fifth went to a university. As might be expected, medicine was one of the most popular career choices—embraced by 42 of the 138 (30 per cent)—but it was just beaten into second place by the armed forces, which attracted 44 (32 per cent) (see Table 6.12).

Interestingly only in seven instances was a career in medicine chosen in the third generation—that is where an army surgeon's son had a father and a grandfather or great-uncle in the profession. Charles Le-Gay Brereton, son of Charles Brereton, no doubt became a doctor so that he could take over the lucrative practice of his father in Beverley and succeed to his position in East Riding society. However after a dispute with his brother-in-law and partner Dr Hartley in about 1867, he retired from the practice at the age of 51, moved away, and was more or

---

[80] www.spaceless.com/fletcher/flet11.htm (Oct. 2005).

[81] Rutherford had been admitted to Cambridge as a sizar in 1831 but never resided: Venn, iv. 506. The third brother, James William, was the deputy district master of Toronto's Loyal Orange Association of British North America in 1849: see http://members.tripod.com/~Roughian/index~144.html (Nov. 2005). He eventually returned to Britain for he married at Kew in 1860 and settled in London: see http://archives.rootsweb.com/th/read/India/2004-09/1094458682 (Nov. 2005); www.ancestry.com (Nov. 2005): *sub* English census 1871 (James W. Muttlebury: 164, Westbourne Terrace, Paddington). James William's son, Frederick Duff (d. 1933), went to Eton and Cambridge and became a famous rowing blue.

less cut out of his father's will.[82] John James Hume and John Hennen followed
their distinguished fathers into the army, unsurprisingly uninterested in setting up
their plate in small-town Ireland and Scotland where their grandfathers had been
in practice. Hume's intention may well have been ultimately to join his father in
his London practice but he was murdered by rebels in Upper Canada in 1838,
only two years after joining up.[83] Charles Fitzroy Macauley and Henry Frederick
Robertson similarly followed their fathers into the army rather than set up in
civilian practice as their great-uncles had done.

Only two families of the seven, moreover, were large and distinguished medical
dynasties. These were the Dunlop Andersons and the Maclagans. Three Maclagan
brothers, Andrew Douglas, Philip Whiteside, and James McGrigor followed their
father, David, and their maternal grandfather, Philip Whiteside, into medicine
and became MDs. The most distinguished was Andrew Douglas, who was professor
of medical jurisprudence in the University of Edinburgh from 1869 to 1896 and
who was knighted for his medical services in 1885. Two of his sons, also, became
doctors and David Maclagan had the distinction of being photographed towards
the end of his life with three generations of Edinburgh medical practitioners.
Philip Whiteside Maclagan joined the army medical service and later settled down
in civilian life as a practitioner in Berwick-on-Tweed. His botanist brother James
McGrigor Maclagan was a surgeon in the Indian Medical Service for four years
before returning to practise in Northumberland and Scotland. He was subsequently medical superintendent of the Morayshire County Lunatic Asylum in
Elgin and later resident physician and surgeon at the Edinburgh Royal Infirmary.
Two of Alexander Dunlop Anderson's sons also studied medicine and at least one
of his nephews. The eldest, Andrew George, abandoned his medical career to
become chairman of the Union Mortgage and Agency Company of Australia,
while his brother, Thomas McCall Anderson, became regius professor of medicine at Glasgow and gained an international reputation and a knighthood for his
contribution to dermatology.[84]

At least eight more sons joined the army medical corps, including Henry Skey
Muir, the son of Henry Muir, who rose to the rank of surgeon-general (the late
nineteenth-century title of the director-general). David Henry Symes Wright, the son
of David Wright, joined the Royal Navy. The brothers William George and Edward
Roberts joined their father in his practice at Sydenham in Kent, William Thomas
Latham was in partnership with his in County Antrim, while Charles William
Gardiner Guthrie worked with his outstanding surgeon father, George James
Guthrie at the Westminster Hospital but was forced to retire early due to ill-health.[85]

No doubt their childhood experience attracted sons to the armed forces, but
in the post-war years obtaining a commission was difficult given the massive

[82] Marjorie Sutherland, *The Brereton Family*, typescript available in East Riding Record Office,
Beverley.   [83] Addison, *Matriculation Albums*, no. 11978.
[84] Tom Gibson, *The Royal College of Physicians and Surgeons of Glasgow* (Glasgow, 1983), 71.
[85] *Lancet*, 10 Jan. (1844), 1003.

reduction. Of the thirty-five families who sent forty-three sons into the army and one into the navy as regular officers, five of the fathers achieved the rank of inspector-general of hospitals, two of physician to the forces, three of apothecary to the forces, two of inspector of hospitals, and three of deputy or assistant inspector of hospitals. Eleven never rose above the rank of surgeon, six of assistant surgeon, and of these, six died young leaving children under the age of 15. The value of the estates of twenty-two fathers is known. Of these, thirteen left £20,000 or more, of whom six had only been army surgeons, and three left children under 14. For instance, Richard Humfrey left £25,000 and John Murray, whose son was only 5 when he died, £22,068, more than enough to buy a commission.

In the post-war army, money alone was not enough to secure a military appointment: influence was vital. John Christopher Alderson, whose father Christopher, a surgeon at Waterloo, died young, came from a prominent East Riding medical family with money, land, and contacts. Samuel Barwick Bruce, the father of Robert Cathcart Dalrymple Bruce, was distantly related to the earl of Elgin and a man of consequence in the North Riding. Robert Dwarris Gibney was equally both well connected and monied with a rich West Indian maternal ancestry. Frederick William Gregory's father had served on the staff of Lord William Bentinck in Italy in 1811. In trying to buy a commission for his son, Frederick Albert Loinsworth, at the time the well-heeled deputy inspector-general of hospitals of the Bombay presidency, quoted his own record of service in the Peninsula with Sir John Moore and Lord Hill, 'which I trust may be considered by His Excellency [the commander-in-chief] to strengthen my position'.[86]

As a result, some poorly placed but well-protected sons still obtained a commission. Edward Nugent Daly, whose assistant surgeon father was drowned at the Cape of Good Hope, was presumably helped to gain an ensignship by his father's brother officers. The same seems to be true of Lewis Augustus Brydon, whose assistant surgeon father died on active service in the West Indies when he was only 2, and John Bickerson Flanagan, whose father seems to have been badly wounded since he applied for relief to the compassionate fund.[87] The route into the army for one son was through the Royal Military Academy at Woolwich and for another thirteen through the Royal Military College, founded in 1807 and based at Sandhurst since 1812.[88] Of these, six probably received a free place as they were orphans whose mothers had been granted widows pensions. This privilege was withdrawn in 1838 on the grounds it was often impossible for such poor scholarship boys to buy commissions.

The prospects for any young officer without wealth and patronage were poor, as the impecunious Richard Webster, not a member of the cohort, found to his cost.[89] He purchased a commission for his two sons in the 34th by borrowing

---

[86] Loinsworth to Major MacDonald, military secretary, Bombay, 25 June 1838, Loinsworth papers, BL, Oriental and India Office, European MS D758.   [87] TNA, WO42/16/125.
[88] One of the fourteen sons who attended Sandhurst did not gain a commission.
[89] Hew Strachan, *Wellington's Legacy: The Reform of the British Army 1830–1854* (Manchester, 1984), 125–30.

money from a friend, but was forced 'to sell out at a great loss', when he was unable to repay the loan. At his wit's end, he then secured one of them an ensignship 'without purchase', but was then faced with the cost of buying his uniform and equipment.[90]

Remarkably at a time of intense competition for promotion, nine sons rose to the rank of lieutenant colonel or above and of these just the well-connected Frederick William Gregory had a father who was not of senior rank. Only one of their fathers had died before they were under 20 years of age, William Markland Lyons, whose father had been apothecary to the forces. The two who became senior officers, General Robert Maclagan and Major General Edward Keate, had not only wealthy but well-connected fathers. David Maclagan was surgeon in ordinary to the queen in Scotland and Robert Keate was surgeon to successive monarchs.

The army may have already been, as it later became, a career for those who lacked ability or inclination to enter other professions, especially those with good connections and a spirit of adventure. The two youngest sons of Alexander Dunlop Anderson did not attend medical classes at the University of Glasgow, not because their father did not have the means but presumably because they lacked ability. His third son and namesake was packed off to Cheltenham College to prepare himself for a military career. He was killed at Peiwar Kotal in Afghanistan in 1878 at the age of 37 with the rank of a major in the 23rd Punjab Bengal Native Infantry (Pioneers).[91] A military career was also highly respectable in the Victorian era given the number of gentry sons who continued to enter the army officer corps. As Habakkuk argued, 'the army provided a career which was acceptable to a man of rank, congenial to the upbringing and natural talents of landed families, and except in time of war, compatible with a social life'.[92] This is just what seems to have attracted sons of members of the cohort to the profession, coupled with the adventure and travel many of them had experienced as children. William St John, the son of Inspector-General Charles St John had been brought up in India. He recorded in his diary the carefree life of the military in Bloemfontein in the early 1850s; his days filled with hunting game and playing billiards.[93]

If the cost of university education inhibited many sons from attending higher education, then it necessarily restricted the numbers receiving ordination in the Churches of England and Ireland, which required their clergy to be graduates. Tellingly, of the fifteen sons of thirteen families who entered the Church, only one of the eight fathers whose wealth at death is recorded left less than £3,000. This was the socially ambitious but financially injudicious George James Guthrie, who sent both his sons to Westminster School and his eldest, Lowry, who was destined for the Church, to Cambridge. Just as in the army, wealth and connection brought

90 WL, RAMC 262/8, no. 27: Webster to Lindsay, 2 Dec. 1825; no. 29, 7 Feb. 1826.
91 *Calendar of Confirmations in Scotland*, 1879. See also n. 94 below.
92 Habakkuk, *Marriage, Debt and the Estates System*, 111.
93 Karel Schoeman, *The Bloemfontein Diary of Lieut. W. J. St John* (Cape Town, 1988).

preferment. William Dalrymple Maclagan, who began his career as an army officer, became archbishop of York.[94] Samuel Peach Boutflower, whose father had influence in the north-west of England and left £3,000, became archdeacon of Carlisle. Talbot Adin Ley Greaves, whose father was an assistant inspector of hospitals and left £8,000, became vicar of Holy Trinity Clifton in Bristol, a leading evangelical parish. Henry George Phillips, whose father had been surgeon to George IV's household and left £16,000, was the incumbent of two good Suffolk livings. John Hemery Carnegie, whose father left £5,000, was vicar of Cranbourne in Dorset, and even Lowry Guthrie was presented to the benefice of Cranleigh in Surrey. These were not the poorly endowed industrial or urban parishes of the struggling clergy.[95] Davy's eldest and only surviving son, Archibald, was educated by his father's good friend Thomas Arnold at Rugby and Trinity College, Cambridge. He became a clergyman in the Church of England and spent much of his life as personal chaplain to the dilettante poet and antiquarian John Byrbe Leicester Warren, the last baron de Tabley of Knutsford, an appointment he probably owed to his family's friendship with Mrs Gaskell. He held a living on the estate, but also inherited the family house in the Lake District.[96]

Although the costs of entry to the bar were even higher than those to the armed services or the Church, success depended more on ability than patronage.[97] Nevertheless Walter Grant James McGrigor, Sir James's second son, and Henry Tudor Davies and Reginald Stevenson Davies, the sons of Henry Davies the well-known obstetrician, could boast impeccable connections to launch them on their careers. Of the thirteen sons from eleven families who became lawyers, three were educated at Cambridge, and one each at Dublin, the Inns of Court, and Oxford. The remainder were presumably apprenticed. Four of the six fathers whose wealth at death is recorded, left £8,000 or more and the other two were pillars of the local community. Robert William Shekelton, whose father left only £300, had strong family links in Dublin society on which to build his career as a barrister, as did his elder brother in medicine. The estate of Joseph Brown (£1,500), the father of Joseph McGrigor Aird Brown, certainly under-represented his wealth, much of which was invested in property in Sunderland, where he practised and served a term as mayor.

It is the accepted view that the learned professions and the armed services were the automatic careers of choice for the sons of the professional and upper middle

---

[94] Thus 16 sons eventually entered the Church, not 15. According to the Archbishop's second wife, Augusta Barrington, William Dalrymple had wanted to enter the Church from the start but his father had not felt he was bright enough. 'His wish from the first was to take Holy Orders, but his father dissuaded him, saying "you have no intellect & will only starve all your life on a curacy, whereas the Duke will give you a commission & you can go and make your fortune in India".' 'Memorials' of Augusta Maclagan, 399, Maclagan family papers (private collection).

[95] B. Heeney, *A Different Kind of Gentleman: Parish Clergy as Professional Men in Early and Mid-Victorian England* (Hamden, Conn., 1975).

[96] www.spaceless.com/fletcher/flet11.htm (Oct. 2005).

[97] Habakkuk, *Marriage, Debt and the Estates System*, 113–14.

class in the nineteenth century.[98] The occupations of the sons of the cohort suggest that this opinion needs to be nuanced. A small number of the surgeons' sons entered the new professions. Four were civil engineers—Robert Henry Bow, James Benjamin Marlow Cruikshank, David Law, and Francis Lightbody—and two entered the developing colonial service: Henry Tudor Davies, who became commissioner of Chinese Imperial Marine Customs and the well-connected Robert William Keate, who had a glittering career ending as governor of Trinidad and later Natal. Sydney James, the second son of William James, became a civil servant, Alexander Wallace an astronomer at the Royal Observatory, and William Alexander Campbell Cruikshank a 'professor' (teacher) of music in Burnley in Lancashire. There were almost certainly more teachers but the profession was largely unregulated until the twentieth century and it is hard to identify individuals. Other sons entered the burgeoning world of business and finance, though here again there must have been many more than has been uncovered.[99] Significantly, on the other hand, very few seem to have entered trade or manufacturing, despite the fact that many of the cohort hailed from such a background. In at least one case, too, a career in industry does not seem to have been planned. William Black inherited his grandfather's textile business in the Scottish borders, only because neither his father, Ebenezer, nor his uncle wished to work in it.[100] To this extent, then, the anti-trade rhetoric of contemporary novelists such as Surtees and Trollope seems to reflect social reality.

There are only three examples of fathers buying property to set up their sons as landed gentlemen. Richard William Batty purchased Broats near Gretna Green, though he took the precaution of sending his son to the University of Glasgow. John Philipps owned the West Farm estate near Barton in Suffolk which he left in its entirety to his fourth son and namesake.[101] In the 1840s William Parrott acquired land in Cape Province for his son Henry Daniel.[102] There were other members of the cohort, who were owners of real estate, but these seem to have been investments rather than intended as a family seat. Robert Brown (not to be mixed up with Joseph) had properties in Faversham and Strood, which he instructed could be sold by his executors.[103] John McRobert had a 45-acre farm in County Down, hardly large enough to be the residence of a country gentleman without other means of support and which in any event he divided equally at his

[98] See for example Perkin, *Rise of Professional Society*, 84, and Hoppen, *Mid-Victorian Generation*, 44.
[99] Since completing the manuscript of this book, the authors have had access to the 1851–1901 census registers for England and Wales through www.ancestry.com (Jan. 2006) and to the 1861 census for Scotland through www.scotlandspeople.gov.uk (Dec. 2005). Among the new sons discovered are three with white-collar rather than professional occupations. The retired army surgeon, Charles Annersley, was practising in Chelsea in 1851: both his sons were clerks, one with an accountancy firm, one in the WO. This would suggest that the less successful practitioners placed their sons in the sub-professions rather than trade, if they could not put them into the professions proper.
[100] NAS, SC40/40/11, and Roxburgh sasines, 1830, no. 2285, 1834, nos. 626–7, 1845, no. 1041, 1853, no. 725, and 1866, no. 504.
[101] TNA, IR 26 1558, fo. 284; Prob 11/1928, q. 358.
[102] NASA, KAB CO LEER 404 801 88 1.   [103] Will: First Avenue House, Calendar, 1865.

death between his four surviving children. Charles Aesculapius Newcomb owned houses in Camberwell, as did Sir Charles Fergusson Forbes.[104] William Greaves, who was the tenant of Mayfield Hall in Staffordshire, purchased farms at Oldbury, near Thornbury in Gloucestershire, along with the 'Rising Sun' public house. On his death this property was split up amongst his widow, daughter, son, and grandchildren.[105]

Although a family's economic position was an important element in determining the range of career choice, the wealthiest members of the cohort did not necessarily direct all their sons into established professions. Admittedly, of the thirteen members of the cohort who had families and left more than £10,000, only Stewart Crawford did not send at least one son to university or place a son in either the learned professions or the armed services. However, among the sons of the twelve who did, there were three in business, three who described themselves as simple gentlemen, and twenty whose occupation is unrecorded, some of whom may also have been living off rents. Indeed, a number of sons of army surgeons who were only moderately well off may also have lived as landless gentlemen in fairly reduced circumstances.[106] Of the 77 sons of 35 fathers who left between £1,000 and £10,000, the occupations of 45 (58 per cent) is unrecorded. On the other hand, even where a son inherited landed property with sufficient income to support an independent lifestyle, this did not necessarily mean that he abandoned his chosen career. George Home, who inherited the family's Whitefield estate in Edinburgh on his father's death in 1875, was an established medical practitioner in Hull and remained there until his death a decade later. It was his brother Eugene who farmed the residue of the family's Manderston estate in Berwickshire.

Seemingly, then, most sons of the cohort ended up in the professions or business or, less certain, lived off rents. Where there was more than one son in the family, care was usually taken to ring the professional changes, doubtless in part a reflection of filial preference. Among the best-documented families are those of Sir James McGrigor (£25,000), David Maclagan (£25,523), John Lightbody (£9,863), and William Cruikshank (estate not known). McGrigor set up his eldest son, Charles Rhoderic, in the lucrative business of acting as an army agent, in effect as a private banker. His second son, Walter Grant James, he sent to Trinity College, Cambridge, from which he graduated and, after toying with the ideas of being an engineer or a churchman, became a barrister. Both sons married daughters of senior military officers, Charles the second daughter of Major General Sir Robert Nickle and Walter the eldest daughter of Vice-Admiral Digby. Charles, however, in monetary terms made the best choice, leaving a fortune of £191,772, while Walter left only a modest competence of £3,258. Maclagan's two eldest sons, Andrew Douglas and Philip Whiteside, and his youngest, James McGrigor, followed him into medicine through the University of Edinburgh, the

---

[104] TNA, Prob 11/1816, q. 317   [105] TNA, Prob 11/2086, q. 25.
[106] Six sons seem to have lived as gentlemen off a private income. Three of these had been to Oxbridge and one, James Humfrey, son of Richard, was a JP in Monmouthshire.

third son Robert joined the Royal Engineers and was to become a general, and the fourth and sixth sons, David and John Thomson, entered the thriving Edinburgh insurance industry. William Dalrymple, the fifth son, studied law at the University of Edinburgh, but then joined the 51st Madras Native Cavalry where commissions did not have to be purchased. He was only two years in India before being invalided out and coming home to go to Peterhouse in Cambridge in preparation for ordination into the Church of England. He held prestigious London Evangelical incumbencies before being consecrated bishop of Lichfield and then archbishop of York.[107] The two eldest Lightbody sons, John and Thomas Dehane, became surgeons, while the youngest Francis was a civil engineer, a new profession closely aligned with business. Of the four sons of William Cruikshank, one joined the army, one became a music teacher, one an engineer, and the last a financial agent.

OTHER DEPENDANTS

It was beyond the scope and resources of this study to research the lives of the 339 daughters of 148 of the families in the cohort, just as it was of the occupations of the 100 odd sons whose profession has not been identified. This would be practical as often their places of residences and their married names are recorded. For the most part they remain invisible during their father's lives. Mary Collier's biography of her father Charles Collier suggests that at least some of them shared in their father's literary and scientific work.[108] She was born in 1841 and lived with him in London after her mother's death in about 1860. Not only did she document his career, particularly his work in Ceylon, she also helped with his philological enquiries and his exploration of the Greek, Latin, Spanish, French, and German languages. Memoirs are probably extant for others but these along with their own life histories await investigation. The only time daughters become really visible was at the time of their father's death, when they are mentioned in testamentary dispositions and named by their widowed mothers in pension applications to the War Office. As was accepted practice amongst the middle class, the members of the cohort divided their property equitably amongst their sons and daughters and often, if they had no surviving children, amongst grandchildren, their siblings, and nieces and nephews.[109]

Charles Whyte, who left £12,000 in 1881, bequeathed £3,000 each to his two daughters, Helen Hawkden Palin and Adela Jane Mackenzie, and to his widowed

[107] His career change cannot have completely pleased his father, who did not pay for him to go to Cambridge but lent him the money (£500) instead. William Dalrymple paid an annual interest on the sum for the rest of his father's life and also an interest on his small army pension: 'Memorials' of Augusta Maclagan, 403, Maglagan family papers (private collection).

[108] *Deputy Inspector General of Army Hospitals, C. Collier.... A Life Sketch by his Daughter, M. A. E. L.* (London, 1870). His literary oeuvre is discussed in Ch. 7.

[109] See for example Amy Louise Erickson, *Women & Property in Early Modern England* (London, 1993), 162–73, and Earle, *English Middle Class*, 311–23.

daughter-in-law, Charlotte Caroline Whyte. He gave only £500 to his surviving son, Frederick English Whyte, and £1,000 to his third daughter, Emily Frances Downes, as they had already benefited from his settlement. He also left his two unmarried sisters £100 each.[110] George Robertson Baillie in a most complicated disposition left his two sons £500 each, three of his daughters £1,333 each, and four £495 each.[111] William Thornton, whose probate valuation was £2,000 but was worth very much more because of his substantial investments in property, left the whole of his real and personal estate to his widow, which was to be divided equally amongst his three daughters on her death. He split the residue of his estate between his two sons Captain Charles Frederick Thornton and William Henry Thornton, a general practitioner who also inherited his medical books, midwifery, tooth, and surgical implements.[112] Joseph Brown left the bulk of his estate, mostly property in Sunderland, to his son Joseph McGrigor Aird Brown on condition that his widow and his three daughters could live with him and his wife. On his widow's death, the property was to be sold and divided amongst the surviving children, if the daughters were married.[113] 'Having already provided for my sons', Thomas Draper bequeathed the two of them specific items of furniture and jewellery and left the residue, valued at some £240, to his improbably named daughter, Emeline Jane Cassandra.[114] Illegitimate children were also provided for. Edward Porteus left his illegitimate son, George, his gold snuff box, breakfast canteen, turquoise ring, silver watch, gold chain and seals, and £1,500 in 3 per cent consoles.[115] Patrick Paterson left his illegitimate daughter an annuity of £50 a year until she was married or aged 21.[116] The unmarried Michael Fogerty not only provided for an illegitimate daughter, but also for two of his mistresses, one in Jamaica and the other in Nottinghamshire.[117]

Daughters also defined themselves and their expectations through marriage. Altogether the occupations of nineteen out of forty sons-in-law is known, representing fifteen families (see Table 6.12). These confirm much the same pattern as those of the cohort's sons: the surgeons were primarily marrying their daughters into the professional middle classes. There were six doctors, five rectors, two lawyers, and three officers in the armed forces, a sugar refiner, a builder, and the comptroller of the General Post Office. Only one of the doctors was in the army. McGrigor's rector son-in-law, Frederick Parr Phillips, was no ordinary cleric, leaving over £180,000.

Childless members of the cohort usually provided for their wives, if they survived them, and then divided their estates between siblings, nephews, and nieces. Bachelors did much the same. John Gogill Leath, who had no children, provided

110 *Probate Calendar England and Wales*, 1881.
111 TNA, Prob 11/1893, q. 217; and IR 26/1473, fo. 206.
112 TNA, IR 26/1785, fo. 220; Prob 11/2053, q. 278.
113 *Probate Calendar England and Wales*, 1868.
114 TNA, IR 26/1863, fo. 710; Prob 11/2120, q. 730.   115 TNA, IR 26/1655, fo. 852.
116 TNA, IR 26/924, fo.1425; Prob 11/1664, q. 609.
117 TNA, IR 26/1674, fo. 418; Prob 11/2003, q. 630.

for his widow and his sister and her two children out of his estate of £11,000.[118] They all lived together in Notting Hill. Likewise the childless widower George Paulet Morris made bequests to a legion of nieces and nephews and great nieces out of his considerable estate. They were not all treated equally, possibly reflecting their circumstances.[119] Sir Charles Fergusson Forbes, who was unmarried, divided the bulk of his £5,000 and leasehold property in Camberwell equally between his five nieces and one nephew but made special provision for the one nephew, William Forbes Laurie, who had followed him into medicine.[120] Joseph Skey, another childless widower, scattered his £20,000 across an extended family of great nieces and cousins, including a doctor husband of a niece, Borrie Sewell, who got £50, and his distinguished surgeon cousin Frederick Carpenter Skey, who cannot have needed the £500 he was left.[121] The unmarried Stephen Panting divided his £20,000 up amongst his solicitor brother, Thomas, who received £3,000, and seven nieces and nephews who received between £1,000 and £1,500 apiece.[122] John Robert Hume, whose wife and two children were both dead, left his £45,000 to his five grandchildren and cancelled all the debts owed to him by his-son-in law, Archibald Campbell.[123] The probably unmarried Samuel Jeyes left his bedroom carriage clock to one niece, his silver plate to be divided between three others, four silver dining room candlesticks to his nephew Philadelphus Jeyes, the inventor of the eponymous fluid, and the residue of his estate (valued at £450) to another nephew Francis Ferdinando Jeyes.[124] Andrew Browne, when he died childless in 1848, left his widow the life interest in his estate of £23,500, willing that on her death the sum should be divided between the son and daughters of his brother, Peter Rutledge Browne, a captain in the 9th regiment on half-pay, who lived at Janesville, near Killough, Downshire. His 12-year-old nephew, Andrew Smythe Montague Browne, did particularly well. He not only was to receive ultimately half the estate but while his aunt was alive he was given £180 from the annual interest for his maintenance and educaton. In the hope that he might follow him and his father into the army, Andrew left him his sword and accoutrements. He was not to be disappointed. Andrew Smythe went to Sandhurst and rose to the rank of major general.[125]

Childless couples or bachelors seem to have more generally helped out with the education of nephews in order to consolidate the professional standing of their extended family. The bachelor Archibald Arnott, who left over £10,000, sent five of his nephews, the sons of his elder brother John and Catherine Shortt, to Edinburgh, his old *alma mater*, to study medicine.[126] The second of the nephews, John, and his uncle's heir, became surgeon-general of the Bombay Medical

---

[118] *Probate Calendar England and Wales*, 1859. This includes the £5,000 in his marriage settlement.
[119] TNA, Prob 11/1884, q. 678.   [120] TNA, IR 27/1930, fo. 214; Prob 11/2151, q. 304.
[121] *Probate Calendar England and Wales*, 1865.   [122] TNA, IR 26/1236, fo. 260.
[123] TNA, Prob 11/2248, q. 206.
[124] First Avenue House, Calendar: Wills and Administrations 1872, I–L, *sub nomine*.
[125] www.user.dccnet.com/s.brown/familytree/BROWNE-Janeville-Montague.htm, and TNA, Prob 11/2074.   [126] James Arnott, *The House of Arnott* (Edinburgh, 1918), 126–32.

Department and an honorary surgeon to the queen. Lawrence, the nephew of the bachelor Stephen Panting and son of his brother Thomas, the Lichfield solicitor, was aided through Shrewsbury and Oxford and became a Church of England clergyman. Probably because his education had been paid for, he did not inherit, unlike his four siblings, a quarter share in the residue of his uncle's £20,000 estate.[127] Henry William Markham's brother, Charles, was a master in Chancery and had six sons, three of whom went into the law and a fourth, William Orlando, into medicine. The fact that Henry William left these nephews nothing in his will out of his substantial estate again more than suggests he had contributed to their education. He left the bulk of his fortune to his sister Elizabeth and his brothers John and Christopher.[128] Similarly, John Mort Bunny in his will left his nephew Joseph, who had followed him into the medical profession, just 19 guineas, almost certainly because he had helped put him through his training.[129]

Other childless surgeons singled out nephews already established in the professions to be their heirs, whether or not they had played any part in their education. Doubtless the intention thereby was to ensure the extension of the family professional dynasty into a further generation. William Laurie, one of the nephews of Sir Charles Fergusson Forbes, became a doctor and was handsomely provided for in his will.[130] George Paulet Morris left a large legacy to his nephew, George Morris, a clergyman at Hamble near Southampton. John Jeremiah Bigsby left his fortune of £9,000 to his nephew, the Reverend Henry Julian Bigsby. Henry Julian was one of three of John Jeremiah's five nephews who attended Oxbridge and entered the Church. Presumably, he believed that Henry Julian, vicar of St Thomas's Southborough in Kent, and son of his younger brother, Charles, also a clergyman, was the most in need of his clerical nephews.[131]

Apart from bequests to members of their families, a few remembered friends and servants in their wills or left money to charity. Alexander Dunlop Anderson left 19 guineas to the family's old nursery maid and £25 to his coachman.[132] Sir Charles Fergusson Forbes gave £50 to his two servants.[133] Samuel Jeyes left all his household furniture and other articles to his housekeeper. William Burgess Morle gave his servant a bedstead and feather bed, blankets, and a leather trunk along with an annuity of £15 a year.[134] John Kinnis bequeathed £100 to the secretary of the Benevolent Fund for the Relief of the Widows and Orphans of Army Medical Officers.[135] George Richard Melin gave £100 to the same fund and very ecumenically £50 each to the Protestant and Catholic Poor of St Mary's parish Youghall.[136] Such benefactions, however, were few and far between, and the impression is that the members of the cohort, even if childless or unmarried, were

---

[127] TNA, IR 26/1236, fo. 260.   [128] TNA, Prob 11/1925.
[129] TNA, Prob 11/2079.   [130] TNA, IR 27/1930, fo. 214, and Prob 11/2151, q. 304.
[131] First Avenue House, Calendar: CRO M3114–15, 3175.
[132] NAS, SC36/51/59, fo. 390.   [133] TNA, IR 27/1930, fo. 214; Prob 11/2151, q. 304.
[134] TNA, Prob 11/2018, qs. 95–6.   [135] NAS, SC70/4/23, fos. 240–74.
[136] TNA, Prob 11/1863, q. 370.

more concerned to provide for their extended families than to contribute to the well-being of the community.

MAKING MONEY AND FORGING
PROFESSIONAL DYNASTIES

A small proportion of the cohort left only a small estate, often those who died relatively young. Most, though, wherever they ended their lives, were comfortably off, and the third who left more than £5,000 were clearly well-to-do. A few owed their material fortune to a lucky inheritance. But the large majority owed their wealth to professional success, either in or out of the army. The largest fortune was left by Michael Lambton Este, whose father, Charles, had left at least £17,000 when he died in 1828. But Michael, it will be recalled, had been left nothing in his father's will on the grounds that he was already provided for.[137] His £60,000 fortune was his own. The most successful, too, came from all corners of the kingdoms of Britain and Ireland. If most of the wealthy died in England, they were not all Englishmen. The Aberdeen merchant's son, McGrigor, who died worth £25,000 demonstrated what a Scot who had dedicated his professional life to the army medical service could make out of a military career. Andrew Browne, whose father was an apothecary in County Mayo and who left his widow £20,000, showed what an Irishman could do if able to enjoy twenty years on half-pay .

The subsequent family histories of the members of the cohort, which have been traced, tends to confirm Corfield's view that the professions consolidated themselves within the middle class in the early years of Queen Victoria's reign.[138] They were self-conciously creating dynasties that in some cases have persisted to the present day, for example, the Maclagans and the Montague Brownes. Although some of the families that can claim to have enjoyed such success were already in some ways privileged before the experience of army service, the opportunities it afforded for patronage and wealth creation allowed many more to exploit the growth in the professions after the French wars, not just for their sons and daughters but for an extended family. Many enhanced their chances of professional success by prudent marriages into affluent professional families. In consequence, they had the wherewithal to launch their sons on a path to similar success by giving them the education and training they needed to enter in their turn the professions (both learned and new) and in some cases the world of finance. Although the largest group of sons followed their fathers into the medical profession, there is little sign that the cohort thought in terms of forging medical dynasties. Their primary aim was to ensure their sons—and their daughters too through marriage—were firmly embedded in a section of the middle class into which they themselves had seldom been born.

---

[137] See p. 270.   [138] Corfield, *Power and the Professions*.

In doing this, they were not necessarily mimicking the behaviour of their peers in the officers mess, but participating in a trend which encompassed the younger sons of the aristocracy and gentry, and was a consequence of Britain's increased economic power and enlarged imperial possessions after the French wars. An extended empire and rapid industrialization at home needed the professional services of growing numbers of public servants, doctors, military officers, lawyers, clergymen, engineers, teachers, and bankers, and had the resources to pay for them. Such openings, which were well paid and secure, were attractive to professional fathers who considered themselves as participating in the movement that Corfield identified.

It is misleading to think of them as Loudon does as 'men of property', owning land with the ambition to become rentiers. This implies assimilation into a gentry class. The way most of them invested and disposed of their fortunes emphatically makes clear that they had no such ambitions. The equitable distribution of estates, long established amongst the middle class, is incompatible with landed estates which by their very nature pass from one generation to another. The wealthy fathers in the cohort could launch their sons and daughters and nieces and nephews into professional society, but it was up to them to use their talents to build on their inheritance. Inevitably, then, the cohort's sons did not always fair as well as their fathers. McGrigor's plutocratic offspring is a curiosity. Only two of the thirty-one sons whose estate valuation has been discovered left more than £20,000, even if ten (again a third) were worth more than £5,000. In some cases, where a son had been placed in the Church, it is tempting to see this as a deliberate social trade-off. Some medical fathers were presumably willing to purchase a higher professional status for their sons at an economic price.

It must be stressed, too, that the cohort seemed little interested in placing their sons in trade or manufacturing, although many hailed from such a background. The cohort was involved in a specifically professional family project. Paradoxically, this was made all the easier by the relatively unprofessionalized character of the British professions in the first part of the nineteenth century. Whereas on the continent, notably in France, the state had begun to lay down stringent rules of entry by certification, both the learned and new professions in Britain continued, for the most part (the clergy was the obvious exception) to rely on a system of recruitment by apprenticeship. It is not surprising then that so few of the cohort's sons went to university. This was an unnecessary expense for many. Future clergy and, of course, medical practitioners might pass through the portals of academe, but sons bound for other professions had no need to grace its halls.

The cohort then could spread its sons around the professions and finance without investing heavily in education, all the more that its members were not terribly interested in the Church. The fact only fifteen sons are known to have taken the cloth—and this is a group particularly easy to identify—would suggest that this was not an option high on a family's list of preferences. This in turn more than hints at the probability that the cohort's professional project was a largely secular one. Coming as they did from different religious backgrounds and often marrying 'out', their frequent readiness to conform to the established Church in their civilian life was not necessarily a sign of deep spiritual commitment. Arguably, in their professional project, the army surgeons had more in common with the Darwins and the Wedgwoods than the Coleridges and Wordsworths, which raises the intriguing possibility that the Victorian professional middle class was itself culturally fractured. Certainly, it will become clear in the following chapter that a significant proportion of the surgeons were children of the Enlightenment, who belonged to a later generation of Gay's 'Party of Humanity'.[139]

[139] Peter Gay, *The Enlightenment: An Interpretation*, 2 vols. (London, 1966–70).

7

Enquiring Minds

MEN OF SCIENCE

What Astral Science was ere Newton rose,
Medicine remained till the last century's close,
And years thereafter,—miserable to see—
A so-called system without clue or key.

Samuel Dickson, *Memorable Events in
the Life of a London Physician*

To live for oneself is unnatural; it is to quit our station in the harmonies of
nature, and therefore to be unhappy; while the active and judicious exercise
of our kindly affections in behalf of our fellow beings is rewarded by a
pleasure, enduring, untroubled and inexpressible.

John Bigsby, *A Lecture on Mendicity*

In 1793 Edward Walsh, an alumnus of Edinburgh University and of Trinity
College Dublin, and a future physician to the forces, published his *Bagatelles, or
Poetical Sketches*, a compendium of verse, epigrams, and translations. By the author's
own concession, the pieces—among them his rendition of the *Marseillaise*—were
of 'unequal merit',[1] a barely visible feature of the contemporary literary landscape
in the year of Thomas Paine's *The Age of Reason* and William Blake's *Visions of the
Daughters of Albion*. Yet Walsh's mere *Bagatelles*, published four years before he
joined the service, are indicative of the reach and scope of a significant proportion
of our cohort's interests beyond their professional careers in medical practice,
including Walsh's own much more substantial reflections resulting from his
experience of the Dutch campaign of 1799.[2] This chapter underlines the extensive
participation of these men of science in the Republic of Letters from the 1780s
through to the 1870s. Walsh's homage to Science as 'Reason's fairest, eldest child'[3]
confirms the cohort's primary field of endeavour, and points to the post-
Enlightenment historical context in which the works of Walsh and his peers are
most profitably located. At the same time, Walsh's tribute to the 'candour of the

---

[1] E. Walsh, *Bagatelles or Poetical Sketches* (Dublin, 1793), advertisement.
[2] E. Walsh, *A Narrative of the Late Expedition to Holland in the Autumn of the Year 1799*
(London, 1800).   [3] Walsh, *Bagatelles*, 13.

public',[4] so evocative of the American Declaration of Independence signatories' 'submitted facts to a candid world', exemplified a zest to learn, inform, and divert in a variety of subsidiary spheres beyond the medical arena. In the following pages we construct a coherent biography of these collected works by pursuing the related themes of motivation, patronage, perceptions of society, and prescriptions for social improvement. In particular, this study of the cohort's publications will hinge on the premise that the scramble for patronage accompanied a distinctive and highly developed sense of societies in motion, and of the authors' own place in that trajectory.

In their collective contribution to medical debate and knowledge, this sub-group of the cohort answered and emulated the word of their master, Sir James McGrigor. As we have seen in Chapter 1, McGrigor vigorously promoted the Gradgrindian collation of data as a key component in the army medical service's role in the diffusion and improvement of medical knowledge.[5] In this respect, McGrigor's own publications represent a useful template. Leading by repeated example from early in the nineteenth century, McGrigor produced detailed accounts and analyses of the military and medical experiences of the British army in India, Egypt, the Peninsula, and the West Indies.[6] Many of the pieces to be studied here follow McGrigor's work in format, tone, and detail. But they will also demonstrate the multiplicity of our cohort's interests within and beyond their medical careers. This diversity is recorded in the surgeons' correspondence, and in their associations with learned societies, but above all in the content of their many publications, the main focus of this chapter.

As we have already seen, some forty or so of the cohort were fellows of the long-established royal colleges of physicians and surgeons.[7] Some thirty—many included in the forty—also belonged to some of the new medical societies, which were springing up in Britain and Europe. One surgeon was a member of the Dublin Obstetrical Society, another the London Vaccine Institution, while Thomas O'Halloran of Count Kerry was affiliated to the medical academies of Barcelona and Madrid. However, the largest number—nine apiece—claimed membership of the Royal Medical Society of Edinburgh (which they had presumably joined when they were students at the University) and the Royal Medical and Chirurgical Society of London.

More interestingly, twenty-two of the cohort—again generally to be found among the previous thirty—further belonged to or had an association with non-medical scientific and cultural societies. Some only had one extra medical interest. Stewart Crawford was a member of the Royal Scientific Institution of Bath, while

---

[4] Walsh, *Bagatelles*, Advertisement.   [5] See Ch. 1, pp. 41–2.

[6] See his *Medical Sketches of the Expedition to Egypt from India* (London, 1804); 'Sketch of the Medical History of the British Armies in the Peninsula of Spain and Portugal', *Transactions of the Medico-Chirurgical Society*, 6 (1815); and *Statistical Reports on the Sickness, Mortality and Invaliding among Troops in the West Indies, prepared from the Boards of the Army Medical Department, and War Office Returns* (London, 1838), which appeared under his auspices.   [7] See Ch. 3.

James Tully had an association with the Ionian Academy, the Greek University in Corfu.[8] George Russell Dartnell, on the other hand, exhibited with the Birmingham Society of Artists from 1867 to 1873, although he was not a member. A highly competent watercolourist, Dartnell is remembered in the present for the landscapes he painted while in service in Canada from 1835 to 1844.[9] A few of the cohort, however, had fingers in many learned pies. The Edinburgh physician David Maclagan was a member of the Scottish Society of Antiquaries, the Edinburgh Society for Nature and Chemistry, the Royal Scottish Society of Arts, and the Royal Society of Edinburgh. The Nottingham born John Bigsby, a naturalist of some importance, who initially practised in Newark before moving to the capital, belonged to a clutch of London societies. He was a fellow of the Linnaean Society, the Geological Society (from 1823), and the Royal Society (from 1869). He was also a member of the Geographical Club and an associate of the American Philosophical Society. He was particularly involved with the Geological Society, where he served as president in 1843, received the Murchison medal in 1874, and inaugurated the biennial Bigsby Medal in 1877.[10]

Nine of the cohort became fellows of the London Royal Society.[11] Their proposers for membership contain some striking names. For instance, John Davy numbered William Blake among his supporters in 1814; and the famous London surgeon, Benjamin Brodie backed Joseph Carpue two years later. McGrigor also became a fellow in 1816, puffed by his sponsors as a 'Gentleman well versed in several branches of Knowledge, and a Zealous promoter of Science'.[12] He in turn helped to elect Collier and Guthrie to the magic circle. Ultimately, too, he was one of five of the nine, along with Bigsby, Carpue, Davy, and Guthrie, who received a posthumous stamp of approval from the society's obituary pages, a conclusive sign of active membership. Given the director-general's aim to give the army medical service a positive public profile, he could not but have approved of the society's tributes to his erstwhile colleagues. Bigsby was praised for his 'long and well-spent life';[13] Guthrie for his constant activity 'in publishing his knowledge and opinions on all the questions which he had opportunity of studying',[14] while Davy was remembered for his 'multifarious labours', his pursuit of 'a regular and methodical course of literary and scientific work up to the latest days of his life'.[15] These admiring glances apply more generally to the prospect of the whole body of publications studied here.

[8] Founded in 1824.

[9] Honor de Pencier, *Posted to Canada: The Watercolours of George Russell Dartnell, 1835–1848* (Toronto, 1987). Many of his watercolours are today in Canadian galleries. The Royal Birmingham Society of Artists has no record of his membership.

[10] See Royal Society Papers (London), Item M/115.

[11] These nine were: John Bigsby, Charles Collier, John Davy, George Guthrie, Joseph Carpue, George Gregory, Thomas Keate, James McGrigor, and George Morris.

[12] Royal Society Biographical Details, available at **www.royalsoc.ac.uk/page.asp?id=1727** (July 2005): citation for McGrigor.   [13] *Proceedings of the Royal Society*, 33 (1881–2),pp. xvi–xvii.

[14] *Proceedings of the Royal Society*, 8 (1856–7), 273.

[15] *Proceedings of the Royal Society*, 16 (1867–68), pp. lxxix–lxxxi.

Excluding manuscripts, university dissertations, and reprints, we have discovered a total of 308 works by 69 of our sample in a variety of fields, published as letters, pamphlets, articles, and books. Of the 69 authors, 46—exactly two-thirds—held MDs, as against only two out of five within the whole cohort.[16] The seven most prolific in the sample produced more than ten works each: they included Davy (39 pieces), Guthrie (26), Dickson (16), Gregory (16), Joseph Brown (15), Collier (12), and McGrigor (11).[17] Overall, the dates of these publications spanned the 106 years from Alexander Thomson's enquiry into the treatment of nervous disorders in 1782[18] through to Bigsby's study of the flora and fauna of the Devonian and Carboniferous eras in 1878,[19] predominantly falling in the sixty years from 1810 to 1870.[20] We can divide the contents of the 308 works into five principal categories: social, topographical, literary, scientific, and medical. Of course, numerous pieces contained elements of more than one of these categories. For instance, Robert Dundas's account of his experiences of Brazil, published in 1852 and classified here as topographical, also contained substantial medical and social elements.[21] Similarly, medical reports on the British army's experience of disease in foreign campaigns often touched on topography, illustrated by McGrigor's study of the health of troops stationed in the West Indies and by Thomas O'Halloran's analysis of the outbreak of yellow fever in Spain.[22] Conversely, topographical works by Davy and by John Williamson based on their experiences of the West Indies had strong social overtones.[23] Similarly, the publications by Michael Este on public baths and by James Macauley on gymnasiums demonstrate the strong affiliation between therapeutic medicine and schemes of social improvement.[24] Despite these intersections, we can allocate a single dominant strain to each piece to give us totals of:

- 4 social works, which presented perspectives on contemporary society, and postulated potential improvements, notably, for instance, the lecture on

[16] 184 out of 454, or 40 per cent.

[17] Five out of the nine who were an FRS were thus prolific authors.

[18] A. Thomson, *An Enquiry into the Nature, Causes and Methods of Cure of Nervous Disorders; in a Letter to a Friend* (London, 1782).

[19] J. Bigsby, *Thesaurus Devonico-Carboniferous: The Flora and Fauna of the Devonian and Carboniferous Periods, the Genera and Species Arranged in Tabular Form: Showing the Horizons, Recurrences, Localities, and Other Facts: with Large Addenda from Recent Acquisitions* (London, 1878).

[20] 223 of the works (72%) were published in this period.

[21] R. Dundas, *Sketches of Brazil: Including New Views on Tropical and European Fever, with Remarks on a Premature Decay of the System Incident to Europeans on their Return from Hot Climates* (London, 1852).

[22] See McGrigor, *Statistical Reports . . . among Troops in the West Indies*; and T. O'Halloran, *A Brief View of the Yellow Fever as it Appeared in Andalusia during the Epidemic in 1820* (London, 1821). This helps to explain O'Halloran's connection with the two Spanish medical academies.

[23] J. Davy, *Five Discourses Delivered before the General Agricultural Society of Barbados* (London, 1849); and *Introductions on the Present State of the West Indies, and on the Agricultural Societies of Barbados* (London, 1849); and J. Williamson, *Medical and Miscellaneous Observations, Relative to the West Indian Islands*, 2 vols. (Edinburgh, 1817).

[24] M. L. Este, *Remarks on Baths, Water, Swimming, Shampooing, Heat, Cold and Vapour Baths* (London, 1812); and J. Macauley, *Observations on Gymnastics, and the Gymnasium* (Dublin, 1828).

mendicity given by Bigsby in 1836[25] and the letter on nutrition by Joseph Brown, addressed to the Member of Parliament Henry Fenwick in 1865.[26]

- 18 topographical works, which reflected the sample's widespread encounter with foreign countries and cultures. These pieces include, for instance, John Hennen senior's *Medical Topography of the Mediterranean*, published in 1830;[27] Adam Neale's recollections of his travels through Germany, Poland, Moldavia, and Turkey (1818);[28] and several works by Davy, such as his studies of Ceylon (1821), of the Ionian Islands (1842), and of the West Indies (1849).[29]

- 46 literary works, including diversions such as Walsh's collection of verse (1793)[30] and Davy's work on angling (1857);[31] histories such as George Power's account of the Muslim occupation of Spain and Portugal (1815);[32] translations such as Charles Collier's rendition of classics by Aristotle (1855) and Thucydides (1857)[33] and Henry Tytler's treatment of Callimachus (1793);[34] and autobiographies including Samuel Dickson's lively recollections (1863)[35] and the posthumously published memoirs of William Gibney (1896)[36] and Charles Boutflower (1912).[37]

- 35 scientific works, not directly related to medicine. These included Bigsby's various pieces on geology and natural history;[38] Davy's numerous experiments and observations on a range of substances and phenomena;[39] Thomas Prosser's

[25] J. Bigsby, *A Lecture on Mendicity, its Ancient and Modern History and the Policy of Nations and Individuals in Regard to it; as Delivered before the Worksop Mechanics' Institute on the 14th of April 1836* (Worksop, 1836).

[26] J. Brown, *The Food of the People: A Letter to Henry Fenwick esq. M. P. with a Postscript on the Diet of Old Age* (London, 1865).

[27] J. Hennen, *Sketches of the Medical Topography of the Mediterranean, Comprising an Account of Gibraltar, the Ionian Islands, and Malta . . . edited by his son John Hennen* (London, 1830).

[28] A. Neale, *Travels through Some Parts of Germany, Poland, Moldavia, and Turkey* (London, 1818).

[29] Davy, *An Account of the Interior of Ceylon and its Inhabitants, with Travels in that Island* (London, 1831); *Notes and Observations on the Ionian Islands, with some Remarks on Constantinople and Turkey, and on the System of Quarantine as at Present Conducted* (London, 1842); and *The West Indies before and since Slave Emancipation, Comprising the Windward and Leeward Islands Military Command* (London, 1854). [30] See above, n. 1.

[31] Davy, *The Angler and his Friend, or Piscatory Colloquies and Fishing Excursions* (London, 1855).

[32] G. Power, *The History of the Empire of the Musulmans in Spain and Portugal, from the First Invasion of the Moors to their Ultimate Expulsion from the Peninsula* (London, 1815).

[33] C. Collier, *Aristotle on the Vital Principle, Translated from the Original Text, with Notes* (London, 1855); and *The History of the Plague of Athens: Translated from Thucydides, with Notes Explanatory of its Pathology* (London, 1857).

[34] H. Tytler, *Works of Callimachus Translated into English Verse; the Hymns and Epigrams from the Greek, with the Coma Berenices from the Latin of Catullus; with the Original Text and Notes* (London, 1793).

[35] Dickson, *Memorable Events in the Life of a London Physician* (London, 1863).

[36] W. Gibney, *Eighty Years Ago, or the Recollections of an Old Army Doctor; his Adventures on the field of Quatre Bras and during the Occupation of Paris in 1815*, ed. by his son Major R. D. Gibney (London, 1896).

[37] C. Boutflower, *The Journal of an Army Surgeon during the Peninsular War* (Manchester, 1912).

[38] Especially his *Thesaurus Siluricus: The Flora and Fauna of the Silurian Period, with Addenda from Recent Acquisitions* (London, 1868); and his *Thesaurus Devonico-Carboniferous*.

[39] See, for instance, his *Lectures on the Study of Chemistry in Connection with the Atmosphere, the Earth, and the Ocean* (London, 1849).

treatise on equine diseases (1790);[40] James Millar's guide to botany (1821);[41] and William Lempriere's lectures on natural history (1830).[42]

- 205 medical works, themselves divisible into 5 further categories:

- 10 therapeutic studies, principally on water cures, spas and baths. These feature pieces by, for instance, Millar (1821),[43] William Macleod (1855),[44] and notably Este (1812);[45] and also Macauley's work on the benefits of gymnasiums (1828).[46]

- 5 anatomical pieces, such as Joseph Carpue's *Description of the Muscles of the Human Body* (1801).[47]

- 32 works on surgery, best represented here in the publications of Guthrie, whose distinguished military and civilian career inspired his major works on military surgery and on ophthalmic operations.[48]

- 43 pieces directly related to episodes, developments, or commitments in the authors' professional careers. These range from the single line of Gibney's signature of a petition sent to the Home Secretary in 1849 by Cheltenham medical practitioners;[49] through reports on specific campaigns or military units, led by McGrigor's contributions;[50] to long-running professional disputes involving George Gregory, sagas played out by Gregory and his adversaries in the pages of the *Lancet*.[51]

- 115 works of Pathology. These included, for instance, pieces on epidemics and fevers by O'Halloran (1821), Brown (1828), and William Bow (1829);[52] studies of cholera by James Gillkrest (1831), James Kell (1834), and

[40] T. Prosser, *A Treatise on the Strangles and Fevers of Horses: with a Plate Representing a Horse in the Staggers Slung* (London, 1790).

[41] J. Millar, *A Guide to Botany, or, A Familiar Illustration of the Principles of Linnaean Classification* (London, 1821).

[42] W. Lempriere, *Popular Lectures on the Study of Natural History and the Sciences, as Delivered before the Isle of Wight Philosophical Society* (London, 1830).

[43] J. Millar, *Practical Observations on Warm and Cold Bathing, and Descriptive Notes of Watering Places in Britain* (London, 1821).

[44] See, for instance, W. Macleod, *Hydro-therapeutics or the Water Cure: Considered as a Branch of Medical Treatment* (London, 1855).   [45] Este, *Remarks on Baths*.

[46] Macauley, *Observations on Gymnastics*.

[47] J. Carpue, *A Description of the Muscles of the Human Body, as They Appear on Dissection* (London, 1801).   [48] See pp. 320–2.

[49] Published in *Lancet*, 53/1339 (1849), 461–2.

[50] See n. 6 above; and, for instance, R. Amiel, *Answers to Queries from the Army Medical Board, on the Epidemic at Gibraltar 1828* (London, 1829).

[51] See, for instance, Gregory's numerous notices on the administration of the smallpox vaccination: in *Lancet*, 31/799 (1838), 497–98; 33/853 (1840), 551; 35/900 (1840), 359; 57/436 (1851), 285–56; 59/1492 (1852), 344; 59/1494 (1852), 391–2; and 59/1496 (1852), 435; and his version of his dispute with George Wigan, also in *Lancet*, 48/1207 (1846), 437; 48/1212 (1846), 572; and 48/1214 (1846), 624–5.

[52] See O'Halloran, *A Brief View of the Yellow Fever*; J. Brown, *Medical Essays on Fever, Inflammation, Rheumatism, Diseases of the Heart & c.* (London, 1828); and W. Bow, *Notions of the Natures of Fevers and Nervous Action* (Edinburgh, 1829).

Dickson (1848);[53] works on ophthalmia by George Power (1803) and Charles Farrell (1810);[54] and reviews of the British army's experience of disease in specific locations by William Lempriere on Jamaica (1799), John Douglas on Upper Canada (1819), and Robert Shean on the East Indies (1865).[55]

These 308 pieces vary greatly in content, substance, and merit but they were all written in the volatile context of the development of the British medical profession in the age of reform. In this respect, an awareness of three related factors must accompany our reading of the publications: the absence of an easily discernible, fixed medical establishment; the contested influence of the College of Physicians, the College of Surgeons, and Apothecaries' Hall; and the inherent tensions of an overcrowded profession. An anonymous polemic against the Royal College of Physicians helps to illuminate this broader picture. Published in 1826, this work insisted that for 'the community [to] derive the greatest sum of good from the exercise of any profession, it is essential that the number of its members should . . . be limited only by the demand';[56] detailed the overcrowding of the medical profession;[57] and damned the Old Corruption of the Royal College of Physicians as 'self-constituted monopolists' detrimental to the meritocratic cause of 'the doctors of physic throughout the British dominions . . . members of the "FACULTY OF PHYSIC ACCORDING TO LAW" '.[58] Though not uniformly contentious, our authors' publications appeared amid the noise and haste of this impolite commercial world. Thus, two critics accused Adam Neale of venality in a controversy over the spa waters at Cheltenham;[59] and the editor of the *Lancet* dismissed a pamphlet on viruses written by David Macloughlin in 1864 as 'a tissue of self-seeking and ignorant nonsense, ill-written, and without anything like ordinary reasoning power'.[60]

The contours of this combative environment are readily apparent in the publications featured here. For instance, Thomas Speer articulated the sense of overcrowding very distinctly in his presentation of the contemporary medical

[53] See J. Gillkrest, *Letters on the Cholera Morbus* (London, 1831); J. Kell, *On the Appearance of Cholera at Sunderland in 1831* (London, 1831); and S. Dickson, *Revelations on Cholera* (London, 1848).

[54] See G. Power, *An Attempt to Investigate the Cause of the Egyptian Ophthalmia, with Observations of its Nature and Different Modes of Cure* (London, 1803); and C. Farrell, *Observations on Ophthalmia and its Consequences* (London, 1810).

[55] See W. Lempriere, *Practical Observations on the Diseases of the Army in Jamaica, as They Occurred between the Years 1792 and 1797* (London, 1799); J. Douglas, *Diseases of the Army during the Campaign in Upper Canada, 1813–1815* (London, 1819); and R. Shean, *Observations on the Most Prevalent Diseases of British Soldiers in the East Indies* (London, 1835).

[56] *An Exposition of the State of the Medical Profession in the British Dominions; and of the Injurious Effects of the Monopoly, by Usurpation, of the Royal College of Physicians in London* (London, 1826), 1.

[57] Ibid. 5. [58] Ibid. 372–3.

[59] See W. Halpin, *Fact versus Assertion, or Critical and Explanatory Observations on Some Erroneous Statements, Contained in Dr. Adam Neale's Pamphlet on the Nature and Properties of the Cheltenham Waters* (London, 1820); and T. Newell, *A Letter to the Editor of the City Gazette upon the Misrepresentations Contained in a Pamphlet Recently Published by Dr. Neale, upon the Subject of the Cheltenham Waters by Thomas Newell, M.D., Surgeon Extraordinary to the King* (London, 1820).

[60] See Lancet, 83/2117 (1864), 368.

profession as 'manifestly overdone... the proportion of its followers manifestly exceeds those for whom it is necessary'.[61] Similarly, Brown bemoaned 'the besetting sins of medical men, jealousy of, and illiberality towards each other,'[62] a phenomenon vividly exemplified even within our cohort in the accusations of plagiarism levelled at Robert Dundas, stigmatized by Dickson as 'ROB-BER DUNDAS'.[63] At the same time, it would be misleading to present these publications as a single, coherent record of the growing pains of the British medical profession in the nineteenth century. Rather, in our overall context, we can see their content as an amalgam of the authors' record of their experiences—at home and abroad—and their engagement with contemporary debates.

IN THE NAME OF HUMANITY?

A strong ethos of the improvement of medicine and society informed these works, expressed in the authors' concern for the disadvantaged, notably the sick, the poor, the ignorant, and the enslaved. But the authors themselves were far from downtrodden, and we cannot disregard mundane individual motives, even in the face of one author's claim, characteristic of these works, that 'if he succeed in imparting a portion of information conducive to the well-being of the community, he shall consider himself amply repaid'.[64] In short, although overall profits would be exceptionally hard to tabulate, we must acknowledge the potential incentives of 'the mercenary spirit' and the 'objectless egotism' refuted by Brown and Dickson respectively.[65] In addition to reprints and subsequent editions, several items, even on their first outing, were collections of previously released material, occasionally incorporating minor amendments. To take four examples: William Bow's study of fevers and nervous action reprised his contributions to the *London Medical and Physical Journal* of 1829;[66] in November 1831 James Gillkrest brought out a set of ten letters on cholera which he had released over the previous three months;[67] John Davy's 'Discourses' of 1849 assembled the five lectures he had given to the General Agricultural Society of Barbados between 1846 and 1848;[68] and only three days elapsed between the delivery and the publication of Gregory's lecture on dropsy in January 1819.[69]

---

[61] T. C. Speer, *Thoughts on the Present Character and Constitution of the Medical Profession* (Cambridge, 1823), 22.   [62] Brown, *Medical Essays on Fever*, 4.

[63] Dickson, *The Destructive Art of Healing, or Facts for Families* (London, 1853), 61; conversely, Dickson's works also contain a notable example of endorsement from within the cohort: see the support given to the chronothermal system by J. R. Hume, reprinted by Dickson in *Fallacies of the Faculty* (London, 1865), 75.

[64] H. Davies, *The Young Wife's Guide during Pregnancy and Childbirth, and the Management of her Infant* (London, 1852), p. vi.

[65] Brown, *Medical Essays on Fever*, 5; Dickson, *Memorable Events*, 5.

[66] Bow, *Notions of the Natures of Fever*.   [67] Gillkrest, *Letters on the Cholera*.

[68] Davy, *Five Discourses Delivered before the General Agricultural Society*.

[69] George Gregory, *A Lecture on Dropsy* (London, 1819).

Of these, Gregory's lecture is the most helpful here in that it leads directly to the much richer theme of philanthropy, and to the authors' promotion of scientific knowledge as the touchstone of the improvement of humanity. Writing in the 'advertisement' to his lecture, Gregory's avowed 'desire of contributing his share towards the improvement of a most important branch of physical science' typified the broad didactic animus coursing through these publications. At the same time, Gregory's preface was unusual in the reminder that he intended his words for the attention of 'the junior members of the profession alone'.[70] In fact, whatever the breadth and depth of their readership, and despite numerous dedications and acknowledgements, the authors seldom explicitly identified a target audience, still less a specific beneficiary. In this respect, the 'Address' published in 1839 by James Barlow was even more exceptional both as a lesson aimed directly at 'medical and surgical pupils, on the studies and duties of their profession' and in the promise that all profits were to be given to 'some Charitable Institution in Blackburn'.[71]

As we will see, the authors engaged in numerous polemics and campaigns within and beyond medicine. Yet in general they cast their philanthropic spirit as the solemn service of a global purpose. From this perspective, the publications read as a collective refutation of La Rochefoucauld's maxim that 'c'est une grande habileté que de savoir cacher son habileté'. Rather, to display and broadcast hard-gained erudition was the prescriptive duty of enlightened men, as Brown made clear. 'An individual, who has been unceasingly occupied in the contemplation of an extensive class of objects, will most probably have discovered some facts regarding them, which had escaped the perspicacity of others; and hence, though perhaps of humble powers and pretensions, may be enabled to contribute his mite to the sum of human knowledge.'[72] According to Este, this precept was the special preserve of the professional classes. 'Every man is duty-bound to contribute his portion, however small, to the mass of general knowledge, especially in a learned profession; and whoever locks up his talent, inconsiderable as it may be, deserves censure as an unworthy member of the society in which he lives'.[73] Most pertinently, in our context, as Brown, Este and many of their colleagues stressed, this imperative applied above all to medicine, where a heightened sense of duty underlined William Wallace's description of medics as 'guardians of the public health, that greatest of blessings', under a moral obligation to maximize every opportunity 'of multiplying their capabilities of being useful';[74] and bolstered Dundas's explanation that the principles he laid down had 'occupied the writer's thoughts for many years, and in many lands . . . [A] profound conviction of their truth . . . of their importance to the preservation of health, and in the treatment of disease, has imposed on him the duty of publishing them.'[75]

---

[70] Ibid., Advertisement.
[71] J. Barlow, *An Address to Medical and Surgical Pupils, on the Studies and Duties of their Profession; to Which is Appended a Case of Caesarean Operation* (London, 1839).
[72] Brown, *Medical Essays on Fever*, 1.   [73] Este, *Remarks on Baths*, pp. xii–xiii.
[74] W. Wallace, *Observations on Sulphureous Fumigations as a Powerful Remedy in Rheumatism and Diseases of the Skin* (Dublin, 1820), 3.   [75] Dundas, *Sketches of Brazil*, pp. v–vi.

To contribute to the sum of human knowledge, to share Gregory's 'reliance on the value of *public* discussion',[76] was necessarily, in places, to initiate or resume personal and professional disputes, another powerful motive behind these publications. In this respect, the combined works of Brown, Dickson, and Henry Robertson offer three excellent case studies of tenaciously pursued and varying agendas. Published in 1828, Robertson's *A Blast from the North*, a fierce polemic against medical education in England, made a particular target of the corruption, monopoly, and nepotism he saw as endemic at Oxbridge and the London College of Physicians and as unjust obstructions to the aspirations of Scottish graduates. In his attack on contemporary practice at Oxford and Cambridge, Robertson wrote that 'the science of Medicine, as a study, is scarcely known by name at either of these Universities'.[77] Similarly, he argued that 'Medicine as a science or a practical art, owes nothing for improvement to the London College of Physicians.'[78] These specific points decorated Robertson's general portrayal of Scottish education as superior to its English counterpart. He illustrated this in stinging verdicts on institutions and personnel, in his refusal to accept Eton as 'preferable to the High School at Edinburgh... or to the grammar school in any of the larger towns of Scotland', and in his condemnation of Samuel Johnson as 'a man so blinded by prejudice that he could not allow it to be said in his presence, that any Scotsman could write the English language, till after Lord Bute had signed the order for his pension'.[79]

Robertson's grievances resurface in the pieces published by the Quaker-raised Joseph Brown of Sunderland, another archetypal occupant of David Knight's 'provincial and dissenting sphere', akin in this respect to Joseph Priestley in Birmingham and John Dalton in Manchester.[80] Brown explicitly aligned himself with 'We provincials'[81] and defended the interests of Scottish medicine from an England he condemned as at once overbearing and negligent in his reference to 'the united empire, of which Scotland is certainly not the least gifted and intellectual portion'.[82] As a distinguished veteran of the Peninsular war and a pioneer in cardiology, Brown contributed regularly to Sir John Forbes's *Cyclopedia of Practical Medicine* and to the *British and Foreign Quarterly Medical Review*.[83] In addition, Brown published four longer works in which he gave full voice to his reflections on developments in medicine and society: *Medical Essays on Fever,*

---

[76] Lancet, 59/1492 (1852), 344.

[77] H. Robertson, *A Blast from the North in Vindication of the Medical Graduates of Edinburgh against the Invidious and Calumnious Aspersions Cast upon their Literary and Professional Education, through the Bye-laws of the London College of Physicians* (London, 1828), 6. [78] Ibid. 16.

[79] Ibid. 12, 20. Scottish literary pride was also evident in the earl of Buchanan's recognition of Tytler as the first native of Scotland to have translated a Greek poet into English: see Tytler, *Works of Callimachus*, p. vi.

[80] *Collected Works of Humphry Davy, Edited by his Brother, John Davy*, introd. David Knight (Durham, 2001), vi. [81] *Medical Essays*, 3.

[82] Ibid. 8.

[83] Forbes (1787–1861) had been a navy surgeon who established himself at Chichester: *DNB, sub nomine.*

Inflammation, Rheumatism, Diseases of the Heart in 1828; *A Defence of Revealed Religion* in 1851; *Memories of the Past and Thoughts on the Present Age* in 1863; and *The Food of the People: A Letter to Henry Fenwick M.P.* in 1865.[84] Published in London but fired off from his practice in Sunderland, these reflected Brown's Quaker upbringing in their expression of an inward call to examine and instruct.

Brown's lucidity served him well in his intricate analysis of social strata and the impact of legislation. As a polemicist he was equally effective. His defence of religion, for instance, rested on the powerful union he forged between patriotism and Christianity. In 1851 he wrote that 'England, it has long appeared to the reflecting, is prosperous and great because she is Christian; should she cease to be Christian, she would be one of the meanest and least among nations.'[85] In 1863 he pursued the same theme, quoting his own earlier work with approval and adding that 'England owes very much of her position, prosperity and even security, among nations, to the fact that Christianity is not merely in a verbal way "part and parcel of the law of the land", but that the pure and lofty morality which Christianity inspires is infused into the acts of her legislature and the proceedings of her government... Man is a religious animal.'[86] Brown's preoccupation with the moral condition of the nation again underpinned his advocacy of improved nutrition for the labouring classes, leading him to declare that 'the food of the people is the basement-story of the edifice of social improvement'.[87] Similarly, moral indignation, particularly at 'the revolting scenes connected with the occupation of *body-snatching*', sustained his participation in the demands for regulation of the use of corpses in anatomy, arguing that the bodies of all executed criminals and of all 'who die unclaimed in public hospitals' should be available to anatomy schools.[88]

As splenetic as Robertson and as prolific as Brown, Dickson centred his substantial output on his development and defence of the chronothermal system. Insisting on 'the periodicity and intermittency of all animal movement, whether in health or in disease', Dickson perceived time and temperature as the keys to pathology. In the chronothermal system, he explained, 'the various movements of the body of a man in health resolve themselves into a unity or harmony of special periodic action'; and 'there can be no important alteration in any of the chrono-metrical or chronal movements of man, without a corresponding thermal change'. For Dickson, therefore, cures for disease must concentrate on 'the regulation of Time or Period, and the regulation at the same time, of Temperature or Heat'.[89] From 1839 to 1865, he produced six editions of his *Fallacies of the Faculty with the Principles of the Chrono-Thermal System*, also translated into French and German

---

[84] Full titles: *Medical Essays on Fever, Inflammation, Rheumatism, Diseases of the Heart & c.* (London, 1828); *A Defence of Revealed Religion, Comprising a Vindication of the Old and New Testaments from the Attacks of Rationalists and Infidels* (London, 1851); *Memories of the Past and Thoughts on the Present Age* (London, 1863); and *A Letter to Henry Fenwick M. P. with a Postscript on the Diet of Old Age* (London, 1865).   [85] *A Defence of Revealed Religion*, pp. iii–iv.
[86] *Memories of the Past*, pp. viii–ix.   [87] *The Food of the People*, 12.
[88] *Medical Essays*, 14.   [89] Dickson, *Memorable Events*, 14–15.

and published in America. Dickson combined his advocacy of the chronothermal system with his campaign against the practice of bloodletting.[90] He gained numerous supporters, even attracting the distinguished admiration of the famous explorer Sir Richard Burton.[91]

In these pieces, professional credo and personal crusade became inextricable, as Dickson railed against his version of institutional and individual corruption. In the first edition of *Fallacies of the Faculty*, Dickson warned prospective medical practitioners that a 'thorny path' awaited them, where success 'is less frequently the reward of patient merit than of superior dexterity in the arts of intrigue, and the skilful appliance of corrupt and secret means'.[92] Similarly, in his preface to the fourth edition six years later, Dickson thanked his allies for their support in his stance 'against the organised opposition of the Schools—the Brodies, the Chambers, the Clarks[93]—who, with their clique of pedantic, sycophantic supporters, conspired to cry me down in my efforts to cleanse the Augean stables of British Medical practice of its filth and corruption'.[94] Finding an appropriate publisher in the Virtue Brothers of London, Dickson's memoirs of 1863 recapitulated his long charge-sheet against old adversaries. In particular, he attacked Sir John Forbes for his belated and partial acknowledgement of the disadvantages of bloodletting; and presented Sir Benjamin Brodie as the personification of 'the gigantic system of corruption which has so long prevailed in medicine'.[95]

Yet for a self-styled outsider, and despite the Rousseauist venom of his prose, Dickson was remarkably conventional in his pursuit of patrons to advance his career, notably Sir James McGrigor and Lord Melbourne. In 1832 Dickson dedicated his work on the cholera epidemic endured by British soldiers in Madras to McGrigor, hailing both the office and the man in his tribute to 'your high situation, and the ability with which you have so long filled it'.[96] Seven years later, Dickson anticipated that the stamp of the Prime Minister's approval—Lord Melbourne's 'high and distinguished auspices'—would enhance the impact of his work *The Unity of Disease analytically and Synthetically Proved.*[97]

Dickson's desire to emphasize and develop links with medical and political grandees brings us to the final and most significant motivation behind these

[90] See, especially, Dickson's *Fallacies of the Faculty, with the Principles of the Chrono-Thermal System of Medicine* (London, 1839; subsequent edns. 1841, 1843, 1845, 1853, 1865); and his *The Forbidden Book: With New Fallacies of the Faculty: Being the Chrono-Thermalist, or People's Medical Enquirer*, 2 vols. (London, 1850–1).

[91] In the notes to his *A Pilgrimage to Al-Madinah and Meccah*, first published in 1893, Burton mentions 'the chronothermal system, a discovery which physic owes to my old friend, the late Dr. Samuel Dickson': see Sir R. Burton, *A Pilgrimage to Al-Madinah and Meccah*, 2 vols. (London, 1986), i. 13.

[92] *Fallacies of the Faculty* (1839), Dedication: 'To the Rising Generation of Medical Practitioners'.

[93] Sir Benjamin Brodie, the *Chambers's Edinburgh Journal*, and Sir James Clark (1788–1870), a former naval surgeon, FRS, and royal doctor.   [94] *Fallacies of the Faculty* (1845), preface.

[95] *Memorable Events*, 103, 270–5.

[96] *On the Epidemic Cholera, and Other Prevalent Diseases of India* (London, 1832), dedication.

[97] *The Unity of Disease Analytically and Synthetically Proved, with Facts and Cases Subversive of the Received Practice of Physic* (London, 1839), dedication.

publications: patronage. Some of our authors included fulsome tributes to appropriate institutions, exemplified in Este's homage to the Military Medical Library at Fort Pitt;[98] in Charles Boutflower's display of enduring loyalty to the 40th regiment which he had served in the Peninsular war;[99] and in Davy's tributes to the Reid School of Chemistry and to the General and District Agricultural Societies in Barbados.[100] But in general the majority of the plethora of dedications, acknowledgements, and encomia offered by the authors, as prefaces and within the texts, were personal. McGrigor himself led the way here. In 1804 he dedicated his *Medical Sketches of the Expedition to Egypt, from India* to three distinguished physicians: Sir Lucas Pepys, Thomas Keate, and Francis Knight.[101] Family tributes, such a mainstay of Edinburgh University medical theses, were now notable absentees.[102] Rather, the most significant recipients fall into four occasionally overlapping categories: military, medical, political, and aristocratic.

Unsurprisingly, the weightiest military figure honoured in these publications was the duke of Wellington. According to Boutflower, who lovingly detailed Wellington's social and military itinerary throughout his memoir of the Peninsular campaign, the duke after the triumph of Salamanca in 1812 was 'almost beyond the reach of rivalry'.[103] Even before he had fully established himself in the Peninsula, the then Sir Arthur Wellesley won public admiration from the army medical service. As early as 1809 Adam Neale eulogized Wellington for his possession of the 'entire confidence and affections of the soldiery', and for his 'combination of rare qualities, as seldom fall to the lot of an individual... With the exception of Nelson, whose fame he bids fair to rival, England has, perhaps, produced no man, since the days of Marlborough, of such innate military acumen.'[104]

George Power in 1815 was even more direct and effusive, and explicit in seeking 'a degree of importance and patronage'. He devoted the opening six pages of his history of the Muslims in Spain and Portugal to his dedication to Wellington, doggedly listing the duke's full array of titles and honours, then acclaiming the man

whose comprehensive mind, genius, and powerful arm, having defended a portion of that Peninsula from the hordes of Gauls who aimed at its subjugation... has been the instrument employed by Divine Providence to preserve and cherish in Portugal the spark of liberty which the overwhelming influence of France, under its late ruler, had nearly extinguished on the Continent of Europe.[105]

---

[98] Este, *Remarks on Baths*, 2nd edn. (London, 1845), inscription inside front cover.

[99] Boutflower, *Journal of an Army Surgeon*, 162.

[100] Davy, *Introductions on the Present State of the West Indies, and on the Agricultural Societies*, pp. ix–x; and *Five Discourses*, 131.

[101] Then physician-general, surgeon-general and inspector-general of hospitals respectively; see McGrigor, *Sketches of the Expedition to Egypt*, dedication.   [102] See Ch. 3.

[103] Boutflower, *Journal of an Army Surgeon*, 149.

[104] A. Neale, *Letters from Portugal and Spain; Comprising an Account of the Armies under their Excellencies Sir Arthur Wellesley and Sir John Moore, from the Landing of the Troops in Mondego Bay to the Battle at Coruna* (London, 1809), 82–3.

[105] Power, *History of the Empire of the Musulmans in Spain and Portugal*, 3–8.

Similarly, Guthrie stationed his salute to Wellington between his tributes to the president and the vice-president of the Royal Westminster Infirmary in the first edition of his *Lectures on the Operative Surgery of the Eye* in 1823.[106]

Guthrie inscribed this volume personally to Sir James McGrigor, emulating the gesture made two years earlier by Thomas O'Halloran, who had presented a copy of his work on the epidemic of yellow fever in Andalusia to McGrigor in 1821, 'with the author's most respectful compliments'.[107] Understandably, McGrigor was the most frequent recipient of the authors' tributes. Here again, praise—and proof of patronage—fell within the texts and in opening dedications. In these pieces, to honour McGrigor was to salute not only his career but also his status; and to take care to emphasize, even revere, an amalgam of public service and private virtue, to broadcast, in Brown's phrases, 'motives of private friendship' and 'reasons of a more public nature'.[108] To praise McGrigor made particular sense as a career move. From an abundance of further candidates, the words of John Hennen, echoed by his son, and of George Gregory provide archetypal examples. These authors addressed McGrigor directly. In his 1818 study of military surgery and hospital administration, Hennen wrote that 'You, sir, in your various official capacities, have uniformly presented to the Medical Officers of the British Army, an invaluable example of zeal tempered by judgement, and of energy combined with prudence, while science has guided both; and to the elevated station which you now fill, you have added the still higher distinction, of being looked up to as the father and friend of your department.'[109] Editing his late father's study of the medical topography of the Mediterranean, Hennen's son applauded McGrigor for 'the paternal interest you have taken in the author's surviving family'.[110] Gregory produced much the same formula in the second edition of his 1825 study on *Elements of the Theory and Practice of Physic*. Encouraged by McGrigor's support for the first edition, Gregory claimed that a 'sense of public duty, as well of private friendship, urges me to place this work under your auspices. When I reflect upon the distinguished station which you have held in the Army for many years, and the efforts you have unceasingly made to uphold the character of the Military Medical Department, to give to its members one common interest and to cement their union with the practitioners in civil life, I am sensible that I should in vain look round for more honourable or efficient patronage.'[111]

Wellington and McGrigor were not alone. For instance, in 1803 Power dedicated his work on Egyptian Ophthalmia to Thomas Young, inspector-general of hospitals to the forces serving in Egypt;[112] in 1853 Guthrie dedicated the fifth

[106] G. J. Guthrie, *Lectures on the Operative Surgery of the Eye* (London, 1823), dedication.

[107] O'Halloran, *Brief View of the Yellow Fever*, inscription.

[108] Brown, *Medical Essays*, dedication.

[109] J. Hennen, *Observations on some Important Points in the Practice of Military Surgery, and in the Arrangement and Police of Hospitals* (Dublin, 1818), pp. v–vi.

[110] Hennen, *Sketches of the Medical Topography of the Mediterranean*, pp. v–vi.

[111] G. Gregory, *Elements of the Theory and Practice of Physic, Designed for the Use of Students* (London, 1825), pp. iii–iv.   [112] Power, *Egyptian Ophthalmia*, pp. iii–iv.

edition of his *Commentaries on the Surgery of War* to the commander-in-chief of the British army, Lord Hardinge;[113] ten years later Brown, in his *Memories of the Past and Thoughts on the Present Age*, hailed Gladstone, then chancellor of the exchequer, as 'the Scholar, the Statesman and the Philanthropist'.[114] Finally, of course, this culture of deference and patronage incorporated a host of aristocrats. Here, these pieces combined social aspiration with a determination to secure— and acknowledge—influential sponsorship in professional missions and medical or social initiatives. Thus, O'Halloran, posted to investigate the outbreak of yellow fever in Spain in 1821 by the grace of the duke of York, included in his report the assurance that 'the sanction of your Royal Highness's name is a guarantee for its obtaining due attention from the public';[115] and when the earl of Chatham arrived as the new governor of Gibraltar in 1822, the local inspector of hospitals William Fraser was quick to alert him that there were 'few matters which could more seriously demand your Excellency's attention than such as concern the health of the troops and inhabitants'.[116] Domestically, in 1845 Este recognized the royal dukes of Kent and Sussex as the founding patrons of his campaign for the introduction of public baths launched in 1812.[117] Similarly, as early as the 1790s, Thomas Prosser had sought to enlist the support of the fourth duke of Queensberry, the notorious 'Old Q', famed for his attempts to develop horse-racing into a science. In his work on farriery, Prosser applauded the efforts of this alchemist of the turf whose 'horses are said to be managed with a great superiority to the common methods, and by your own immediate directions'.[118]

The strain of reverence in these pieces is undeniable, never more blatant than in Joseph Carpue's paean to the prince regent in his study of lithotomy[119] published in 1819, where the author extolled '[t]he gracious permission which your Royal Highness has given me to lay at your Royal Highness' feet the following work... the anxious solicitude your Royal Highness expressed for the first operations performed in this manner since its revival in England... the deep interest your Royal Highness takes in the causes of suffering humanity, and the protection your Royal Highness gives to every attempt that is made for its amelioration'.[120] But to see these dedications as merely time-serving would be to disregard the

---

[113] G. J. Guthrie, *Commentaries on the Surgery of War in Portugal, Spain, France and the Netherlands, from the Battle of Roliça, in 1808, to that of Waterloo, in 1815*, 5th edn. (London, 1853), dedication.　　　　　　　　　　　　　　[114] Brown, *Memories of the Past*, frontispage.

[115] T. O'Halloran, *Remarks on the Yellow Fever of the South and East of Spain; Comprehending Observations Made on the Spot, by Actual Survey of Localities, and Rigorous Examination of Fact at Original Sources of Information* (London, 1823), dedication.

[116] W. Fraser, *A Letter Addressed to His Excellency the Right Honourable Earl of Chatham, K. G., Governor of Gibraltar... Relative to the Febrile Tempers of that Garrison* (London, 1826), 1.

[117] Este, *Remarks on Baths*, (1845), dedication.

[118] Prosser, *A Treatise on the Strangles and Fevers of Horses*, pp. i–ii.

[119] The surgical removal of a calculus, especially from the urinary bladder.

[120] J. A. Carpue, *A History of the High Operation of the Stone, by Incision above the Pubis; with Observations on the Advantages Attending it; and an Account of the Various Methods of Lithotomy, from the Earliest Periods to the Present Time* (London, 1819), pp. iii–iv.

authors' genuine enthusiasm for their patrons and superiors: for example, the admiration of Wellington expressed by Boutflower and Gibney appears in works committed to the public domain only after their deaths. For the majority, the stamp of living luminaries confirmed the sense of prestige the authors derived from their military and medical careers, the hard-won warrant to comment on contemporary enterprises of pith and moment within and beyond medicine. Furthermore, the intriguing corollary of servility was an acute awareness and delineation of social strata, largely acquired through long years of military service.

CONSERVATIVE PROGRESSIVES

'Dissect, dissect, dissect' was the instruction burnt into Dickson's memory from his student days in Edinburgh and Paris.[121] This section explores the readiness of the authors of the cohort to extend this maxim to their readings of society within and beyond Britain. The starting-point here must be the accounts that they have left of their travels around the globe, especially in the light of the belief expressed by the traveller, army officer, and ex-veteran of the Peninsular campaign, Joseph Moyle Sherer, that the English at least were unsympathetic observers. The 'English ... will not bend with good humour to the customs of other nations ... wherever they march or travel, they bear with them a haughty air of conscious superiority, and expect that their customs, habits and opinions should supersede ... those of all the countries through which they pass'.[122]

    At first glance, this assertion seems to be borne out by our authors' memoirs and travelogues. Although William Gibney declared that 'one must not judge national peculiarities',[123] he was happy to describe the French as a 'frivolous' nation, 'never knowing their own minds two minutes together',[124] and recoiled in horror at the offer of a cordial embrace from a French brandy-seller.[125] Boutflower similarly dismissed the Spanish as a people undeserving of 'the sacred blessing of Freedom';[126] while John Williamson, encountering a Portuguese regiment in Funchal in 1798, was quick to condemn the 'appearance of degeneracy and conscious inferiority in them, as well as in the lower classes of the community'.[127] Moreover, these characteristics were all presented in noxious contrast to 'the sterling sense and perseverance of Britons' honoured by Brown,[128] the 'liberal and enlightened British public' glorified by Dundas,[129] and 'the soundness of the English character' invoked by Bigsby.[130]

---

[121] *Memorable Events*, 13.
[122] J. Sherer, *Recollections of the Peninsula* (London, 1823), 36–7.   [123] Gibney, 132.
[124] Ibid. 121.   [125] Ibid. 245.   [126] Boutflower, *Journal of an Army Surgeon*, 95.
[127] Williamson, *Medical and Miscellaneous Observations, Relative to the West Indian Islands*, i. 9–10.
[128] Brown, *Medical Essays*, 6.   [129] Dundas, *Sketches of Brazil*, 386.
[130] J. Bigsby, *A Brief Exposition of those Benevolent Institutions, often Denominated Self-Supporting Dispensaries; with a View to Recommend them to the Patronage and Support of the Public* (Newark, 1832), 9.

Closer reading of our authors' writings, however, reveals a greater sensitivity towards other nations. Above all, exposure to the societies they encountered in their military careers intensified the authors' perceptions of the interplay between race, social class, and political institutions. To start with three small but telling instances: Boutflower, stationed at Badajoz in 1809, attended a funeral and observed that 'only the wealthy are permitted to lie near the altar';[131] Romaine Amiel, reporting to the Army Medical Board in 1829, confirmed that the epidemics in Gibraltar 'always commenced in the filthiest spot, among the lower and more disorderly class of inhabitants';[132] and James Kennedy observed in Jamaica that the 'white inhabitants never associate with the Creoles; the latter, whatever be their wealth, cannot enter a ballroom'.[133]

The observations of Davy on the West Indies, Dundas on Brazil, and Walsh on the Dutch Republic provide more extensive examples. A distinctive socio-political scenario formed the backdrop to these three portraits. In the clearest-cut instance, writing at a time of 'struggle between free labour and slave labour' in the mid-nineteenth century,[134] Davy dissected the components of the society of mid-nineteenth century Barbados very precisely. Davy's advocacy of racial equality, his prospect of a future 'when the distinction of colour—established during slavery—will be abolished',[135] sharpened his focus. Thus, he was able to distinguish between 'the African', that is 'a labourer', formidable in his 'power of endurance and resistance', and 'the planter, the proprietor, to allude to another and higher class', marked by their 'industry and intelligence … denoted in the high state of culture of the land'; and subsequently between these landowners, 'the higher order of the white West Indians', and 'the working class, who are too commonly steeped in vice connected with intemperance, and are altogether a degraded and diseased set, and that in body and mind'. In this forensic analysis, Davy also incorporated the further category of the 'European immigrant of the class of day labourers', from Portugal for example, and ill-suited, in his view, to the Caribbean climate.[136]

As a witness of Brazilian independence and its aftermath in the 1820s, Dundas was in a position, lecturing in Liverpool thirty years later, to chronicle 'a series of remarkable political and social changes', when he considered the multiple consequences of the leap from 'the strict and simple forms of despotic government … to one almost of licence, including household suffrage, popular legislative assemblies (imperial and provincial), open courts of law, trial by jury, local justices, and a national guard elected on popular principles'. Dundas's assessment,

[131] Boutflower, *Journal of an Army Surgeon*, 25.
[132] Amiel, *Answers to Queries from the Army Medical Board*, 5.
[133] J. Kennedy, *Conversations on Religion with Lord Byron and Others, Held in Cephalonia, a Short Time Previous to his Lordship's Death* (London, 1830), 435.
[134] Davy, *Introductions on the Present State of the West Indies*, p. xvii. Davy had been living in the West Indies for three years prior to publishing his book in 1854.
[135] Davy, *Five Discourses*, 148.
[136] Davy, *Introductions on the Present State of the West Indies*, pp. xix–xxiii.

though brief and incidental to the main thrust of his work, nonetheless constituted a sophisticated and measured reading of a society in upheaval. Thus, while
he regretted the expenditure of resources on war and inter-provincial disputes,
ill-administered laws and 'lax morality', Dundas applauded improvements in
education, commerce, and agriculture. In his view, too, the Catholic priesthood
had 'utterly lost its prestige, unless, perhaps with the very lowest classes of the
community'. Finally, he detailed 'some of those evils too commonly attendant
on increased wealth, luxury and indolence... that "wear and tear" so painfully
characteristic of highly civilised society', specifically, an increase in cerebral and
nervous disorders, and in diseases of the lungs and heart.[137]

The studied ambivalence of Dundas contrasted sharply with Walsh's unequi-
vocal indictment of the Dutch 'revolutionary transit' of the late 1790s. Published
in 1800, Walsh's work contained a routine military account of the British expedition to Holland in 1799 but also a cogent conservative appraisal of the consequences of the complicated journey from William V to the Batavian Republic by a
man who had quickly lost his earlier enthusiasm for the 'Marseillaise'.[138] Walsh
conceded that there had been 'less bloodshed, outrage and change of property'
in Holland than in contemporary revolutions, attributing this in part to the 'less
impassioned character' of the people. But for Walsh the consequences of the transfer 'from the old to the new order of things' had been 'highly calamitous and
ruinous to the Dutch nation... their navy has been annihilated, their colonies
possessed and their commerce destroyed by their old allies whilst their wealth and
moveable property, at home, have fallen a prey to the requisitional plunder of their
new friends'.[139]

Even half a century apart, and despite the ethnographical variety of their
subjects, the reflections of Davy, Dundas, and Walsh are comparable in the
assumption, even insistence, that moral order must underpin society. This imperative was implicit in Dundas's reference to the dangers inherent in the 'sudden
and premature concession of political principles to a people yet in the infancy
of civilisation',[140] and in Walsh's applause for 'the complete suppression and
repression of insurrection' in late 1790s Britain, presumably particularly in his
native Ireland;[141] and explicit in Davy's conclusion that 'the condition of a
community is most strongly marked by its moral and intellectual state... that
society... in which morals are purest, the virtues most active... must compara-
tively stand high in influence, happiness and prosperity'.[142]

Furthermore, this theme is equally visible in the considerations of British
society encountered in the works of Davy's peers, best illustrated by Brown,

[137] Dundas, *Sketches of Brazil*, 349–50.
[138] See S. Schama, *Patriots and Liberators: Revolution in the Netherlands 1780–1813* (London, 1977).   [139] Walsh, *A Narrative of the Late Expedition to Holland*, 17–18.
[140] Dundas, *Sketches of Brazil*, 349.
[141] Walsh, *A Narrative of the Late Expedition to Holland*, 19.
[142] Davy, *Five Discourses*, 146.

Bigsby, and Thomas Speer. Immediate historical context helped Speer to under-line the bond between morality and social order. Writing in the 1820s, and unafraid of vivid metaphor, Speer reflected that the wars, revolutions, and 'politi-cal tumults' of the previous thirty years constituted 'the true school for the public mind to keep moving and turning in, true moral volcanoes, laying waste all around their craters and creating fresh, green and lively productions with their widely-hurled lava... the storm has subsided, but the waters still heave'.[143] Speer listed the consequences of these convulsions to include diminished respect for 'antiquity and ancient institutions', contending that 'the sacredness of the pulpit holds less in awe, the dignity of the Bench holds less in terror... moral and social order seem shaken',[144] even in an England where 'moral energy and activity form such prominent traits'.[145] At a distance of thirty years, in places Speer's work reads as a minor but highly informed reprise of Edmund Burke's *Reflections on the Revolution in France*. For instance, where Burke in 1790 had defended political institutions 'in a just correspondence and symmetry with the order of the world',[146] Speer understood the medical arena of the 1820s as particularly suscep-tible to 'the change of mind and modes of thinking', having moved 'at even a more rapid rate than its colleague institutions'.[147]

As we have seen, Brown saw organized religion as a fundamental safeguard to social order, his work driven by 'the conviction that Infidelity is spreading throughout our country, and threatening to destroy all that is valuable in its character'.[148] Less zealous than Brown in this respect, Bigsby nonetheless heralded the salutary influence of churches, chapels, schools, and bible and missionary societies, noting that 'few things are so beneficial to the individual as a deep sense of the religious wants of others'.[149] However, Bigsby's portrait of the moral climate was broader. In 1826 he wrote of the importance of 'the dissemination of know-ledge to the welfare of the whole frame and body of society', of an 'intellectual culture' geared to 'direct the mind to a knowledge of all the obligations which man owes to his fellow men', extolling 'the friend of rational liberty, the lover of social order';[150] and six years later, in the year of the Great Reform Act, was sanguine enough to believe that 'the majority of the commonalty... have a great sense of self-dependence, and are provident, industrious and orderly... imbued with a considerable feeling of their sacred and moral obligations'.[151]

Bigsby was as sedulous as Davy in his analysis of social classes, distinguishing, for example, between 'the labourer in the open air, and the labourer in the workshop, or artisan', and even introducing the three subdivisions of those 'who

---

[143] Speer, *Thoughts on the Medical Profession*, 2–3.   [144] Ibid. 7–8.   [145] Ibid. 15.
[146] E. Burke, *Reflections on the Revolution in France* (1790; London, 1986), 120.
[147] Speer, *Thoughts on the Medical Profession*, 106.
[148] Brown, *A Defence of Revealed Religion*, iii.
[149] Bigsby, *Self-Supporting Dispensaries*, 12 (note).
[150] J. Bigsby, *Observations Addressed to the Inhabitants of Newark and its Neighbourhood, on the Establishment of a Mechanics' Institution* (Newark, 1826), 13–14.
[151] Bigsby, *Self-Supporting Dispensaries*, 9.

are just able to support themselves, whether well or ill', those 'who are only able to support themselves when well' and those 'who are unable to support themselves whether well or ill ... the English paupers'.[152] Similarly, in 1865 Brown demarcated 'the upper classes ... the middle class ... highly skilled artisans ... in a state of transition ... passing from the labouring into the middle class ... [and] the labouring class'.[153] As early as 1790, Prosser had articulated a similar readiness to compartmentalize society in his work on farriery, explaining that 'the health and preservation of a valuable horse are interesting to a gentleman, as instrumental to his pleasure and amusement, so is the matter interesting to a person of inferior rank, on account of the animal's intrinsic value; and indeed many of the *middling rank* have so large a proportion of their property in horses that they are frequently ruined by them'.[154] There was, certainly, an apprehensive aspect to these readings of society, a dread of the unruly, notable, for instance, in Boutflower's sense of 'melancholy' at 'how the Lower Orders of People are led away'[155] and his alarm at the assassination of the prime minister Spencer Perceval in 1812, when he feared 'this diabolical act as the precursor of much woe and bloodshed to England'.[156] Similarly, Williamson applauded the 'lower class of inhabitants' at Ryde on the Isle of Wight as 'decent; the cleanliness of their houses and persons extremely prepossessing' while deploring their counterparts in nearby Portsmouth, where the 'indecency going on in the streets is extremely unpleasant'.[157]

However, it would be a severe distortion to present social fear as the defining characteristic of these works. Rather, we must stress and examine the more compelling common denominator of the sharp compassion of the healer's art, applicable to society and public health domestically and abroad. To read Williamson on late eighteenth-century Jamaica and Davy on mid-nineteenth-century Barbados is to witness the age of improvement evolve from the patrician to the progressive. On his arrival in Jamaica, Williamson declared himself 'agreeably surprised' at the 'liberal policy and principles of conduct towards the negro labourers',[158] particularly the 'liberal and humane intention of proprietors, in securing medical attendance to their negroes',[159] backed up by the 'humanity of medical practitioners towards their negro patients ... a duty which every proper feeling calls on them to discharge with scrupulous fidelity'. Williamson felt no unease in the 'degree of exultation' he sensed at his frequent introduction 'to new friends, on account of negroes reporting to their masters or mistresses the kindness with which they had been treated by him under sickness'.[160] In short, for Williamson, the black Jamaicans, in happy thrall to their masters, their 'zealous and kind protectors', 'enjoyed as much freedom as it would be well for them to do'.[161] Where Williamson had acquiesced to, and even largely endorsed, the status quo in

[152] Bigsby, *Self-Supporting Dispensaries*, 12–13.   [153] Brown, *The Food of the People*, 1.
[154] Prosser, *A Treatise on the Strangles and Fevers of Horses*, 2.
[155] Boutflower, *Journal of an Army Surgeon*, 46.   [156] Ibid. 136.
[157] Williamson, *Medical and Miscellaneous Observations*, i. 2–3.   [158] Ibid., p. v.
[159] Ibid. 64.   [160] Ibid. 52–3.   [161] Ibid., ii. 92.

Jamaica, Davy subsequently experienced, foresaw and advocated substantial change in Barbados.

As we have seen, Davy championed a Barbados which ceased 'to associate with colour any ideas of superiority or inferiority'[162] and greeted the abolition of slavery in 1833 as 'a great evil got rid of'.[163] Contrasting the histories of 'The Society for the Improvement of Plantership', founded in 1804, and the 'St. Phillip's District Agricultural Society', formed in 1843, Davy struck the vital distinction between the *Plantership's* treatment of blacks 'as stock', where 'much the same rules were inculcated for their amelioration as for any other species of stock', and the St Phillip's Society's understanding of the 'condition of the labourers as men, as thinking, responsible moral beings, a part of the community'.[164] Davy's agenda for the future welfare of Barbados hinged on a gradualist and paternalistic emphasis on education, the source for the labourer to add to his 'bodily good qualities... certain mental ones, such as skill, improved intelligence, and honesty... he is fully equal to the making of such attainments... judiciously directed... equally for his own good, as a moral agent, and for the good of society'.[165] But Davy did not preach full equality between blacks and whites. Where he prescribed 'a religious, moral, industrial education to the inferior class, the labouring body', and 'encouragement to the coloured man to raise himself in the social scale by merit', he reserved 'a scientific education to the higher class—the proprietory class, the directing mind'.[166]

Davy's attention to class harmony, his deference to 'the sound principle' that proprietors and labourers 'cannot be disunited without injury to both classes',[167] is transferable directly back to Britain. Indeed, Davy explicitly indicated this himself by quoting from William Wordsworth's poem *The Excursion*, published in 1814, and including the lines:

> The discipline of slavery is unknown
> Amongst us; hence the more do we require
> The discipline of virtue; order else
> Cannot subsist, nor confidence, nor peace.[168]

Among our cohort, this philosophy found detailed expression in many of the specific recommendations for improvements in public health made by Bigsby, Brown, Este, and Macauley. These pieces fulfilled the physician's duty to publish discussed above, honouring Bigsby's imperative to target 'the public mind through the medium of tracts, lectures and newspapers'.[169] The public's right to know necessarily implied the opportunity to act on their improved knowledge: as

---

[162] Davy, *Introductions on the Present State of the West Indies*, p. xxiii.   [163] Ibid. p. xviii.
[164] Davy, *Five Discourses*, 138–40.
[165] Davy, *Introductions on the Present State of the West Indies*, p. xx.   [166] Ibid., p. xxiii.
[167] Davy, *Five Discourses*, 140.
[168] *Introductions on the Present State of the West Indies*, 21. John's brother Humphry had proof-read the 1798 *Lyrical Ballads*. John had nursed William in his last illness.
[169] *A Lecture on Mendicity*, 41.

Brown put it, from 'the really enlightened a deserving man has nothing to dread'.[170]
Sharing the standard conviction that 'Doctor Preventive is better than Doctor
Cure',[171] they targeted the poor and labouring classes, though not exclusively. For
instance, in his promotion of the benefits of gymnasiums, published in 1828,
Macauley bemoaned the lack of exercise taken by the gentry, professional men,
merchants, and college students but indicted the working classes in particular,
considering that regular visits to gymnasiums would be 'the most desirable change
that could be effected in the manner of rearing them'.[172] For Macauley, physical
exercise guaranteed mental fortitude: gymnastics offered children 'exercises so
well calculated... to add strength and vigour to their bodies, and thus prepare
them for the exertion of those mental faculties, with which in these countries they
are so abundantly gifted'.[173]

Este's involvement in the campaign for public baths bore much the same stamp,
in the spirit of the inaugural committee's design of 1812 that the baths would provide
'health and comfort to the community at large, and to the diseased poor in particular'.[174] By 1845 he was able to list the foundation of numerous municipal baths,
in Liverpool, Manchester, Birmingham, Glasgow, and Edinburgh for example, their
facilities 'opening to the humbler classes great sources of health and enjoyment'.[175]
Este followed Davy in the understanding that physical and spiritual welfare were
inseparable, for the individual and for the community: thus he invoked 'the old
proverb, "Cleanliness is next to Godliness" '; and celebrated further initiatives in
Scotland, activated by the duke of Buccleuch, Lord Kinnaird, and Sir George
Mackenzie, as indicative of 'a sympathy between the wealthier classes and the
more humble... an earnest desire in the affluent to promote the happiness of their
poorer brethren'.[176] At the same time, this brand of paternalism did not preclude
the prospect of self-help systems, hinted at by Este in his approval of the pioneering example of the baths in Liverpool, already almost 'self-supporting',[177] and
given further expression by Brown and especially Bigsby.

Brown, steeped in the interrelated concerns of housing, nutrition, and temperance
in his native north-east, went so far as to define 'a paternal government' as 'the
greatest and most emasculating evil that can befall a country'.[178] He found
another great source of malaise in the thirty-one-year lifespan of the 1815 Corn
Law, 'this famine law as it was not inaptly styled',[179] responsible for a generation
of malnutrition among the labouring class and their families, with the result that,
by the mid-1860s, there remained the 'plague-spot, the skeleton in the closet of
England... HER PEOPLE ARE UNDERFED'.[180] Again, poor nutrition had lasting
physical, moral, and social consequences: in Brown's analysis, the 'physical evils
resulting from deficient nutriment are extremely deplorable, and suggestive of
apprehensions of gloomy portent to the state... to reflective minds the moral ills

[170] Brown, *Medical Essays*, 29.   [171] Macauley, *Observations on Gymnastics*, 24.
[172] Ibid. 12–20.   [173] Ibid. 5.   [174] In Este, *Remarks on Baths* (1812), 83.
[175] Este, *Remarks on Baths* (1845), dedication.   [176] Ibid. 46.   [177] Ibid.
[178] Brown, *The Food of the People*, 34.   [179] Ibid. 19.   [180] Ibid. 1.

which are its probable results will appear still more dark and fearful... not only must I live well, but I must live tolerably well, if I am to be a working and useful bee, and not a mere drone, or wasp, in the human hive'. As Brown continued, this applied particularly in youth: 'Withhold in early life the food required to impart adequate physical strength for labour or much active exertion, and you form in all probability a being who must be useless or noxious to society, for scarcely to being thus reared is any moral principle imparted.'[181] Aside from his contempt for the Corn Laws, and the recommendation for increased nitrogenous products in the people's diet, Brown did not itemize specific policies beyond his broad commitment to free trade in corn and all produce, asking 'Can nations be occupied in more Christian work than the conferring of mutual benefits doubly blessing all, for all are at once both givers and receivers?'[182]

Brown expressed his attachment to the goal of self-help in the cryptic formula that the solution to poor nutrition was 'not Feed the sheep, but give the sheep pasture whereon to feed themselves'.[183] Bigsby, who shared Brown's belief in the strong correlation between poor housing and intemperance, was much more specific when he condemned the administration of the old Poor Laws as 'a grievous calamity...founded in opposition to the only true principle on which the labouring classes can be made easy in their minds, their persons, and in their dwellings—which is, that of causing them to depend upon and help themselves... rather than on the uncertain supplies of charity, or the wretched pittance dealt out with grudging hand by the overseer of the parish'.[184] Bigsby's works on the formation of a mechanics' institution at Newark and on self-supporting dispensaries encapsulate several of the same themes in social improvement. First, his celebration of a primary benefit of living in '*enlightened times*', the dissemination of knowledge 'among *all classes* of the community...no longer claimed by the *sage* only as his peculiar possession, but...the heritage of *man as man*',[185] prefigured Davy's hopes for the potential progress of the ex-slaves of Barbados. Second, Bigsby's reference to the prospect of 'a moral revolution in the working community'[186] confirms these authors' sense of a profound bond between physical and spiritual welfare. Finally, his rationale for the self-supporting dispensaries provides another example of the authors' preoccupation with class harmony: the dispensary, Bigsby explained, would enjoy 'the favour of the labouring population, together with the zealous and disinterested patronage of the upper classes'.[187]

It would be misleading to present this panoply of publications as so many components of a common agenda: Boutflower, for instance, felt that if 'the lower Orders' were to 'compare their lot with other countries, they would be sensible of the numerous Blessings and Privileges they enjoy',[188] his stance the antithesis of Bigsby's endorsement of a labouring class motivated by the 'prospective feeling' of future

[181] Ibid. 12–13.   [182] Ibid. 19.   [183] Ibid. 13.
[184] Bigsby, *Self-Supporting Dispensaries*, 11, and *Mechanics' Institution*, 12.
[185] Bigsby, *Mechanics' Institution*, 3–4.   [186] Bigsby, *Self-Supporting Dispensaries*, 6.
[187] Ibid. 5.   [188] Boutflower, *Journal of an Army Surgeon*, 34.

welfare recommended by his colleague 'Dr Smith'.[189] Still, even the most progressive among the cohort's authors in their examination of Bigsby's 'great Science of Social Happiness'[190] strike a pronounced conservative tone in their emphasis on a stable social order, cemented by private virtue and religion, and in their endorsement of cultural continuity, visible in numerous classical and historical references. Conservatism, patriotism, and deference were understandable products of a prolonged encounter with the hierarchy and discipline of army life, just as the theme of self-help matched the trajectory of the authors' careers.

PUBLISHING PROFESSIONALS: PERSONAE GRATAE?

Cantlie in his 1970s study of the army medical service believed that military medical writers of the early nineteenth century had exerted a profound influence on the profession in a wide variety of areas—surgery, tropical diseases, pathology, hygiene, preventive medicine, and post-mortems. He noted in particular the prominence of Hennen and Guthrie in the application of lessons learnt to civilian practice.[191] At the time contemporaries made a similar boast that the army was a good school of medicine. Guthrie himself hailed the salutary phenomenon of professional baptisms under fire. In his widely respected *Treatise on Gun-Shot Wounds* he recalled 'having seen young men sent out from England to the Peninsula, incapable of performing any military surgery, become able operators, in a short time, from the practical lessons inculcated in our dissecting rooms, in our hospitals, and on the field of battle'.[192] More generally, Speer distinguished between the capabilities of surgeons who had served in the army and navy, 'the greater part of whom have seen disease', and novice medics 'perfectly inexperienced and raw in all branches'.[193] On the other hand, this chapter has suggested that army surgeons did more than just hone their medical skills in their years of service, by demonstrating the readiness of a section of the cohort to engage in the manifold conflicts and tensions of their era beyond their breveted specialism in surgery and medicine. However disparate their careers and formal education, collectively these authors produced an extensive repository of experience and erudition, where their formidable discursive weaponry enabled them to set their arguments in historical, prospective, and comparative contexts.

This breadth of perspective was evident, for instance, in Brown's work on nutrition, where he referred approvingly to Malthusian theory, recollected eighteenth-century England as a land of plenty, and contrasted the topography of

---

[189] Bigsby, *Self-Supporting Dispensaries*, 34.   [190] *Lecture on Mendicity*, 1.
[191] Sir Neil Cantlie, *A History of the Army Medical Department*, 2 vols. (Edinburgh, 1974), ii. 389–99.
[192] G. J. Guthrie, *A Treatise on Gun-Shot Wounds, on Inflammation, Erysipelas, and Mortification, on Injuries of Nerves, and on Wounds of the Extremities Requiring the Different Operations of Amputation* (London, 1815), pp. v–vi.   [193] Speer, *Thoughts on the Medical Profession*, 100.

mid-Victorian London with Haussmann's *grands boulevards* in Paris.[194] Similarly, Walsh spooled his analysis of 1790s Holland as far back as the Reformation.[195] The treasure-trove of antiquity provided an irresistible sourcebook here, evidence that in their early years the authors had received a good classical education.[196] Among many, Barlow and Macauley each quoted Horace;[197] where Brown quoted Virgil, Este quoted Cicero;[198] and where Power quoted Lucretius, Dickson quoted Hippocrates.[199] Thus, as Bigsby concluded, 'in oratory and poetry, and sculpture and architecture, the remains of Greece and Rome *still* serve as models for our delighted imitation... the sages of antiquity are even now referred to for the profundity of their observations and the truth of their moral maxims'.[200] Speer inadvertently highlighted the preponderance of these references in his assertion that 'we need not go back to the days of Plato and Aristotle to learn the contempt and ridicule which... they threw upon physic when the number of doctors became too great at Athens'.[201]

In the main too late, too poor, and ultimately too professional for the Grand Tour, these authors had made the best of their service abroad to gain more than just a patina of gentlemanly *bon ton*. Their works indicate a substantial immersion in contemporary and distant cultures. Gibney, who was enraptured by the collections in the Louvre, albeit 'stolen goods from all parts of the world', estimated that he would require three volumes to cover his encounter with post-Waterloo Paris. Boutflower had passed leisure hours in the Peninsula reading William Robertson's *History of Charles V* and Germaine de Staël's *Corinne*.[202] Where Dickson invoked Rousseau, Power consulted Volney.[203] And where Neale marvelled at an Albrecht Dürer portrait of St Jerome, Wallace wondered at the 'magic influence' at work in the sculptures of Canova and Thorwaldsen.[204]

In this respect, the *Conversations on Religion with Lord Byron and others* undertaken by James Kennedy and the *Essay on the Principles of Education* written by Charles Collier provide two very striking final examples of the cohort's elevated cultural and educational standards.[205] Collier recruited ancients and moderns in

[194] Brown, *The Food of the People*, 15–16, 35.

[195] Walsh, *A Narrative of the late Expedition to Holland*, iii.   [196] See Ch. 3.

[197] Barlow, *An Address to Medical and Surgical Pupils*, frontispage; Macauley, *Observations on Gymnastics*, frontispage.

[198] Brown, *The Food of the People*, frontispage; Este, *Remarks on Baths* (1845), frontispage.

[199] Power, *Egyptian Ophthalmia*, 15; Dickson, *The Unity of Disease Analytically and Synthetically Proved*, frontispage.   [200] Bigsby, *Mechanics' Institution*, 2–3.

[201] Speer, *Thoughts on the Medical Profession*, 23.

[202] Gibney, 232; Boutflower, *Journal of an Army Surgeon*, 9.

[203] Dickson, *On the Epidemic Cholera*, frontispage; Power, *Egyptian Ophthalmia*, 1–9. Volney was a member of the Idéologues, a group of materialists and social reformers who dominated Parisian intellectual life about 1800. His most famous work was his *Méditations sur les revolutions des empires* (1791).

[204] Neale, *Letters from Portugal and Spain*, 106–8; Wallace, *A Physiological Enquiry Respecting the Action of the Moxa*, 5.

[205] J. Kennedy, *Conversations on Religion with Lord Byron* (London, 1830). Kennedy's work is familiar to Byron scholars: see, for example, Paul Douglass, 'Byron's Life and His Biographers', in D. Bone (ed.), *The Cambridge Companion to Byron* (Cambridge, 2004), 18.

his treatise: Aristotle, Quintilian, and Plutarch, followed by Montaigne, Milton, Locke, and Rousseau.[206] Kennedy's attempts to convert Byron—'not the poet of virtue'[207]—to the gospel truth of the Scriptures offer the poet's biographer the beguiling prospect of 'the renowned poet of ungodliness... locked in gentle, bantering argument with an evangelical preacher'.[208] In our context, the profusion of Kennedy's learning provides the most significant aspect of the account. This enabled him, for instance, to counter anticlericalism in Hume, Voltaire, and Gibbon with transrationalism from Milton, Newton, and Pascal.[209] Even more revealing was the autodidactic fervour Kennedy displayed in the preparation of his work, the extensive diet of reading he prescribed for himself to justify his intention to 'present a view of the external, but chiefly of the internal evidence of Christianity, such as they appear to a well-educated layman'.[210] Yet Kennedy did not favour erudition over duty. When his widow published the *Conversations* in 1830, she included excerpts from her husband's agonizing correspondence written shortly before his death from the yellow fever he had treated among British troops in Jamaica in September 1826. These letters record Kennedy's determination, only a fortnight from the grave, not to 'flinch from such duty... I could not leave in the midst of such sickness, when medical men are so few.'[211] This is a helpful reminder that, for all their range and diversity, these publications were primarily an offshoot of the authors' military and medical careers.

In this perspective, where McGrigor presides as the dominant personality in the cohort, Guthrie emerges as the most substantial man of science, the weight of his career evident in his imposing body of publications, dating from 1811 to 1853. Their contents confirm Guthrie's significance in three key areas: as an effective contributor to public debate, and as an expert in ophthalmia and surgery. On all three counts Guthrie operated in London, at the eye of Brown's 'storm which apparently agitates the metropolis'.[212] As a professor of anatomy and surgery to the Royal College of Surgeons, Guthrie was an influential voice in the campaigns which culminated in the passing of the Anatomy Act in 1832. In the late 1820s and early 1830s, he lobbied Parliament directly in open letters to the home secretary and to Lord Althorp. The Act's creation of the post of inspector of anatomy fulfilled Guthrie's advocacy of greater cooperation between medical experts and politicians and introduced a system of licensing for all anatomists, again at the insistence of Guthrie and other notable medics.[213]

Guthrie's works on ophthalmia reflect one of the central concerns and achievements of his civilian career. Even before Waterloo, he had attended lectures in

[206] C. Collier, *An Essay on the Principles of Education, Physiologically Considered* (London, 1856), 30.
[207] *Conversations on Religion with Lord Byron*, 330.
[208] F. MacCarthy, *Byron: Life and Legend* (London, 2002), 469–70.
[209] *Conversations on Religion with Lord Byron*, 54.   [210] Ibid. 430–1.
[211] Ibid. 441–2.   [212] *Medical Essays*, 3.
[213] G. J. Guthrie, *A Letter to the Right Hon. the Secretary of State for the Home Department, Containing Remarks on the Report of the Select Committee of the House of Commons on Anatomy* (London, 1829); and *Remarks on the Anatomy Bill, in a Letter Addressed to Lord Althorp* (London, 1832).

London at the capital's Infirmary for Diseases of the Eye (later Moorfields), where the surgeons were William Lawrence (1783–1867) and the former East India Company doctor, Benjamin Travers (1783–1858).[214] Between 1819 and 1834 he published treatises on artificial pupils and cataracts and three editions of his *Lectures on the Operative Surgery of the Eye*.[215] The appearance of these works ran parallel with Guthrie's instrumental role in the foundation and development of the infirmary, established as the Royal Westminster Ophthalmic Hospital in December 1815.[216] They accompanied Guthrie's tangible contributions—professional and financial—to the early successes of the hospital. Through the first fifteen years of the hospital's history, Guthrie donated £142;[217] through the same phase the hospital recorded 604 successful treatments of cataracts and formations of artificial pupils, a figure which rose to 1,958 by 1851.[218] Guthrie dedicated the second edition of his lectures to the patrons, president, vice-president, and governors of the infirmary 'to whose kindness and liberality the institution is indebted for its origin and support'.[219] The appreciation was mutual: in the month of Guthrie's death in May 1856, a special meeting of governors and managers hailed 'the valuable services he has rendered to this Hospital from its first formation, extending over a period of nearly forty years . . . his skill, high reputation and untiring energy in promoting its interests'.[220]

Finally, Guthrie's works on the treatment of gunshot wounds in particular and military surgery in general testified to his expertise and innovation in the field, where his appetite for the lessons of conflict even led him to regret that 'we had not another battle in the south of France, to enable me to decide two or three points of surgery which were doubtful'.[221] Though denied this opportunity, Guthrie had derived and refined his skills through his charge of the wounded at numerous battles and sieges in the Peninsular war, and from his presence at the military

[214] Eye diseases were a particular bane of the army. While in Egypt, the soldiers had been struck down by a particularly virulent infection. Later in the Peninsula, it was believed by some surgeons that malingerers had learnt to produce the symptoms of the disease. See Martin Howard, *Wellington's Doctors: The British Army Medical Service in the Napoleonic Wars* (Staplehurst, 2000), 175–7. For Travers and Lawrence, see *DNB*, *sub nominee*.

[215] See his *Treatise for an Operation for the Formation of an Artificial Pupil* (London, 1819); *On the Operation for Extraction for a Cataract from the Eye* (London, 1834); *On the Certainty and Safety with which the Operation of the Extraction of a Cataract May be Performed* (London, 1834); and the three editions of his *Lectures on the Operative Surgery of the Eye* (London, 1823, 1827, and 1830).

[216] Institute of Ophthalmology Library (London): *Rules for the Government of the Royal Westminster Ophthalmic Hospital . . . with a List of the Governors and Subscribers and the Report of Receipt and Expenditure for the Year 1831, Corrected to July 1832* (London, 1832), 1.

[217] Ibid. 24.

[218] Ibid. 3; and *Rules and Regulations of the Royal Westminster Ophthalmic Hospital . . . with a List of the Governors, Subscribers & c. to June 1851; and the Treasurer's and Surgeon's Report to the End of the Year 1850* (London, 1851), 14.

[219] *Lectures on the Operative Surgery of the Eye*, 2nd edn. (1827), dedication.

[220] *Report of the Royal Westminster Ophthalmic Hospital, Charing Cross, Founded in 1816 for the Relief of Indigent Persons Afflicted with Diseases of the Eye, with a List of the Governors, Subscribers & c. to April 1856, and the Treasurer and Surgeon's Report to the End of the Year 1855* (London, 1856), 6.

[221] *Commentaries on the Surgery of War*, v.

hospitals in Brussels and Antwerp in the aftermath of Waterloo. He drew heavily on this experience in his further works, notably in the five editions of his *A Treatise on Gunshot Wounds*, later republished as *Commentaries on the Surgery of War*.[222] As late as 1846, in yet another study of surgical practice, Guthrie was able to reflect that the established treatment for wounded arteries dated back to the methods he had helped to pioneer in the Peninsular and Napoleonic wars.[223] In short, here again Guthrie's publications cemented his eminent status, encouraging the Royal Society obituarist to note that he had 'justly earned the highest reputation among the British military surgeons of his time; and all his writings prove that they were to him fields not only of action but of study'.[224]

In action and especially in print, Guthrie incarnated the aspect of our authors' advance with the army presented in this chapter. In one sense, we can read these collected works as the title deeds of a burgeoning corps of medical professionals in nineteenth-century Britain, as evidence of their right to be respected and taken seriously by an educated lay world, especially by fellow optimists and improvers. The cohort's authors were helping to make medicine something more than the marketplace squabbled over by the loose community of quacks, celebrated by the late Roy Porter.[225] In this respect, of course, our authors' contribution was dynamic but not unique. Many other practitioners who had never been near the armed services made important contributions to the development of medical science and practice. It would be extravagant to identify the army as the dominant source of an emerging confederacy of medical professionals. There again, as a subgroup of the professionalizing medical community, they made an impressively large contribution. Over 15 per cent of the cohort were published authors. A survey of the publications of Edinburgh MDs who graduated in the two years 1812–13 would suggest that a maximum of only 10 per cent of learned physicians, the most obvious subgroup from which medical authors would emerge, ever went into print.[226]

The publications studied in this chapter, then, have demonstrated the notable extent to which our cohort matched the conviction, assigned to Tertius Lydgate by George Eliot, that the medical profession presented 'the most perfect interchange between science and art' and offered 'the most direct alliance between intellectual conquest and social good'.[227] What united many, if not all, of the

[222] *A Treatise on Gun-shot Wounds* (London, 1815, 1820, 1827); and *Commentaries on the Surgery of War* (London, 1853, 1855).

[223] G. J. Guthrie, *On Wounds and Injuries of the Arteries of the Human Body, with the Treatment and Operations Required for their Cure Illustrated by 130 Cases Selected from the Records of the Practice of the Most Celebrated Surgeons in Europe and America* (London, 1846), 1.

[224] *Proceedings of the Royal Society*, 8 (1856–7), 273.

[225] Roy Porter, *Health for Sale: Quackery in England, 1660–1850* (Manchester, 1989).

[226] Twelve authors out of 120 doctors—and of these, four were army doctors: see *Nomina eorum qui gradum medicinae doctoris in academia Jacobi sexti Regis quae Edinburgi est, adepti sunt* (Edinburgh, 1846), 44–7.

[227] George Eliot, *Middlemarch*, ch. 15. Lydgate had studied in Paris but had never been in the army. The novel is set in Coventry in the 1830s.

cohort's authors was their fusion of profession and discovery.[228] We can encapsulate this combination in Bigsby's belief that he inhabited an epoch where the principles of mechanical and chemical science were 'never so well understood, nor the laws of social life so well investigated',[229] and in Speer's assertion that 'the pride of profession has succeeded the pride of commerce'.[230] In short, these works attest the authors' confidence that they had witnessed and articulated the definitive rejection of 'the old uninquiring times'.[231]

[228] Wallace, *A Physiological Enquiry*, 4.   [229] Bigsby, *Mechanics' Institution*, 3–4.
[230] Speer, *Thoughts on the Medical Profession*, 35.   [231] Ibid. 105.

8

Reflection

METHODOLOGY

Any rigorous study of a microcosm of society, such as this, inevitably prompts the question, and so what? This is always difficult to answer objectively from a particular perspective after years of laborious research. We would argue from our experience of detailed prosopographical enquiry over the last decade that we are experiencing a paradigm shift certainly in social history, but perhaps also in other parts of historical discourse, making 'what was familiar appear strange and what was natural seem arbitrary'.[1] Our claim rests on the ability to explore collective biography drawing on resources that are available in increasing volume across the Internet. Many of these have only been released during the course of our research, for example the wills proved in the Prerogative Court of Canterbury (PCC) and commissary courts in Scotland, the union catalogue of the United Kingdom's research libraries, and the Access to Archives database.[2] Such resources are not just available at a national level, but also locally and particularly, for example wills proved in the diocesan court at Chester in the Chester wills database, and the lists of officers who served at any time with the Gloucester Regiment and their place of death.[3] These are mirrored by equivalent resources in other countries, such as the on-line catalogue of the National Archives of South Africa and the Australian Medical Pioneers Index.[4] The majority of these resources represent the making available of existing physical catalogues on-line. In some instances the underlying resources can also be accessed, as is the case with the PCC wills and those proved in Scotland. Although these were obviously searchable in the past, finding information was both frustrating and time consuming. Moreover the way in which the physical indexes were constructed made it almost impossible to search by occupations or professions, or by place. This inevitably constrained prosopographical research, especially where no genealogies were readily available. Until recently, the most accessible family trees were those to

---

[1] Cited in P. Burke, *A Social History of Knowledge from Gutenberg to Diderot* (Cambridge, 2002), 2.
[2] Available at www.nationalarchives.gov.uk/documentsonline (July 2005), www.scottishdocuments. com/content/default.asp (July 2005), www.copac.ac.uk (July 2005), and www.a2a.org.uk (July 2005).
[3] www.cheshire.gov.uk/Recordoffice/Wills/Home.htm (July 2005) and members.tripod.com/ ~Glosters (July 2005).
[4] Available at www.medicalpioneers.com (July 2005) and www.national.archives.gov.za (July 2005).

be found in the pages of the peerages and landed gentry. This may help explain why there has been so much interest by historians in the aristocracy and gentry, typified by Lawrence Stone, *The Crisis of the Aristocracy, 1588–1641*, J. V. Beckett's *The Aristocracy in England 1660–1914*, and Sir John Habakkuk's *Marriage, Debt, and the Estates System: English Landownership 1650–1950*.[5] Even studies that ostensibly have a wider focus draw heavily on examples from the aristocracy and gentry, for example William Rubinstein's early work on large fortunes.[6] This makes all the more remarkable the work of historians who investigated the middle and professional classes before the advent of on-line catalogues, such as Leonore Davidoff and Catherine Hall, and Peter Earle.[7]

Although the existence of these catalogues has made this investigation possible, they are by no means the only resources available on the Internet that we have drawn on to amplify our study. Archivists have been aware for some time of the growing enthusiasm for family history, and historians owe the conversion of many on-line catalogues to this constituency. Both the National Archives at Kew and the National Archives of Australia place family history at the top of their lists of research interests on their home pages.[8] Archives produce and contribute to a multitude of guides to help the family historian, such as Amanda Bevan's *Tracing Your Ancestors in the Public Record Office*,[9] Cecil Sinclair's *Tracing Your Scottish Ancestors*,[10] and John Grenham's *Tracing Your Irish Ancestors*.[11] The National Archives has published specialist guides for those researching family members in the armed services, which are invaluable tools in navigating the complex War Office and Admiralty series.[12] These conventionally published guides are supplemented by a plethora of on-line guides and resources. In the United Kingdom the most extensive is GENUKI, which provides comprehensive information about resources available either on-line or physically in every part of the United Kingdom and Ireland.[13] The website of the Church of the Latter Day Saints, Family Search (IGI) gives access to a large number of records of baptisms, marriages, and censuses in the United Kingdom and many other parts of the world, particularly North America.[14] We used this resource relentlessly in building the genealogies of the members of the cohort.

As for every user, the Internet has rendered the epistemic family history communities much more tractable, and, as a result, they have become more

[5] (Oxford, 1967); (Oxford, 1986); (Oxford, 1994).

[6] W. D. Rubinstein, *Men of Property: The Very Wealthy in Britain since the Industrial Revolution* (London, 1981).

[7] L. Davidoff and C. Hall, *Family Fortunes: Men and Women of the English Middle Classes, 1780–1850* (London, 1987; rev. edn., London, 2002); Peter Earle, *The Making of the English Middle Class: Business, Society and Family Life in London, 1660–1730* (London, 1989).

[8] www.nationalarchives.gov.uk/default.htm (July 2005), and www.naa.gov.au (July 2005).

[9] 6th edn. (London, 2002).   [10] (Edinburgh, 1990).   [11] (Dublin, 1992).

[12] Simon Fowler, *Army Records for Family Historians*, Public Records Office Readers' Guide No. 2 (London, 1992); William Spencer, *Army Records for Family Historians* (London, 2000); Bruno Pappalardo, *Tracing Your Naval Ancestors* (London 2003).

[13] www.genuki.org.uk (July 2005).   [14] www.familysearch.org (July 2005).

fragmented and narrowly focused and at the same time locationally more dispersed. This has made it possible for extended family networks around the globe to discover each other and communicate in real time in a way that was never possible before. This excites the anthropologist Alexander Stille, who in his otherwise gloomy book, *The Future of the Past: How the Information Age Threatens to Destroy our Cultural Heritage*, concluded euphorically: 'Genealogy Web sites rank just after pornography sites as the most popular venues on the World Wide Web, . . . suggesting that the desire for finding one's historical roots ranks just after erotic pleasure among humankind's deepest needs'.[15] Be that as it may, engagement with such communities of family historians, analogous to the *équipes* of the Annales school of a pre-digital age, can be richly rewarding as they exchange information that previously would have been almost be impossible for the historian to unlock. They are encountered serendipitously using search engines. It is true that those with unusual patronymics or combination of names are easier to locate, but that does not make these resources any the less valuable. In some instances such groups are making available in digital form whole family histories or transcriptions of family papers. A search for Loinsworth (the patronymic of two members of the cohort) results in a remarkable series of letters of Thomas Goldie Scott (not in the cohort), surgeon to the 79th Cameron Highlanders (written between 1842 and 1859), which are being patiently transcribed by a descendant, Hamish Goldie-Scott.[16] These contain some quite wonderful insights, such as this description of Sir Robert Sale, the putative hero of the Afghan campaign:

I met Sir Robert as I came up the hill, and found him thrashing a few of the native workmen, and knocking them right and left. I was sure of him as soon as I saw him, and asked a soldier if it was the great man. So I went up and introduced myself to him, and after taking a good look at me, he gave me a hearty shake of the hand; "I am delighted to see you, Scott. Just come eh? We are all in a bustle here, you see boy". He thereupon set to again to thrash the natives, so I made off.[17]

The key to unlocking the Irish antecedents of Sir William Beatty, Nelson's surgeon at Trafalgar, was making contact with the Beatty family history group, which provided the evidence that the entry in the *Victory*'s crew-list, which gave his place of birth as Scotland, was incorrect.[18] Some historians affect to distrust such research, disparagingly dismissing it as amateur. Our experience both in the quality of the results and the guides provided is quite the reverse. As with any historical scholarship, the output of others needs to be approached sceptically, but by careful triangulation results can be easily verified. Although most (but not all) such resources are brutally reductionist, they cannot be criticized for being positivist as they lack context, because their focus is so particular.

---

[15] A. Stille, *The Future of the Past: How the Information Age Threatens to Destroy our Cultural Heritage* (London, 2002), 330.

[16] www.dgs.btinternet.co.uk/Files/DIARYII.doc1Loinsworth&hl5en (July 2005).

[17] Thomas Goldie Scott to his father, Kussowli, 4 May 1843.

[18] www.beattydna.org and homepages.rootsweb.com/~bp2000/summaries2.htm (July 2005).

When we began this research it would have been almost unthinkable that a word or phrase entered into a search engine with global reach would yield satisfying results. Our first significant discovery that convinced us of its utility was Lisa Rosner's engaging biography of Alexander Lessassier, *The Most Beautiful Man in Existence: The Scandalous Life*, which was found on a pornography website.[19] Others followed including John Brine's biography of William Lane Milligan and the diaries of Lt. William St John, son of Deputy Inspector St John;[20] and Margaret Mason's remarkable on-line history of the Mason family with details of John Davy's marriage and family.[21] By the end of the project, there was something compulsive about searching for individual members of the cohort on the web and surprise if the results were incompatible. This certainly made what was familiar appear very strange indeed. We are not arguing that traditional modalities of discovery will disappear; they will not as not everything can ever be on-line. We will continue to consult lists and indexes, but the more of these that appear on-line along with other resources the greater the possibilities of contingencies that will advance understanding. In much the same way as printing advanced the distribution of knowledge, so the Internet allows such contingencies to occur irrespective of the physical location of the underlying information. This is exciting and opens up new possibilities for prosopographical research such as this, which, because of the nature of service in the armed forces, obviously transcends national boundaries. Its potential applies equally, but less obviously, to much European family history, to that of most other professions, and to the wide republic of letters.

Taken together these novel avenues of enquiry allow collective biography to become more systematic and dynamic with better coverage of antecedents and descendants. In the past the social history of regions, class, or occupational groupings in the period under study in this book have relied heavily on individual cases to develop a hypothesis. Edward Hughes began his *North Country Life in the Eighteenth Century* with the dismal tale of Sir William Chaytor as 'an extreme example of society on the wane'.[22] Davidoff and Hall began their study of the middle class with the story of James Luckock, a Radical Birmingham jeweller, whose 'narrative fits neatly into the established picture of radical politics, religious dissent and manufacturing enterprise typical of the existing account of the provincial middle class'.[23] In discussing the income and expenditure of general practitioners, Loudon relied heavily on the example of Matthew Flinders of Donnington in Lincolnshire.[24] He, also, depended a good deal on the extraordinary biographical

[19] Lisa Rosner, *The Most Beautiful Man in Existence: The Scandalous Life of Alexander Lesassier* (Philadelphia, 1999).
[20] John Brine et al., *Looking for Milligan: The Fascinating Search for William Milligan a Pioneering Doctor of the Swan River Colony c.1795–1851* (Perth, 1991); Karel Schoeman, *The Bloemfontein Diary of Lieut. W. J. St John* (Cape Town, 1988).
[21] web.archive.org/web/20041012000935/www.spaceless.com/fletcher/flet1.htm (October 2005).
[22] Edward Hughes, *North Country Life in the Eighteenth Century: The North East 1700–1750* (Oxford, 1952), 1–11. [23] Davidoff and Hall, *Family Fortunes* (edn. 1987), 13–18.
[24] Irvine Loudon, *Medical Care and the General Practitioner, 1750–1850* (Oxford, 1986), 103–9.

memoirs of Richard Smith junior, an eccentric Bristol practitioner who had strong personal preferences for those he included.[25] They all used these examples because they were accessible: in Chaytor's case because he was imprisoned in the Fleet for debt, Luckcock because he wrote an autobiography, and Flinders because he left 'meticulous financial records'. The main drawback of this approach is that it relies heavily on the judgement of the individual historian, and inevitably overlooks those who only leave shallow footprints on the pages of history. But in a situation where the historian possesses at best only partial quantifiable data and at worst none at all, this is inevitable if analysis is to be anything other than anodyne or superficial.

The *annalistes* sought to correct this approach by assembling *équipes* to gather masses of data from an extraordinary range of archives, and by so doing exposed themselves to criticism of 'naïve positivism'.[26] There has always been a suspicion amongst British historians of cliometrics, typified by Peter Burke, who in 1990 wished to write the obituary of the *Annales* school without pausing to consider the transforming effect of the computational technology.[27] Those who have whole-heartedly adopted such an approach have been few. The pioneering work of Pat Hudson on industrialization[28] and W. D. Rubinstein on wealth holding and creation[29] have been very much the exception.

The difficulty with any quantitative approach to social and economic history is that it demands commitment, time, and, for ambitious projects, resources. Although it has not yet been used for this purpose, the Oxford *DNB*, published in 2004, has been constructed to allow such analysis and for its data to be linked dynamically to other resources.[30] The Arts and Humanities Research Council-funded Clergy of the Church of England database from 1540 to 1835 at King's College, London, will provide a second resource for the investigation of a pivotal profession.[31] 'Throughout the period the Church of England was the single most important employer of educated males in England and Wales', and even at the end still represented two-thirds of all the clergy.[32] The construction of this database

---

[25] These are preserved in BRO: Loudon, *Medical Care*, 319.

[26] George Huppert, 'The *Annales* Experiment', in Michael Bentley (ed.), *Companion to Historiography* (London, 1997), 880.

[27] P. Burke, *The French Historical Revolution: The 'Annales' School 1929–1989* (Stanford, Calif., 1990).

[28] P. Hudson, *The Industrial Revolution* (London, 1992).

[29] Rubinstein, *Men of Property*; W. D. Rubinstein, 'The Role of London in Britain's Wealth Structure, 1809–99: Further Evidence', in John Stobart and Alistair Owens (eds.), *Urban Fortunes, Property and Inheritance in the Town, 1700–1900* (Aldershot, 2000).

[30] Available at www.oxforddnb.com (July 2005). Despite this good intention, the quality of the entries for the medical profession is variable and essential details for any aggregate studies, such as wealth at death, is often missing.

[31] Available at www.theclergydatabase.org.uk (July 2005).

[32] 'The Church of England between 1540 and 1835 and its Records', www.lambethpalacelibrary. org/holdings/Guides/clergyman.html (July 2005). A. Burns, K. Fincham, and S. Taylor, 'The Historical Public and Academic Archival Research: The Experience of the *Clergy of the Church of England Database*', Archives, 27 (2002), 110–19; for access to the work as it stands at present see: www.theclergydatabase.org.uk/.

exemplifies the way in which the academy can benefit from the experience in use of sources by family historians working in the localities. As the directors readily acknowledge: 'These research assistants often possess a formidable grasp of the history and records of their locality, from which the Project has benefited enormously.'[33] In Australia the Australian Medical Pioneers Database, which contains references to over 3,000 doctors from the 1700s to 1875, was built by an enthusiast, Dr David Richards, with the assistance of a band of volunteer contributors.[34]

EXISTING APPROACHES TO THE HISTORY OF THE MEDICAL PROFESSION: LIMITED HORIZONS

As we pointed out in the introduction, no one has undertaken a quantitative study of any profession, although the completion of the Clergy of the Church of England project will make this possible in the case of the most prestigious.[35] For the medical profession there is a parallel collective biography study to ours, but for a later period, nearing completion at the University of Glasgow, based on 2,000 medical students who began their studies at the universities of Edinburgh and Glasgow around 1871.[36] There have also been similar, but nothing like as extensive, studies based on other cohorts of medical students, notably Lisa Rosner's investigation of the nearly 17,000 Edinburgh students and apprentices from 1760 to 1810, and on a much smaller scale Derek Dow and Michael Moss's study of the 5,000 or so students enrolled at Glasgow from 1802 to 1830.[37] In addition use of lists of students and graduands has provided the basis for much collective medical and scientific biography, particularly in assessing the impact of great teachers and researchers, such as Hermann Boerhaave, Justus von Liebig, and Lamarck.[38] One of the drawbacks of such an institutional approach is that in the absence of systematic professional directories or registration until the middle of the nineteenth century, it is difficult to discover details of later careers or to be certain that someone with the same name is in fact the same person. This can

---

[33] 'The Collection and Processing of Data', www.lambethpalacelibrary.org/holdings/Guides/clergyman.html (July 2005). [34] Available at www.medicalpioneers.com (July 2005).

[35] see Intrd.under 'The Project'.

[36] This project is directed by Professor Anne Crowther and Dr Marguerite Dupree, their book *Medical Lives in the Age of Surgical Revolution* is forthcoming.

[37] Lisa Rosner, 'Students and Apprentices: Medical Education at Edinburgh University, 1780–1810' (Ph.D. thesis, Johns Hopkins University, 1986) [Ann Arbor: University Microfilms Internations, 1988c1985], and Derek Dow and Michael Moss, 'The Medical Curriculum at Glasgow in the Early Nineteenth Century', *History of Universities*, 7 (1988).

[38] Sabine Heller investigated Boerhaave's Swiss students in *Boerhaaves Schweizer Studenten: Ein Beitrag zur Geschichte des Medizinstudiums* (Zurich, 1984). Jacob Volhard as early as 1909 included a list of Liebig's pupils in his biography, *Justus von Liebig* (Leipzig, 1909). The tradition continued with W. H. Brock's *Justus von Liebig: The Chemical Gatekeeper* (Cambridge, 1997). Pietro Corsi, *Genèse et enjeux du transformisme, 1770–1830* (Paris, 2001), 333–65: list also available on the Internet.

be just as problematic for students of great teachers, as many tried to give the impression that they had been taught by a Boerhaave or Liebig when in fact they had not. The other uncertainty is that until the medical curriculum stabilized in the later nineteenth century, and disciplines, such as botany and chemistry, became subjects in their own right with associated degrees, it is almost impossible to discover which students were intent on entering the medical profession and which had other career plans. Equally difficult is plotting the cursus of study when, certainly amongst a large proportion of students, something equivalent to the German *peregrinatio* was commonplace, and not just in medicine. It is not sufficient to dismiss the occasional students as mere auditors, as Rosner does, because they may either have been attending lectures, particularly chemistry, to further other careers as Dow and Moss showed, or because they had or were intending to attend other courses elsewhere.[39]

The most common approach to the study of medical teaching is through the curriculum and the regulations governing the award of degrees. This can be misleading. Although the MD was the most awarded degree until the late nineteenth century, its significance can be overstressed in an age when taking a degree was not the principal reason for university attendance. Moreover, unlike the MA, it was a higher degree in the British Isles awarded, as we have shown in Chapter 3, frequently many years after the recipient had begun practice, and often as a formality, with the notable exception of Edinburgh, where a thesis was a mandatory requirement. In addition, regulations governing the taking of degrees, which had origins in the medieval syllabus, appears by the eighteenth century to have been more honoured in the breach than the observance. Medical students were supposed to have taken the foundation arts degree before progressing to higher study, but few did. Flagrant abuse, such as that at the universities of Aberdeen and St Andrews, which awarded medical degrees without any examination or 'any personal knowledge of the candidates', led to tightening of regulations early in the nineteenth century, but this was more often out of self-defence than for the good of the profession as a whole.[40] Furthermore, changes to the regulations did not necessarily mean they were translated into practice. There is enough contemporary evidence therefore to deter most historians from seeking to draw comparisons between developments in medical education and professional formation, although undoubtedly there were advances in the first part of the nineteenth century, particularly in surgery, in the principal centres of medical training, Dublin, Edinburgh, London, and to a lesser extent Glasgow. It would also be wrong to assume that certification of class attendance was simply a formality. It was not. *Viva voce* examination and peer group assessment was often robust, but it did not

[39] Lisa Rosner, *Medical Education in the Age of Improvement: Edinburgh Students and Apprentices 1760–1828* (Edinburgh, 1991), 104–18, and Dow and Moss, 'Medical Curriculum', 248–9.

[40] J. Coutts, *A History of the University of Glasgow, from its Foundation in 1451 to 1909* (Glasgow, 1909), 542–3.

equate to the utilitarian professional examinations that were to become a feature of the late nineteenth century.[41]

The much more common approach to the study of professional formation is through the histories of medical corporations. A. M. Carr-Saunders and P. A. Wilson relied heavily on the histories of corporations in their pioneering study of the professions, published in 1933.[42] Penny Corfield's treatment of the medical profession has a strong institutional focus.[43] This is not to say that the medical corporations were irrelevant in the development of a strongly cohesive identity. They were, but in their membership and locale, they represent metropolitan or civic elites, and do not reflect the wider profession in town and country, or more importantly in the developing empire. Loudon's treatment of medical associations in the context of the family doctor reveals the extent of the tension between the commonwealth of medicine and the old corporations.[44]

Although it is self-evident that many men who practised medicine or held medical qualifications had interests or even professional lives that extended far beyond medicine, studies that are narrowly professionally focused fail to encapsulate this aspect of their lives. At best men such as Charles Darwin or William Henslow, both of whom had MDs, are described as scientists, at worst their scientific interests or contribution to the republic of letters is overlooked. This failure to capture 'whole lives' becomes more acute when trying to locate the medical man, such as the Bristol surgeon and member of the cohort, John Howell, with his multifarious interests and engagements, within the context of his family or society at large.

Such neglect is not surprising. There are almost no studies that attempt to examine family strategies against the background of emerging professional opportunities. This is even true for the landed, the one group whose fortunes have been closely surveyed by historians. It has become a truism that younger sons of the aristocracy and the gentry entered the Church, but as families grew in size from the late eighteenth century there would be too many younger sons to fill even the expanding number of benefices. Given the contraction in the size of the armed services after 1815, the officer cadre cannot have taken up the slack either. In fact, a glance through the genealogies in the peerage and landed gentry seems to suggest that there were clearly defined multiple strategies in some families in approaching the professions, a son in the armed services, another in the East India Company, another in the law, another in the Church, another in medicine, and some even in trade. The Mackenzies of Scatwell provide one such example. Sir John of Tarbat, the first baronet (b. 1626), had six sons: George the eldest became 1st Earl of Cromarty; John the second died young; Roderick the third became a senator of the College of Justice (a judge); Alexander of Ardloch the

[41] H. J. Perkin, *The Origins of Modern English Society, 1780–1880* (London, 1969), 258–9.

[42] A. M. Carr-Saunders and P. A. Wilson, *The Professions* (Oxford 1933).

[43] P. J. Corfield, *Power and the Professions in Britain, 1700–1850* (London, 1995), 153–7.

[44] Loudon, *Medical Care*, 267–301.

fourth married land; Kenneth the fifth has no professional designation; and James the sixth was an MD.[45] John Habakkuk laid to rest the myth of the unprovided younger sons of the aristocracy and gentry in his masterly *Marriage, Debt, and the Estates System: English Landownership 1650–1950*, but the evidence from family genealogies is that many sons had careers, which would suggest that they were not prepared simply to live on their competences.[46] And this was probably not new. J. H. Hexter for an earlier period has shown that there was direct interaction between the landed elite and expanding commercial centres, with younger sons pursuing urban careers to build fortunes.[47]

The education of children of the aristocracy and gentry is again rarely discussed, and even where occasionally it is, as in Toby Barnard's recent study of the Irish aristocracy, not in the context of any future career.[48] This is despite the fact that as John Brewer has shown increasingly during the eighteenth century even for appointments in the public service patronage was necessary but not sufficient without some proof of ability.[49] Siblings of the aristocracy were not above holding such positions, which could be lucrative.[50] Charles Leadbetter, the author of *The Royal Gauger*, the eighteenth-century bible of the excise service, recommended that prospective candidates concentrate on passing the tough entry exams before seeking the support of a patron.[51] Given the extent of patronage in aristocratic hands, the lack of interest in the extended families of the aristocracy and gentry is all the more surprising.

This can partly be explained by the lack of exploration of patronage networks, even though there is an abundance of evidence amongst the papers of aristocratic families. It, also, certainly owes something to the notion that the professional and commercial classes were 'rising' and filling the careers that were increasingly open to talent. Corfield expresses this point of view when she writes: 'Social rank was not abolished; but it was becoming more diversified and accessible.'[52] So, too, does Christopher Brooks in his study of 'apprenticeship, social mobility and the middling sort, 1550–1800'. Although he shows that a substantial number of entrants to London and provincial guilds came from gentry origins, he qualifies this finding by pointing out that many came from the borderline between gentry and yeoman stock. In the case of the London Company of Barbers Surgeon between 1658 and 1660, 23 per cent claimed to be from such a background, while in the case of the Apothecaries between 1680 and 1681 25 per cent. A decade later

---

[45] *Burke's Peerage* (London, 1936), *sub nomine*.   [46] (Oxford, 1994), 97–117.
[47] J. H. Hexter, 'The Myth of the Middle Class in Tudor England', *Explorations in Entrepreneurial History*, 2/3 (1950), 128–40.
[48] John Habakkuk, *Marriage, Debt and the Estates System* (Oxford, 1994), ch. 2; Toby Barnard, *Making of the Grand Figure: Lives and Possessions in Ireland 1641–1770* (New Haven, 2004).
[49] John Brewer, *The Sinews of Power: War, Money and the English State, 1688–1783* (London, 1989).
[50] See for example L. A. Clarkson and E. M. Crawford, *The Ways to Wealth: The Cust Family of Eighteenth-Century Armagh* (Belfast, 1985).
[51] Charles Leadbetter, *The Royal Gauger*, 3rd edn. (London, 1750), pp. xii–xiii and 212–14.
[52] Corfield, *Power and the Professions*, 212.

the proportions were 21 per cent and 34 per cent respectively.[53] Loudon in his discussion of the background of general practitioners reached a similar conclusion from an analysis of the backgrounds of medical practitioners in Bristol and the West of England, apothecaries in London, and the roll of the Royal College of Physicians and Surgeons of London. From his small samples he opined: 'Thus medical practice at the level of the surgeon-apothecary was open to men from a wide social background; but very few were the sons of the aristocracy or the richer landed gentry. Most were the sons of medical practitioners, non-medical professionals and the minor gentry.'[54] All of this may be true, but it overlooks the obvious fact that, within a very diversified professional class, both within and between professions, there were those with strong familial bonds to the old elite, not just obviously among the clergy but among lawyers and doctors.[55]

Such evidence of professional backgrounds, as exists, is drawn entirely from English examples and there is no corresponding research in Ireland, Scotland, or Wales. The current interest in British identity naturally prompts the questions of national differences. Did the problems of marginal agriculture in Ireland, Scotland, and Wales before the French wars lead landed families to adopt different strategies from their counterparts in England? There has been some work on the national composition of the army by J. E. Cookson, but even he is forced to speculate about the background of the officer cadre.[56] Although Scots and Irish 'on the make' were a well-known feature of society in London and other English cities, Loudon did not explore this phenomenon. Corfield touches on it by quoting the 'hardly scientific' survey of the 'geographical distribution of British intellect' by the young Conan Doyle in 1888, in which he showed that every part of the United Kingdom contributed to the mid-Victorian British intelligentsia. She recognizes the self-evident contribution of the non-native English in England and more importantly in the empire, but does not go on to ask if their very mobility contributed to an emerging sense of British identity.[57] This is a difficult question to answer and demands some assessment of their contribution to the republic of letters and to the political landscape, and not only of their position but that of their children in wider society.

Although the impact of the French wars and accompanying rise in public expenditure is readily acknowledged in promoting the industrial and commercial growth of the United Kingdom, its effect on society and the professions has scarcely been examined. Patrick Colquhoun, writing in 1816, had no doubt of its impact: 'The long war, in which this country and the continent have been engaged, may be said to have given a new character to the state of society in every

---

[53] In Jonathan Barry and Christopher Brooks (eds.), *The Middling Sort of People: Culture, Society and Politics in England 1550–1800* (London 1994), 58–61.

[54] Loudon, *Medical Care*, 30–4. [55] To be fair, Corfield recognizes this.

[56] John E. Cookson, *The British Armed Nation* (Oxford 1998), 126–7. 'By these figures [i.e. the sheer number of officers during the French wars], the small gentry and other families of quite modest wealth in Scotland must have provided huge numbers of officers'.

[57] Corfield, *Power and the Professions*, 216–17.

part of Europe.'[58] Corfield concedes that the army is a profession, but she only refers to this career choice in passing.[59] Despite Cookson's assertion that the officer cadre, at least in Scotland, was drawn from the middling sort, there are few references to the military in treatments of the middle class. Peter Earle in an essay on 'the middling sort in London', refers to the fact that, 'Virtually all military men down to the rank of sergeant (and often corporal) styled themselves gentlemen on documents, however miserable their half-pay or no pay.'[60] It is difficult to know on what he based such a sweeping generalization, which overlooks the fact that half-pay was equivalent to a modern pension, payment for doing nothing. Although not secure unless an officer was lucky enough to be transferred to the retired list, it established an important principle that was to develop in the course of the nineteenth century into the concept of retirement from active work.[61] The system was admittedly confused, capricious, and inequitable, but sixteen years after Waterloo there were still over 9,000 officers drawing half-pay.[62] Many no doubt had taken civilian jobs to supplement their income or retired to agricultural properties, but their half-pay must have represented a cushion against hardship. This can be clearly seen when some officers were faced with the harsh alternative of losing it or returning to active service.[63] The hapless General Elphinstone would never have found himself in his early seventies in Afghanistan in 1846, if he had not needed the money. Half-pay, particularly in less advantaged communities in the post-bellum depression, must have had a significant impact on the economy, and contrary to the impression of its meagreness it does seem to have allowed some officers to live modestly as gentlemen.

The emergence of a retired officer class that extended beyond the aristocracy and gentry to those from less privileged social backgrounds cannot fail to have had ramifications for leisure pursuits from the chase to the library. The strong social networks that characterized army service translated into civilian life and were maintained through regimental affiliations. It is often assumed that the middling classes in the early nineteenth century were broadly Whig in outlook with a strong dissenting flavour, but this officer cadre was more likely to be Tory and, Scotland apart, Anglican. It is a mistake to conclude that this would necessarily equate with reaction. The progressive Tory was a feature of many pre-reform conurbations, particularly manufacturing centres, such as Glasgow and Manchester. Many would have served in Ireland and come to sympathize with calls for Catholic Emancipation. Many with overseas experience would have been broadly in support of free trade. Not being drawn exclusively from the 'old corruption', they had nothing to lose from reform. It is hard to know how they fitted into society. Being

---

[58] Patrick Colquhoun, *A Treatise on the Wealth, Power and Resources of the British Empire* (London, 1815), 427.					[59] Corfield, *Power and the Professions*, 25, 191, 215, and 224.
[60] Barry and Brooks, *Middling Sort*, 149.
[61] See for example L. Hannah, *Inventing Retirement* (Cambridge, 1986).
[62] Hew Strachan, *Wellington's Legacy: The Reform of the British Army, 1830–1854* (Manchester, 1984), 114.					[63] This is discussed in *United Services Magazine* (1844), no. 11, 356–8.

present at Waterloo gave them a social cachet that lasted until the end of their lives, but whether being a colonel or captain accounted for as much as it was to do later in the nineteenth century is difficult to tell. It was a new phenomenon. Just as problematic is to judge how far military experience shaped officers' career expectations for their children, or whether widening possibilities of government service shaped their children's careers. Although in the immediate post-war period the opportunities for military careers were restricted, later in the century, with the termination of the East India Company monopoly and the expansion of empire, there was an embarrassment of choices in almost every part of the globe. We know very little about intergenerational patterns of employment except the widely held, but almost certainly mistaken, assumption that sons followed in their father's footsteps in the professions as much as in industry and commerce. Loudon believed in the 'well-recognised tendency for sons to and nephews to medical men to follow their relatives' footsteps', even though this was hardly borne out by his limited statistical surveys.[64]

WHAT DOES THIS STUDY SUGGEST?

It is always tempting to conclude too much from a single study based on an admittedly small sample of members of the medical profession, who opted from whatever motive to serve in the army during the French wars. However, the sources from which it is drawn do have some unique features, not to be found with the same degree of richness elsewhere. The survey conducted by McGrigor must be one of the first in-depth enquiries into a group of employees, and, because of the range of questions asked, has a dynamic not replicated elsewhere. It is the only source, as far as we know, that contains so much detail about origins, apprenticeship, and the educational cursus. Because of the wealth of personal detail kept by the War Office and the paymaster-general, it was relatively easy, if time consuming, to supplement this core data to build a very detailed account of the cohort's military careers and subsequent places of residence. By using other resources, such as local, national and professional directories and the increasing number of on-line resources already referred to in this chapter, it was possible to build family profiles for a large proportion of the cohort. Although a small number, it is much larger and broader based than those used by other historians who have tried to shed light on the complex interactions and conjunctions that resulted in the professional groupings and what we have come to think of as the middle class. Moreover, because of the composition of the army, the cohort in its origins within the United Kingdom transcends national boundaries, extends well beyond the social elite to embrace the yeomen and mercantile classes, and confessional divides, and in its destinations embraces the wider world.

[64] Loudon, *Medical Care*, 14.

Our findings confirm that the origins of the medical profession were diverse, but suggest there are real differences between the countries that made up the United Kingdom. It was more likely that a doctor from England would have a merchant or a member of the professions as a father than a doctor from Ireland and Scotland, where many were drawn from the ranks of the minor gentry. Much evidence suggests, as we conclude in Chapter 2, that the majority were in some way more disadvantaged than their peers entering the medical profession (lack of funds, position in a family, and so on) and only finally opted for a military career because other avenues closed. However, for most, no firm choice of career was made until either the end of their training or well into it. To this extent the cohort's educational experience can be taken as representative.

As only a handful of army surgeons came from medical dynasties, there is little sign of sons following fathers into medicine, although this may not be true more widely of entrants to the profession. There is some evidence of a strategic approach to professional opportunities with the cohort's siblings pursuing other careers, but, significantly, its members were generally the only ones to enjoy the benefit of higher education and to enter the learned professions. More surprising were the number who were not initially members of the established Churches, even if several, perhaps even most, prudentially converted later to gain advancement. This is an area in which records in the United Kingdom, when compared with the rest of Europe, are unusually silent, but can be discovered from baptismal and marriage registers. There is much to be done to unravel the confessional history of the professions and the networks they supported.[65]

In the progression through apprenticeship to medical classes, our army surgeons followed a well-worn path, at least amongst those who had ambitions to rise above the mass of the profession. Much more revealing was the pattern of attendance at classes, bearing out contemporary advice to would-be medical students and the tentative conclusions of other studies. Not unexpectedly Edinburgh's importance as a centre of medical education is confirmed; so too is the central importance of the London teaching hospitals and the unaffiliated medical teachers in the capital, such as Joseph Carpue. Less expected was the peregrination of students around the London, Edinburgh, and Dublin triangle. This had been hinted at by other studies, but on nothing like the scale that this study suggests. Although Glasgow was the most important medical school outside this metropolitan triangle, it paled in comparison, but was definitely well in front of other competitors at home and abroad. There is also enough evidence to confirm the reported interest in contemporary French hospital medicine and pathological anatomy with a number of the cohort imitating colleagues in the wider profession in hurrying to the Paris Hospitals after the Battle of the Nations and then Waterloo.[66]

[65] See for example Sahni D'Cruze, 'The Middling Sort in Eighteenth Century Colchester: Independence, Social Relations and the Community Broker', in Barry and Brooks, *Middling Sort*, 181–207.

[66] For the chief secondary works on the Paris school and its attraction to British medical students, see Ch. 4, n. 50.

The most remarkable feature of the cohort's attendance at medical classes is its members' persistence. The presence of 'mature' students had been noted by Dow and Moss in their study of early nineteenth-century Glasgow but, again, they had never suggested that many practitioners returned to the classroom after initial training.[67] This has the hallmark of modern professional development, but may have had as much to do with collegiality and patronage. The other interesting feature is the importance the cohort attached to obtaining formal medical qualifications, particularly MDs and membership of the Royal College of Surgeons. This can be explained in some instances by regulations governing promotion and preferment, but not all, suggesting that an MD was a useful cachet in building a civilian practice.

Occasionally there are glimpses of patronage at work in the background of medical education. Medical teachers, such as Carpue in London and Thomson in Edinburgh, appear as significant brokers in securing appointments, but behind them are often real patrons whose guiding advice had to be sought and approval given before a final career choice was made. Their relationship to the medical students can often only be guessed at, a local grandee from their place of birth, a friend of the family, a relative, and so on. Frequently there seems to be no direct financial relationship, but more of smoothing a young man's path by making the right introductions. For those who made a success of their military careers and, perhaps more importantly, caught the eye of the duke of Wellington or one of his staff, patronage, or at least the expectation of it, influenced career decisions and prospects long after army service had ended. Throughout the United Kingdom, those who had served at Waterloo occupied a special place in the community, and often exploited it to their advantage.

Although for some service in the army was brief, for others it was long and varied. A substantial number saw service in several theatres of war and in many different countries. They emerge not as the stereotypical bores and sawbones of contemporary satire, but, with a few exceptions, as thoroughly professional. Given the quality of their pre-service education, it is not surprising that the majority turned out to be good doctors in a contemporary understanding of the term. But the fact that so many were able to fulfil their potential must owe much to Sir James McGrigor. The director-general was determined to raise the public profile of the army medical service after the biting public criticism and lampooning of the board in the wake of the Walcheren fiasco. The huge reduction in the army after 1815 gave him his chance. The questionnaire that formed the point of departure for this study gave him a proper idea of the educational attainments and service record of the men who were under his stewardship and made it possible to set high-level entry qualifications for future entrants. More importantly, the returns allowed him to root out the incompetent, as well as those he disliked, and to encourage men with scientific interests, long before this became a desirable attribute of the medical practitioner at large. Consequently, it is only to be

[67] Dow and Moss, 'The Medical Curriculum', 244–8.

expected that these men when on overseas service, particularly in countries that were largely unexplored, should have shown a lively interest in its geography and natural history. What remains unknown is how far such interests extended to other members of the officer cadre, or whether the army surgeon with his books and microscope was an anomaly. There is much to suggest that he had companions with interests that extended beyond science into the humanities, particularly local languages and cultures. The White Mughals with their native wives and dress and love of Indian culture and language hardly fit the image of army officers conjured up by Lawrence Sterne in *Tristram Shandy*.[68]

Some surgeons, once they had left the service, self-consciously retired to live on their half-pay and whatever competence they might have. These men are detectably harbingers of a new phenomena of retirement in the middling classes, embracing a life of leisure, that before was confined to the aristocracy and gentry and their dependants. Arguably the possibility of retirement is a defining characteristic of the modern profession. This phenomenon was not confined, moreover, to those with property to return to, but extended to others from relatively disadvantaged backgrounds who had served for many years in the army, such as John Davy. Most of the cohort, however, had to establish themselves in civilian practice. Their ability to flourish and gain much sought-after hospital appointments depended on the critical combination of their army experience, recognition by the outside world of McGrigor's commitment to education and training, and patronage.

Whether retired or in civilian practice, these men, along with their fellow officers, would have represented something new on the streets of Britain. There had been those who had returned from a life abroad before, but never so many and with such varied experience, who could talk not just about battles won and lost, but about countries and places many of their contemporaries could only have guessed at. Many members of the cohort took advantage of their allure to become fully engaged in their host communities. Besides their medical work, they actively pursued their broader intellectual interests and often contributed to the emerging voluntary organizations and adult education in the provision of social welfare. Again it is not known if this was a wider phenomenon amongst the officer class. Did all those younger sons of the gentry who are listed as major generals and colonels do more than indulge themselves when they left the services?

The most striking feature of the surgeons' civilian lives is their mobility, not just in search of civilian employment but also in choice of a place of retirement. Few went home, and usually only if they had something to go home to, occasionally a family practice but more commonly land. Because of the difference in background of those from Ireland and Scotland, more returned to their roots in those countries than in England, but these are a minority. A large proportion chose to settle in England, particularly if they had achieved senior rank in London either to

[68] William Dalrymple, *White Mughals: Love and Betrayal in Eighteenth-Century India* (London, 2004).

practise or, presumably, to be near the friends they had made in the army. Although educated men had been mobile before, the scale of this mobility would seem to be unprecedented in medical practice, particularly away from metropolitan centres and resort towns such as Bath. It was more common in the Church, where young ordinands in search of preferment had to take whatever they could find in whatever diocese. This is likewise a portent for the future, as mobility has become a characteristic of all professional life, both in work and in retirement.

For this period there has been relatively little research into the wealth of the middling classes. Perhaps the most surprising finding of this study is how much money many of the cohort left that cannot be linked to any patrimony. A third left more than £5,000 net of the value of any real estate they may have owned. In present-day purchasing power this was an equivalent to a share portfolio of £350,000, an exceptional sum.[69] It would not be an exaggeration to describe the richest—the Estes of this world—as plutocrats. Many made themselves rich through their civilian practice, but fortunes were also left by surgeons who had spent their whole adult life in the army. This suggests, contrary to the general impression, that army service, though expensive, could be lucrative.[70] Although part of the explanation must be that there was little need to spend money on foreign service, it is not sufficient to explain the impressive wealth of some medical officers. This must be linked to the opportunity to provide care for the wives and families of their colleagues and to indulge more generally in civilian practice while stationed abroad. Sometimes, as in the case of those with long service in India and Ceylon, riches would also seem to have derived from activities completely unconnected with their profession.

The most visible source of non-medical income was through writing and publication. Running as a strand through the careers of 15 per cent of the cohort is literary endeavour, spanning the serious and the popular, medicine, natural history, geography, travel guides, leisure pursuits, and even literature. This was an astonishing discovery and locates these men, quite unexpectedly, within the wider republic of letters and the world of popular literature. In the case of John Davy contact with the world of the literati was particular close. Although it is impossible to be certain, the scale of this engagement with the contemporary literary and scientific world must be exceptional, reflecting the richness and diversity of the surgeon's experience. They had a lot to write about, and were encouraged, certainly in their scientific endeavours, by McGrigor. Their oeuvre was also symptomatic of the contemporary preoccupation with the supposed benefits of spa waters and sea bathing. Their ability to get their works into print was also new, a consequence of the technological advances made during the war, and the improvements in distribution stemming from the coming of the railways and the steamship. They emerge as men, even if usually Tory in their outlook, who were dedicated to

---

[69] £5,000 in 1850 at 2002 prices: see **www.eh.net/hmit/ppower/bp**: Miami university prices index (Jan. 2006).   [70] Strachan, *Wellington's Legacy*, 112.

progress and symptomatic of it. Such progressive Toryism was a feature of many of Britain's professional communities.[71]

The choices of career of their sons and the sorts of family into which their children (both sons and daughters) married is telling, suggesting that the surgeons were not committed simply to consolidating their position within the broad middling classes, but that they were engaged in a peculiarly professional project. They aimed to place their family in future generations, not just within medicine, but in the officer cadre proper or the more 'genteel' professions, such as the law and the Church, or white-collar professions serving the industrial elite. This poses challenging questions about the definition of the middling class in the era of the industrial revolution as closed and self-sustaining. The family dynamics of the cohort, which we would argue is as representative of a profession's behaviour as those used in other studies such as Davidoff and Hall or Corfield, suggests that this is a mistaken view. It would appear at the very least that the mercantile and manufacturing middle class needs to be differentiated from its professional counterpart, as Perkin intuited long ago.[72]

The characteristics of this professional middling class, however, may need to be rethought. Whether defined by occupation or wealth, this professional middling class appears to be fluid and dynamic with considerable mobility both social and geographic: it lacks a neat profile, just as its separate professional components lack a common distinctive identity. The range of wealth alone indicates it was much more granular than a catch-all nomenclature suggests or Hoppen's notion of the membership of an 'exclusive' middle class.[73] At the same time, it was not necessarily modern, a class of individuals whose success depended on education, ability, and effort. As this study makes clear, a successful career in the army medical service still depended highly on patronage, extending down from the grandees of the old corruption, but also entwining the men of the new meritocratic elite.

Of course, it would be foolhardy to reach any firm conclusions from this study alone, but it does provide pointers towards a redefinition of the complex layering of nineteenth-century society with an internal dynamic that cannot simply be characterized by concepts such as the 'rising middle class'. The results of this study show that some surgeons simply maintained a flat social trajectory or even declined. Others did rise but not just within the middling classes; two families at least entered the ranks of the landed elite as defined by Burke's *Landed Gentry*. It is, though, worth asking what exactly this meant in the context of such a pluralized society. Did it set them and their children apart from their peers, or was the distinction more subtle, a social cachet that by the end of the century was more quaint than useful?

Historians are often prompted by studies such as these either to claim too much or to seek for greater amplification. Although we are confident that such enquiries

[71] K. Theodore Hoppen, *The Mid-Victorian Generation 1846–1886* (Oxford, 1998), 44.
[72] Perkin, *Origins of Modern English Society*, 252–70.
[73] Hoppen, *Mid-Victorian Generation*, 42.

are now much more practical than in the past, we would hesitate from indulging in calls for further research to add weight to our general conclusions. We have approached the considerable body of evidence that we have accumulated with caution, but given its catholic composition, it is difficult to argue that the sample cohort can be skewed. It might be claimed that in the early nineteenth century members of the army medical service were socially very much on the margins of the British medical community, but this can scarcely be argued by the end of the McGrigor era. There seems little reason to doubt, then, that our findings have a wider applicability. At the very least they provide statistical scaffolding for a reassessment of the emergence of the medical profession during the critical period of the French wars and before the introduction of 'utilitarian' examinations as the threshold for entry. More broadly, they help to locate the medical profession and the professions *tout court* in the wider milieu of the middling classes.

Arguably, too, our findings help to place the professional middling class within the context of the evolving notion of Britishness. It is very difficult to tell if the surgeons thought of themselves as British, but many of them in their education and experience were undeniably shaped by a British experience, even if they claimed to be English or Scottish or Irish. The majority born outside England, moreover, were not just being Anglicized, although many clearly settled in England and married English women. The fact that a substantial minority of their sons (20 per cent) were directed towards the British army (as regular and medical officers) emphasizes that a large proportion perceived their families as living and moving in an imperial context. The fact, too, that many families, such as the Maclagans, came to have branches in two or more parts of the United Kingdom suggests again that the surgeons were constructing British dynasties and helping to knit the countries of the Union together.

This being so, then this study has also shown why sociological accounts of professionalization, which have concentrated on individual professions, can only reveal part of the reality of being a member of a profession in this or any period. The dynamic we have been able to bring to the study of the cohort more than suggests that the conception of the professions as divisible is mistaken. Of course their individual expertise had and has to be, but to focus on that aspect alone overlooks the extent the professions interacted within families and in the wider society. What we seem to be observing in the first half of the nineteenth century through the prism of the army medical service is the construction of a professional class that is self-sustaining, but nevertherless open at the margins, which in its perceptions is British, urban, progressive, and ambitious for wealth and status.

APPENDIX 1

Description of the Database

The data is held in a relational database. Each army surgeon was allocated a unique identifier that holds the datasets together. The core table contains the life data for each doctor, date and place of birth, and date and place of death. Other tables include details of apprenticeship, educational cursus, army and civilian careers, places of service and civilian residence, publications, marriage, parents, children, and other relatives, and so on. Every entry is fully referenced. The intention is to make the database available on the Internet, funds permitting. The authors will continue to add to it so as to address other questions. Requests for access, and any additional information about members of the cohort or other doctors (not in the cohort) referred to in the book should be sent to Professor Laurence W. B. Brockliss, Magdalen College, Oxford, OX1 4AU.

APPENDIX 2

List of Doctors in the Sample

DID	First Name	Surname	P Birth 1	P Birth 2	Y B	P Death 1	P Death 1	YD
236	George	Adams		England	1783	Morayshire	Scotland	1838
131	George Frederick	Albert		England	1771	Berkshire	England	1853
182	Christopher Richard	Alderson	Yorkshire		1787	Yorkshire	England	1829
132	James	Alexander	Aberdeenshire	Scotland			Scotland	
183	Thomas	Alexander	Berwickshire	Scotland	1802	Greece	Europe	1823
356	George	Allman	County Cork	Ireland				
67	Romaine	Amiel	France	Abroad	1772	Gibraltar	Europe	1847
3	Andrew	Anderson	Selkirkshire	Scotland	1784	Midlothian	Scotland	1860
68	Alexander Dunlop	Anderson	Renfrewshire	Scotland	1794	Lanarkshire	Scotland	1871
409	Philip	Anglin	Jamaica	Abroad	1801	Honduras	C. America	1842
235	Alexander	Angus	Lanarkshire	Scotland			Scotland	1832
66	Charles	Annesley	County Down	Ireland	1783			
4	John	Armstrong	County Fermanagh	Ireland		Nova Scotia	Canada	1827
5	Archibald	Arnott	Dumfriesshire	Scotland	1772	Dumfriesshire	Scotland	1855
184	John	Arthur	County Dublin	Ireland	1781	London	England	1853
410	Thomas	Atkinson	County Mayo	Ireland	1802	County Mayo	Ireland	1875
10	Thomas	Backhouse		Ireland	1792			1847
137	George Robertson	Baillie			1768	London	England	1838
362	William	Balmain			1787			
69	William	Bampfield			1781	County Armagh	Ireland	1845
291	James	Barlow			1784	County Dublin	Ireland	1852
190	Samuel	Barnard			1772	London	England	1827
238	John	Barr	Lanarkshire	Scotland	1784			1832
138	Garrett	Barry	County Cork	Ireland				
289	Richard William	Batty	Cumberland	England	1767	Dumfriesshire	Scotland	1829
75	John Henry	Beaumont	London	England	1763	Devon	England	1824
360	Thomas	Beavan	Herefordshire	England	1804	Herefordshire	England	1843
290	John	Bell			1794	Co. Tipperary	Ireland	1836
240	Titus	Berry	Suffolk	England	1779	London	England	1868
71	John Jeremiah	Bigsby	Nottin'hamshire	England	1792	London	England	1881

8	Ebenezer	Black	Roxburghshire	Scotland	1782	East Lothian	Australasia	1857
239	James	Blair	County Donegal	Ireland	1789		Sea	1824
134	Pasquale	Bocca						1847
241	Charles	Boutflower	Middlesex	England	1782	Lancashire	England	1844
189	William Forrester	Bow	Midlothian	Scotland	1794	Midlothian	Scotland	1868
191	Alexander	Boyd	Perthshire	Scotland		Guiana	S. America	1822
357	Charles	Brereton	Yorkshire	England	1789	Yorkshire	England	1872
359	William Irvin	Breslin		Ireland				
413	Alexander	Broadfoot	Wigtownshire	Scotland	1780	Kent	England	1837
74	Robert	Brown	Northumberland	England	1780	Kent	England	1865
6	Joseph	Brown	Perthshire	Scotland	1784	County Durham	England	1868
187	John William	Brown	Aberdeenshire	Scotland	1791		India	1823
135	David	Brown				Malta	Europe	1825
361	George	Brown			1802		Scotland	1870
7	Frederick	Brown	Berkshire	England	1787	Berkshire	England	1866
73	William	Browne					India	1828
237	Benjamin Haywood	Browne	Gloucestershire	England	1771	Gloucestershire	England	1832
11	Andrew	Browne			1777	France	Europe	1848
358	Alexander	Browne	Kirkc'brightshire	Scotland	1801	Kirkc'brightshire	Scotland	1872
72	Samuel Barwick	Bruce	Barbados	Abroad	1786	London	England	1852
188	James	Brydon	Angusshire	Scotland	1797	Bahamas	W. Indies	1832
133	James	Buchan	Midlothian	Scotland	1770	Midlothian	Scotland	1834
292	John Mort	Bunny	Berkshire	England	1783	Berkshire	England	1848
136	Samuel	Burd	Midlothian	Scotland	1788	Midlothian	Scotland	1838
70	Joseph	Burke				County Dublin	Ireland	1838
242	Henry Barnard	Burman	Hertfordshire	England	1784	Jamaica	W. Indies	1830
9	William Henry	Burrell	Midlothian	Scotland	1795	Devon	England	1866
185	William Robert	Burrowes				Jamaica	W. Indies	1823
186	Edward Warner	Burton				Shropshire	England	1820
411	Edward William	Burton	County Dublin	Ireland	1809	County Dublin	Ireland	1850
412	William Gibson	Byrne	County Dublin	Ireland	1805	County Dublin	Ireland	1855
139	William	Byrtt	County Antrim	Ireland	1786	County Antrim	Ireland	1845

Appendix 2 (*Cont.*)

DID	First Name	Surname	P Birth 1	P Birth 2	Y B	P Death 1	P Death 1	YD
243	Thomas William	Cahill						1826
141	William	Campbell	Argyllshire	Scotland	1794	Fife	Scotland	1871
140	Alexander	Campbell	Perthshire	Scotland	1807	Hong Kong	China	1853
414	Alexander	Campbell	County Armagh	Ireland	1792	London	England	1867
14	James	Campbell	County Wexford	Ireland	1786	Jamaica	W. Indies	1836
295	James Hunton	Cardiff	County Donegal	Ireland		B. Guiana	S. America	1823
78	Thomas	Carey				London	England	1826
348	Michael	Carmac						
368	John	Carnegie	Midlothian	Scotland	1779	Dorset	England	1859
294	Joseph Constantine	Carpue	London	England	1764	London	England	1846
297	John	Carter			1782		Isle of Man	1850
365	Henry Collis	Carter	County Dublin	Ireland	1782		Africa	1848
415	Martin	Cathcart	Co Londonderry	Ireland	1784	C. Londonderry	Ireland	1857
351	William	Cathcart				Antigua	W. Indies	1821
12	William	Chambers					Dominions/US	1833
246	James	Christie	Aberdeenshire	Scotland	1787	Aberdeenshire	Scotland	1838
293	Surtees William	Clarence	Essex	England	1787	Essex	England	1856
15	Charles	Clarke	Stirlingshire	Scotland	1792	Lancashire	England	1865
142	Thomas	Clarke	County Dublin	Ireland	1783	London	England	1857
247	John Frederick	Coates				County Wicklow	Ireland	1848
363	Edward Frederick	Coates						
76	Pennel	Cole	Shropshire	England	1750	Worcestershire	England	1833
194	Charles	Collier	London	England	1785	London	England	1870
364	James	Connell	County Dublin	Ireland	1803			
366	Robert	Constable			1770	Co. Tipperary	Ireland	1830
296	John	Cossins	Dorset	England	1770	Dorset	England	1826
79	Alexander	Coulson			1780	France	Europe	1856
245	Jonathan	Courtney	Hampshire	England	1773	Cape G. Hope	Africa	1843
13	Isaac	Cousins		Ireland		Jamaica	W. Indies	1819

ID	Forename	Surname	Origin	Country	Year	Place	Country	Year
77	Henry	Cowen	County Cavan	Ireland	1786	Somerset	Sea	1824
367	Stewart	Crawford	County Tyrone	Ireland	1772	Lanarkshire	England	1847
193	James	Cross	Lanarkshire	Scotland	1791		Scotland	1870
416	William	Cruickshank	Aberdeenshire	Scotland	1805		India	1858
192	Hugh	Cunningham	Co. Londonderry	Ireland	1795			1826
244	Alexander	Cunningham	East Lothian	Scotland	1784	Midlothian	Scotland	1865
145	Tully	Daly			1790		Sea	1829
417	James	Damerum						1834
199	George Russell	Dartnell	County Limerick	Ireland	1799	Warwickshire	England	1878
17	James	Davidson	Midlothian	Scotland	1796	Midlothian	Scotland	1868
143	Daniel Owen	Davies	Cardiganshire	Wales	1787	Cardiganshire	Wales	1855
248	Henry	Davies	London	England	1782	London	England	1862
196	John	Davy	Cornwall	England	1790	Westmorland	England	1868
302	William	Dawson	Somerset	England	1795	London	England	1861
18	Oliver	Dease				County Dublin	Ireland	1821
195	John Martyn	Dermott	Northamptonshire	England	1789		Ceylon	1819
249	John	Dethick	Nottinghamshire	England	1790			
299	Henry William	Develin			1788	County Tyrone	Ireland	1854
144	Mitchell	Devitt	County Mayo	Ireland	1795	County Sligo	Ireland	1844
419	Crawford	Dick	Ayrshire	Scotland	1803	Ayrshire	Scotland	1836
82	John	Dick			1773	County Wicklow	Ireland	1848
420	Samuel	Dickson	Midlothian	Scotland	1802	London	England	1869
353	George	Dickson			1772			
16	Thomas	Dillon	County Kildare	Ireland	1789	County Galway	Ireland	1879
81	John Hawkins	Divir	County Donegal	Ireland	1792	Co. Donegal	Ireland	1839
200	William	Doherty				Honduras	C. America	1824
418	Gideon	Dolmage			1806			1868
298	John	Douglas	Roxburghshire	Scotland	1788	Roxburghshire	Scotland	1861
197	Thomas	Draper			1775	Devon	England	1850
80	Charles	Ducat	Perthshire	Scotland	1768	Sussex	England	1864
300	William	Dudgeon				County Down	Ireland	1826
301	Michael Lawless	Duigan	County Dublin	Ireland	1787		Ireland	1837

Appendix 2 (*Cont.*)

DID	First Name	Surname	P Birth 1	P Birth 2	Y B	P Death 1	P Death 1	YD
369	Robert	Dundas	Ayrshire	Scotland		County Cork	Ireland	1827
198	George	Dunlop	Renfrewshire	Scotland	1795	Canada	Canada	1848
370	William	Dunlop		Scotland	1778	Midlothian	Scotland	1841
19	John	Easton	Aberdeenshire	Scotland	1805			1878
372	William Cruickshank	Eddie	Cumberland	England		Hong Kong	China	1847
421	Joseph	Edmondson			1804			
83	Henry	Edwards			1780			
371	Clement	Ekins		England		Barbados	W. Indies	1832
422	Robert	Ellson	Cheshire	England	1800	Lancashire	England	1849
303	John Richard	Elmore	London	England	1790	London	England	1856
250	Michael Lambton	Este	London		1779	London	England	1864
201	David	Ewing			1793	Colombo	Ceylon	1843
425	William John	Fagg				Kent	England	1832
85	Joseph	Farnden			1790			1843
305	Charles	Farrell		Ireland	1779	Canada	Canada	1855
147	John James	Fawcett	Hampshire	England	1789	County Galway	Ireland	1827
252	John	Ferguson		Scotland	1783		Ireland	1857
253	William	Ferguson	Jamaica	Abroad	1795	Ayrshire	Scotland	1846
424	George	Ferguson	Stirlingshire	Scotland	1804		Sea	1846
21	Thomas	Fiddes	Co. Fermanagh	Ireland	1788	Midlothian	Scotland	1836
87	Moore Francis	Finan			1774		Sea	1824
84	John	Fisher	Somerset	England	1788		India	1827
146	Percy	Fitzpatrick					England	
148	John Bickerson	Flanagan	Devon	England	1785	County Dublin	Ireland	1846
304	Michael	Fogerty			1792	London	England	1844
306	Charles Fergusson	Forbes	Essex	England	1779	London	England	1852
373	John	Forrest	Stirlingshire	Scotland	1804	Somerset	England	1865
202	Thomas	Forster			1781		Australasia	1856
423	Andrew	Foulis						
20	William Wemys	Fraser		England	1781	Cheshire	England	1832

86	Fraser	Peter	Midlothian	Scotland	1789	Midlothian	Scotland	1831
374	Fraser	John	Midlothian	Scotland	1802	Lanarkshire	Scotland	1867
22	French	James	Lanarkshire	Scotland	1789	London	England	1837
251	Fry	William Dowell	London	England	1784			
376	Gallagher	Michael			1788			
203	Galliers	William	Stirlingshire	Scotland	1775	Stirlingshire	Scotland	1861
151	Gibb	William Richardson	County Meath	Ireland	1787	Lanarkshire	Scotland	1855
24	Gibney	William	Co. Londonderry	Ireland	1794	Somerset	England	1872
428	Gibson	James Brown			1804	Italy	Europe	1868
204	Gilder	James				Gambia	Africa	1821
150	Gill	Christopher				Jamaica	W. Indies Dominions/US	1824
427	Gillice	John	Banff	Scotland	1802	Banff	Scotland	1843
23	Gillkrest	James	County Dublin	Ireland		London	England	1853
88	Glasco	John	County Wicklow	Ireland	1783	France	Europe	1869
149	Goodison	William		Ireland	1785			1836
254	Gordon	Theodore	Aberdeenshire	Scotland	1786	Sussex	England	1845
308	Gowen	James						1834
58	Graham	Edward Smith	Co. Fermanagh	Ireland	1791	Isle of Man	Isle of Man	1847
377	Graham	John	Barbados	Abroad	1783			1862
307	Grant	John	Inverness-shire	Scotland	1771	Morayshire	Scotland	1860
426	Grant	John Donald	London	England	1804			
89	Grattan	Copeland	County Dublin	Ireland	1793			1850
375	Greaves	William	Staffordshire	England	1773	Gloucestershire	England	1848
309	Gregory	George	Kent	England	1790	London	England	1853
255	Guthrie	George James	London	England	1785	London	England	1856
432	Hadaway	Samuel Maitland	Midlothian	Scotland	1805	London	England	1881
206	Hagartye	Daniel			1793	St Helena	St Helena	1825
153	Hall	Thomas	County Tyrone	Ireland	1796	London	England	1866
152	Halpin	Oliver	County Dublin	Ireland	1776	Belgium	Europe	1838
91	Harper	William			1777	Lancashire	England	1843
90	Harrison	William	County Dublin	Ireland	1777		Africa	1824

Appendix 2 (*Cont.*)

DID	First Name	Surname	P Birth 1	P Birth 2	Y B	P Death 1	P Death 1	YD
26	Henry	Hart	County Durham?	England?	1789	London	England	1854
92	James	Henderson	Lanarkshire	Scotland	1791	Jersey	Ch. Islands	1871
379	John	Hendrick	Co. Londonderry	Ireland	1793	County Galway	Ireland	1855
28	John	Hennen	County Mayo	Ireland	1779	Gibraltar	Europe	1828
380	John	Hennen	Kent	England	1800	Kent	England	1871
93	Robert Hobart	Hett	Lincolnshire	England	1790	Kent	England	1827
259	Richard Henry	Heurtley			1764	Middlesex	England	1832
311	John Gray	Hibbert	Somerset	England	1783	Jersey	Ch. Islands	1841
258	West	Hill			1742	Wiltshire	England	1834
312	John Perkin	Hill	Essex	England	1781	London	England	1818
29	John	Hodson	Warwickshire	England	1804	Midlothian	Scotland	1855
429	Horatio Nelson	Holden						
347	William Summers	Holland						1807
313	Edward	Hollier			1790	London	England	1863
205	Samuel	Holmes	Co. Londonderry	Ireland	1788	C. Londonderry	Ireland	1829
378	Alexander George	Home	Dominica	Abroad		Midlothian	Scotland	1875
314	John	Horne						1828
257	John	Howell	Cambridgeshire	England	1777	Sicily	Europe	1857
25	John Robert	Hume	Renfrewshire	Scotland	1782	London	England	1857
256	Richard	Humfrey			1772	Gloucestershire	England	1843
433	William Charles	Humfrey	County Carlow	Ireland	1802	Malta	Europe	1862
431	Thomas	Hunter				London	England	1880
27	James Steele	Huston	County Down	Ireland	1791	County Dublin	Ireland	1839
310	David	Hutcheon	Angusshire	Scotland		British Guiana	W. Indies	1809
430	George James	Hyde	London	England	1801	Hampshire	England	1835
435	Samuel	Ingram	Wiltshire	England	1799	Gloucestershire	England	1842
260	Thomas	Jackson			1777	London	England	1846
30	John	James				Canada	Canada	1823
261	Issac	James				Malta	Europe	1825
207	Henry	James				St Lucia	W. Indies	1824

No.	First name	Surname	Place of birth	Country of birth	Year of birth	Place	Country	Year
349	William	James			1774	London	England	1852
97	David	Jearrad				Midlothian	Scotland	1829
434	Henry James	Jemmett	London	England		Warwickshire	England	1832
154	Samuel	Jeyes	Middlesex	England	1778	Yorkshire	England	1872
31	George	John			1767	Honduras	C. America	1839
96	James	Johnston	County Galway	Ireland	1780	Corfu	Europe	1823
95	George	Johnston	Berwickshire	Scotland	1785			1833
382	Edward	Johnston	Co. Monaghan	Ireland		Barbados	W. Indies	1862
32	John	Johnston	Dunfriesshire	Scotland		Co. Donegal	Ireland	1825
315	Basil	Johnston			1783	County Wicklow	Ireland	1825
316	Francis	Jones		Ireland	1774	London	England	1828
381	Charles	Jordan			1777	London	England	1839
317	Robert	Keate	Somerset	England	1780	County Dublin	Ireland	1857
209	James Butler	Kell	County Cork	Ireland	1807		Ceylon	1845
436	Luke	Kelly	Co. Roscommon	Ireland	1790	Jamaica	W. Indies	1842
208	Hugh	Kelly						
354	John	Kemp				London	England	1811
33	James	Kennedy	Angusshire	Scotland	1793	Somerset	England	1827
156	Thomas	Kidd	Northumberland	England	1777	County Antrim	Ireland	1849
383	John	Kidston	Midlothian	Scotland	1766	Midlothian	Scotland	1834
155	Alexander	Kindell			1782			1850
262	John	Kinnis	Fife	Scotland	1794			1852
211	Thomas	La Cloche			1771	Jersey	Ch. Islands	1864
319	William	Latham			1786			
210	David Jugurtha	Law	Fife	Scotland	1785	Sierra Leone	Africa	1824
265	Rhynd	Lawder	County Monaghan	Ireland	1776	London	England	1836
100	John Gogill	Leath	Norfolk	England	1784	London	England	1859
35	Francis	Leigh	County Armagh	Ireland	1764	Gibraltar	Europe	1839
263	William	Lempriere	Jersey	Abroad	1787	Somerset	England	1834
94	Alexander	Lesassier (afterwards Hamilton)	Midlothian	Scotland			Afghanistan	1839

Appendix 2 (*Cont.*)

DID	First Name	Surname	P Birth 1	P Birth 2	Y B	P Death 1	P Death 1	YD
437	Lewis	Leslie	Aberdeenshire	Scotland	1802			1834
99	John	Lewis					Scotland	1852
384	Andrew	Ligertwood	Aberdeenshire	Scotland	1784	Aberdeenshire	Scotland	1851
159	John	Lightbody	Lanarkshire	Scotland	1786		Scotland	1866
98	David	Linn	County Antrim	Ireland	1784	County Antrim	Ireland	1827
438	Thomas Galbraith	Logan	Lanarkshire	Scotland	1808	London	England	1896
157	Frederick Albert	Loinsworth	County Dublin	Ireland	1783		India	1842
34	Augustus Lewis	Loinsworth			1787		Sea	1839
158	John	Lorimer	Dumfriesshire	Scotland	1788	London	England	1839
264	William Bewicke	Lynn	London	England	1786	Surrey	England	1878
318	William	Lyons	County Galway	Ireland		Canada	Canada	1834
37	Michaiah	Mabey			1775	Canada	Canada	1835
389	Peter	Macarthur	Nairnshire	Scotland	1775	South Australia	Australiasia	1861
108	William	Macartney	Co. Fermanagh	Ireland	1791		Ireland	1833
322	James William	Macauley	County Dublin	Ireland	1789	County Dublin	Ireland	1873
441	Kenneth	McCaskill	County Antrim	Ireland			India	1841
161	Hugh	McClintock	Co. Londonderry	Ireland	1793	Jersey	Ch. Islands	1841
217	Henry	McCreery	County Kilkenny	Ireland	1786		India	1838
105	William	McDonell	Banff	Scotland			Sea	1822
387	James	MacDougle	Northumberland	England	1779	London	England	1843
444	Gregor	MacGregor	Co. Londonderry	Ireland		Tasmania	Australasia	1835
215	Duncan	MacGregor	Perthshire	Scotland			India	1821
320	James	McGrigor	Inverness-shire	Scotland	1771	London	England	1858
213	Archibald	MacIsaac	Argyllshire	Scotland	1787			
325	Edward	McIver			1791	County Dublin	Ireland	1845
386	James	Mack			1757	Hampshire	England	1839
326	Alexander	McKee			1782	C. Londonderry	Ireland	1832
321	Donald	McKinlay	Perthshire	Scotland			Sea	1843
266	Peter	McLachlan	Renfrewshire	Scotland	1796			1832
107	Alexander	McLachlan				Cape G. Hope	Africa	1824

No.	Forename	Surname	Place	Country	Year	Place	Country	Year
106	David	Maclagan	Midlothian	Scotland	1785	Midlothian	Scotland	1865
388	George Gordon	McLean	Aberdeenshire	Scotland	1795	Aberdeenshire	Scotland	1868
267	William	Macleod	Inverness-shire	Scotland	1784			
104	David	MacLoughlin	Canada	Abroad	1792	London	England	1870
162	Robert Andrew	McMunn	County Donegal	Ireland	1785			
212	Donald	McNeil	Inverness-shire	Scotland	1781	Jersey	Ch. Islands	1824
164	William	Macnish						1866
116	John	McRobert	County Cork	Ireland	1786	Hampshire	England	1837
324	Eugene	McSwyny	Aberdeenshire	Scotland	1798	France	Europe	1840
272	John	Mair	Midlothian	Scotland	1787	Canada	Canada	1877
40	John MacGregor	Mallock	Northamptonshire	England	1785	India	India	1832
214	Henry William	Markham				Wiltshire	England	1840
385	George	Martin				Co. Limerick	Ireland	1847
39	William	Maurice				Gloucestershire	England	1852
270	George Richard	Melin	County Cork	Ireland	1788	Warwickshire	England	1836
102	Alexander	Melville	Newfoundland?	Abroad	1792	Angusshire	Scotland	1855
271	Alexander	Menzies	Midlothian	Scotland	1783	India	India	1823
101	Frederick	Micklam				Warwickshire	England	1826
165	John	Millar	County Antrim	Ireland	1789	Lanarkshire	Scotland	1850
41	James Dickie	Millar	Ayrshire	Scotland	1791	Tasmania	Australasia	1839
440	James	Millar	Midlothian	Scotland	1785			1869
216	William	Milligan	County Cavan	Ireland	1795	London	England	1851
166	James	Moffitt	Queen's County	Ireland	1789	Devon	England	1856
391	John	Molyneaux	County Dublin	Ireland	1801	County Cork	Ireland	1839
323	Charles	Montagu				London	England	1809
109	Thomas	Moore	County Meath	Ireland	1781	County Meath	Ireland	1833
44	Robert	Moorhead	Co. Monaghan	Ireland	1791			
392	James Rowland	Morgan					Ceylon	1825
442	Nathaniel	Morgan	London	England	1793	Cape G. Hope	Africa	1842
163	William Burgess	Morle			1779	Somerset	England	1845
38	William	Morrah				Barbados	W. Indies	1821
355	George Paulet	Morris	London	England	1759	London	England	1837

Appendix 2 (*Cont.*)

DID	First Name	Surname	P Birth 1	P Birth 2	Y B	P Death 1	P Death 1	YD
42	William	Morrison				Malta	Europe	1824
160	Henry	Muir	Lanarkshire	Scotland	1792	Lanarkshire	Scotland	1858
268	William	Munro	Inverness-shire	Scotland	1783			1839
390	John Poyntz	Munro	Sutherlandshire	Scotland	1803			
103	John	Murray	Fife	Scotland	1771	Midlothian	Scotland	1846
43	Denis	Murray	County Limerick	Ireland	1793	Co. Wexford	Ireland	1860
269	Thomas	Murray			1781	Jersey	Ch. Islands	1834
443	Adam Walker	Murray	Midlothian	Scotland	1805			
439	John	Murtagh	County Longford	Ireland	1802			1880
36	James	Muttlebury	Somerset	England	1773	Canada	Canada	1832
273	Adam	Neale	Midlothian	Scotland	1778	France	Europe	1832
327	Charles Aesculapius	Newcomb	London	England	1783	London	England	1832
328	William	Newton	Lancashire	England	1786	Sussex	England	1844
346	John Hayne	Newton			1765	France	Europe	1848
445	John	O'Brien	Kent	England	1805	London	England	1841
110	James	O'Connor			1769	Somerset	England	1857
329	John	O'Donnel			1793			1875
218	Daniel	O'Flaherty	County Kerry	Ireland	1775	India	India	1825
45	Thomas	O'Halloran	County Kerry	Ireland	1792	County Cork	Ireland	1832
111	Edward	O'Reilly	County Meath	Ireland		Cape G. Hope	Africa	1825
274	William Pinkstan	O'Reilly	County Meath	Ireland	1784	Barbados	W. Indies	1835
393	James Alexander	Ore	Nairnshire	Scotland	1802	India	India	1843
167	Hugh	Orr	Ayrshire	Scotland	1793	Trinidad	W. Indies	1839
62	Edward	Owen			1784	Jamaica	W. Indies	1831
219	Stephen	Panting	Shropshire	England	1767	Shropshire	England	1830
278	William	Pardey			1787	Canada	Canada	1832
330	John	Parke	County Dublin	Ireland				
275	William	Parrott	Sussex	England	1782	Cape G. Hope	Africa	1850
46	Patrick	Paterson	Orkney	Scotland	1771	London	England	1822
112	William	Paton	Fife	Scotland	1775	Fife	Scotland	1844

No.	Forename(s)	Surname	Birthplace	Country	Year	Place of death	Country	Year
276	George	Peach	Leicestershire	England	1778	Dorset	England	1856
395	Samuel	Peacock	Lancashire	England	1778	County Dublin	Ireland	1835
47	Thomas Montgomery	Perrott	Sussex	England	1787		England	1840
331	John	Phillips			1785	London	England	1851
333	Edward	Pilkington	Kent	England	1810	Denbighshire	Wales	1855
447	Chilley	Pine	Devon	England	1788		Russia	1867
220	Samuel Ayrault	Piper	County Dublin	Ireland	1804	Surrey	England	1849
446	David Charles	Pitcairn			1775	Gambia	Africa	1843
168	Edward	Porteous				Italy	Europe	1824
169	George	Power			1782	County Cork	Ireland	1840
221	Thomas	Price				Essex	England	1813
332	John	Price				St Lucia	W. Indies	1827
277	Thomas	Prosser	County Kerry	Ireland		County Cork	Ireland	1823
113	Maurice Fitzgerald	Quill						
63	William	Ramsay				Cape G. Hope	Africa	1820
48	George	Redmond	County Wexford	Ireland	1767	Co. Wexford	Ireland	1832
335	Gabriel Rice	Redmond	Dumfriesshire	Scotland		St Lucia	W. Indies	1828
117	Francis	Reid	Perthshire	Scotland	1790	Perthshire	Scotland	1864
115	John	Riach		Scotland		County Dublin	Ireland	1828
334	John	Rice		Scotland			Sea	1830
49	George	Richmond				London	England	1843
171	Thomas Hughes	Ridgway	Pembrokeshire	Wales	1783	Sierra Leone	Africa	1824
222	Malcolm	Ritchie	County Down	Ireland		Ayrshire	Scotland	1845
50	John	Robb	Ayrshire	Scotland	1776	Kent	England	1849
52	William	Roberts		Scotland	1779		India	1838
170	Patrick	Robertson	Perthshire	Scotland	1789	Perthshire	Scotland	1849
118	James	Robertson	Peebleshire	Scotland	1803			1881
450	William	Robertson	Aberdeenshire	Scotland	1804		Scotland	1855
448	Peter	Robertson	Perthshire	Scotland	1774			
279	Henry	Robertson			1758	France	Europe	1830
398	Alexander	Robertson				Perthshire	Scotland	
449	James Henderson	Rolland	Angusshire	Scotland	1802		Sea	1848

Appendix 2 (*Cont.*)

DID	First Name	Surname	P Birth 1	P Birth 2	Y B	P Death 1	P Death 1	YD
51	Thomas	Rolston				Malta	Europe	1826
397	Thomas	Ross						1831
396	George	Rowe						1843
223	Robert	Rule			1772	Guernsey	Ch. Islands	1829
114	George Henry	Rutledge	County Sligo	Ireland	1790	Madras	India	1833
401	Thomas	Sandell	Wiltshire	England	1792	Suffolk	England	1835
400	Backshall Lane	Sandham			1777	Sutherland	Scotland	1848
54	Robert	Scott	County Down	Ireland	1787			
124	James	Scott	Midlothian	Scotland	1775			
172	John	Scott	Selkirkshire	Scotland	1793			
56	Samuel	Scott	Cambridgeshire	England		Midlothian	Scotland	1825
227	James	Sharp				Demerara	S. America Dominions/US	1825
225	Robert	Shean	Hampshire	England	1797			
337	John	Shean				Bahamas	W. Indies	1816
57	Robert	Shekleton	County Louth	Ireland	1793	County Dublin	Ireland	1867
399	Louis Machin	Sheppard					India	1826
339	James	Shorland	Gloucestershire	England	1783			
226	Francis	Sievewright	Midlothian	Scotland	1773	Midlothian	Scotland	1872
336	Jeronimo	Simoens			1791			
452	John Hartley	Sinclair	County Armagh	Ireland	1803	Sussex	England	1874
174	Joseph	Skey	Worcestershire	England	1774	London	England	1866
224	John Francis	Smet				Devon	England	1840
53	James	Smith			1785		India	1846
55	John Gordon	Smith	London	England	1792	London	England	1833
122	John	Smith			1792		India	1816
453	William	Smith	Morayshire	Scotland	1806	Stirlingshire	Scotland	1855
281	William	Smyth			1781			1855
338	Thomas Charlton	Speer	County Dublin	Ireland		Somerset	England	1878
282	John Hanmer	Sprague	Somerset	England	1784			1865

No.	Forename	Surname	Birthplace	Birth country	Birth year	Death place	Death country	Death year
228	Charles	St John	County Longford	Ireland	1789	Bengal	India	1853
173	Edmund	Starkie				Kent	England	1841
123	George	Steed		England	1781		England	1853
340	Thomas Gordon	Stephenson	Aberdeenshire	Scotland	1789	Lancashire	England	1842
121	Alexander	Stewart		Scotland	1788	London	England	1863
119	Thomas	Stobo	Lanarkshire	Scotland				
120	James Coulter	Strachan	Perthshire	Scotland		Newfoundland	Canada	1827
451	John Murray	Strath	Midlothian	Scotland	1805	West Indies	W. Indies	1843
454	James	Stuart	Dumfriesshire	Scotland	1807	Hampshire	England	1856
175	John Fitzgerald	Swindell		Scotland		Nova Scotia?	Canada	1819
280	James Fynmore	Symes	Devon	England				
402	John	Taylor			1770	Colombo	Ceylon	1850
229	Robert	Thin	Midlothian	Scotland	1794			1819
283	Joseph	Thomas				Gloucestershire	England	1843
126	William Dyer	Thomas	Gloucestershire	England	1777	Surrey	England	1837
284	Charles	Thompson	Westmorland	England		County Cork	Ireland	1829
61	Andrew	Thompson	Co. Monaghan	Ireland		County Monaghan	Ireland	1828
403	William	Thomson		Scotland		Lancashire	England	1831
125	Alexander	Thomson	West Lothian			Wigtownshire	Scotland	1820
176	John	Thornton		Scotland	1775			1856
177	William	Thornton	County Durham		1777	London	England	1847
455	James Anthony	Topham		England	1797	County Durham	England	1841
456	Robert	Torrie						
285	James	Trigge	County Tyrone			India	India	1826
59	George	Trimble	County Sligo	Ireland	1784	Co. Monaghan	Ireland	1834
60	William	Trumble	County Galway	Ireland		Honduras	C. America	1822
127	James Dillon	Tully	Midlothian	Ireland	1785	Jamaica	W. Indies	1827
342	Robert	Turnbull		Scotland	1793	New S. Wales	Australasia	1842
343	William	Turner			1779	Devon	England	1867
352	Henry William	Tytler	Angusshire	Scotland	1752	Midlothian	Scotland	1808
350	William	Usher			1774			1867
345	Thomas	Wahab	County Down	Ireland		Nova Scotia	Canada	1839

Appendix 2 (*Cont.*)

DID	First Name	Surname	P Birth 1	P Birth 2	Y B	P Death 1	P Death 1	YD
181	Charles	Waite	Lincolnshire	England	1773	Essex	England	1833
179	John Harding	Walker	Jamaica	Abroad	1785			1848
404	Thomas	Walker		Scotland	1784	West Lothian	Scotland	1860
64	William	Wallace			1770		?Ireland	1844
457	William	Wallace	Buckinghamshire	England		Midlothian	Scotland	1864
286	Edward	Walsh	Co. Waterford	Ireland	1767	County Dublin	Ireland	1832
230	Philip	Walter				Devon	England	1823
287	James Low	Warren	Orkney	Scotland	1791	Hampshire	England	1871
178	John Benjamin	Waterson	Co. Monaghan	Ireland	1791			
458	George Ross	Watson	Angusshire	Scotland	1807	County Mayo	Ireland	1832
128	John William	Watson	Midlothian	Scotland	1792	Somerset	England	1858
344	James	Whitelocke			1768	France	Europe	1841
233	Luke	Whitney				Greece	Europe	1825
129	Charles	Whyte	Angusshire	Scotland	1795	Gloucestershire	England	1881
232	William	Williams	Caernarfonshire	Wales	1789			
180	David	Williams	Carmarthenshire	Wales	1792			1853
405	William	Williams	Cornwall	England	1764			1833
406	Thomas	Williams	County Cork	Ireland	1802	London	England	1859
407	James	Williams	Worcestershire	England	1771	Worcestershire	England	1840
130	John	Williams			1785	Italy	Europe	1841
234	William	Williams	Denbighshire	Wales		St Vincent	W. Indies	1827
231	John	Williamson				Jamaica	W. Indies	1825
65	James	Williamson	Banff	Scotland	1784	Banff	Scotland	1833
408	David	Wright			1788		Europe	1837
288	William Henry	Young	Yorkshire	England	1787	Somerset	England	1879

Key: DID: Doctor's Identification Number (in database); P Birth 1: County of Birth (or overseas country or region); P Birth 2: Country of Birth or born abroad; YB: Year of Birth; P Death 1: County (or overseas country or region) of Death; P Death 2: Country (or region or continent) of Death; YD: Year of Death

Manuscript Sources

The foundation of this study are the questionnaires completed by surviving army medical surgeons in the years immediately after Waterloo, and regularly updated for the remainder of an officer's career. These are held in the National Archives in series War Office (WO) 25/3904–11. Although they are now bound together, they appear to have been originally stored loose, and there does not seem to be any obvious logic to the order in which they were subsequently bound. The information culled form this source was enlarged by the use of personal information held in other War Office and Paymaster-General record series. These are well described in Simon Fowler, *Army Records for Family Historians*, Public Record Office Readers' Guide No. 2, 1992 (revised by William Spencer in 2000). Details of wealth at death for those with estates in England who died before 1858 were located in the Prerogative Court of Canterbury (PCC) series, now on-line at the National Archives. Thereafter they were traced in the registers of confirmed estates held in First Avenue House, London, and the values found in the Inland Revenue (IR) and probate (Prob) series at the National Archives. The location of probate records in other jurisdictions is explained on pp. 257–8. Although manuscript material relating to individual army doctors, some not in the cohort, has been cited extensively, no other comprehensive series have been used. Records of matriculation, graduation, fellowships, and memberships are printed, and, in any event, were used largely to corroborate information contained in the questionnaires.

Bibliography

ACKERKNECHT, ERWIN, *Medicine at the Paris Hospital, 1794–1848* (Baltimore, 1967).

ADDISON, W. INNES, *The Matriculation Albums of the University of Glasgow from 1728 to 1858* (Glasgow, 1913).

AESCULAPIUS, *The Hospital Pupil's Guide, being Oracular Communications Addressed to Students of the Medical Profession* (London, 1818).

AMIEL, R., *Answers to Queries from the Army Medical Board, on the Epidemic at Gibraltar 1828* (London, 1829).

ANDERSON, PETER JOHN, *Officers and Graduates of University & King's College Aberdeen MVD-MDCCCLX* (Aberdeen, 1893).

ANDERSON, ROBERT, *Universities and Elites in Britain since 1800* (London, 1992).

ANDREW, DONNA T., *Philanthropy and Police: London Charity in the Eighteenth Century* (Princeton, NJ, 1989).

Army List.

ARNOTT, JAMES, *The House of Arnott* (Edinburgh, 1918).

Bagshaw's Kent Directory.

BANCROFT, E. N., *A Letter to the Commissioners of Military Enquiry Continuing Some Animadversions on Some Parts of the Fifth Report . . .* (London, 1808).

BANKS, J. A., *Victorian Values: Secularism and the Size of Families* (London, 1981).

BARLOW, J., *An Address to Medical and Surgical Pupils, on the Studies and Duties of their Profession; to which is Appended a Case of Caesarean Operation* (London, 1839).

BARNARD, TOBY, *Making of the Grand Figure: Lives and Possessions in Ireland 1641–1770* (New Haven, Conn., 2004).

BARRY, JONATHAN, and BROOKS, CHRISTOPHER (eds.), *The Middling Sort of People: Culture, Society and Politics in England 1550–1800* (London, 1994).

BARTRIP, W., *Mirror of Medicine: A History of the British Medical Journal* (Oxford, 1990).

Belfast Directory.

Belfast Newsletter.

BELL, JOHN, *Memorial Concerning the Present State of Military and Naval Surgery* (Edinburgh, 1800).

BENTLEY, MICHAEL (ed.), *Companion to Historiography* (London, 1997).

BERG, MAXINE, *Luxury and Pleasure in Eighteenth-Century Britain* (Oxford, 2005).

BICKFORD, J. A. R., and Bickford, M. E., *The Medical Profession in Hull, 1400–1900* (Hull, 1983).

BIGSBY, J. J., *Observations Addressed to the Inhabitants of Newark and its Neighbourhood, on the Establishment of a Mechanics' Institution* (Newark, 1826).

—— *Notes on the Geography and Geology of Lake Huron, 1824* (London, 1827).

—— *A Brief Exposition of those Benevolent Institutions, often Denominated Self-Supporting Dispensaries; with a View to Recommend them to the Patronage and Support of the Public* (Newark, 1832).

—— *A Lecture on Mendicity, its Ancient and Modern History and the Policy of Nations and Individuals in Regard to it; as Delivered before the Worksop Mechanics' Institute on the 14th of April 1836* (Worksop, 1836).

BIGSBY, J. J., *Seaside Manual of Invalids and Bathers* (London, 1841).

—— *Lectures on the Study of Chemistry in Connection with the Atmosphere, the Earth, and the Ocean* (London, 1849).

—— *The Shoe and Canoe, or, Pictures of Travel in the Canadas, Illustrative of their Scenery and of Colonial Life with Facts and Operations on Emigration, State Policy, and other Points of Public Interest* (London, 1850).

—— *A Brief Account of the Thesaurus Siluricus with a Few Facts and Inferences* (London, 1867).

—— *Thesaurus Devonico-Carboniferous: The Flora and Fauna of the Devonian and Carboniferous Periods, the Genera and Species arranged in Tabular Form: Showing the Horizons, Recurrences, Localities, and Other Facts: with Large Addenda from Recent Acquisitions* (London, 1878).

BINFIELD, C., and HEY, D. (eds.), *Mesters to Masters: A History of the Company of Cutlers in Hallamshire* (Oxford, 1997).

BLACK, J., *Eighteenth Century Europe: 1700–1789* (London, 1990).

BLANCO, RICHARD L., *Wellington's Surgeon-General: Sir James McGrigor* (Durham, N.C., 1974).

BLOMFIELD, J., *St George's, 1733–1933* (London, 1933).

BONE, D. (ed.), *The Cambridge Companion to Byron* (Cambridge, 2004).

BONHOTE, COLONEL H., *Historical Records of the West Kent Militia* (London, 1909).

The Border Magazine.

BORSAY, P., *The English Urban Renaissance: Culture and Society in the Provincial Town, 1660–1770* (Oxford, 1989).

BOUTFLOWER, CHARLES, *The Journal of an Army Surgeon during the Peninsular War* (Manchester, 1912).

BOUTFLOWER, DOUGLAS SAMUEL, *The Complete Story of a Family of the Middle Class Connected with the North of England (1303–1930)* (Newcastle, 1930).

BOW, W., *Notions of the Natures of Fevers and Nervous Action* (Edinburgh, 1829).

BOWER, A., *The Edinburgh Student's Guide* (Edinburgh, 1822).

BREWER, J., *The Sinews of Power: War, Money and the English State, 1688–1783* (London, 1989).

BRIGGS, A., 'Middle-Class Consciousness in English Politics, 1780–1846', *Past and Present*, 9 (1956), 65–74.

BRINE, JOHN, et al., *Looking for Milligan: The Fascinating Search for William Milligan a Pioneering Doctor of the Swan River Colony c.1795–1851* (Perth, 1991).

British Medical Journal.

BROCK, W. H., *Justus von Liebeg: The Chemical Gatekeeper* (Cambridge, 1997).

BROCKLISS, LAURENCE, and EASTWOOD, DAVID (eds.), *A Union of Multiple Identities: The British Isles, c.1750–c.1850* (Manchester, 1997).

—— and JONES, C., *The Medical World of Early Modern France* (Oxford, 1997).

—— CARDWELL, JOHN, and MOSS, MICHAEL, *Nelson's Surgeon: William Beatty, Naval Medicine and Trafalgar* (Oxford, 2005).

BROWN, J., *Medical Essays on Fever, Inflammation, Rheumatism, Diseases of the Heart & c.* (London, 1828).

—— *A Defence of Revealed Religion, Comprising a Vindication of the Old and New Testaments from the Attacks of Rationalists and Infidels* (London, 1851).

—— *Memories of the Past and Thoughts on the Present Age* (London, 1863).

—— *The Food of the People: A Letter to Henry Fenwick esq. M. P. with a Postscript on the Diet of Old Age* (London, 1865).

[BRUCE, SAMUEL BARWICK], *Short Memoir of S. B. Bruce Esquire* (York, 1841).

BUCHANAN, M. S., *History of the Glasgow Royal Infirmary, from its Commencement in 1787 to the Present Time* (Glasgow, 1832).

Bulletin of the History of Medicine.

BURKE, E., *Reflections on the Revolution in France* (1790; London, 1986).

BURKE, P., *The French Historical Revolution: The 'Annales' School 1929–1989* (Stanford, Calif., 1990).

—— *A Social History of Knowledge from Gutenberg to Diderot* (Cambridge, 2002).

Burke's Landed Gentry (London, 1871, 1886, 1952 edns.).

Burke's Landed Gentry of Ireland (London, 1912 and 1958 edns.).

Burke's Peerage (London, 1936).

BURNS, A., FINCHAM, K., AND TAYLOR, S., 'The Historical, Public and Academic Archival Research: The Experience of the Clergy of the Church of England Database', *Archives*, 27 (2002), 110–A.

BURRAGE, M., and THORSTENDAHL, R. (eds.), *Professions in Theory and History: Rethinking the Study of the Professions* (London, 1990).

—— *The Formation of the Professions: Knowledge, State and Strategy* (London, 1990).

BURTCHAELL, G. D., *Alumni Dublinenses: A Register of the Students, Graduates, Professors and Provosts of Trinity College in the University of Dublin (1593–1860)* (Dublin, 1935).

BURTON, EDWARD, *A Catalogue of the Collection of Mammalia and Birds in the Museum of Fort Pitt Chatham* (London, 1838).

BURTON, Sir R., *A Pilgrimage to Al-Madinah and Meccah*, 2 vols. (London, 1986).

By-Laws, Ordinances, Rules, and Constitutions of the Royal College of Surgeons in Ireland (Dublin, 1785).

BYNUM, W. F., 'Medicine at the English Court', in Vivian Nutton (ed.), *Medicine at the Courts of Europe 1500–1837* (London, 1990).

—— and PORTER, R., *William Hunter and the Eighteenth-Century Medical World* (Cambridge, 1985).

BYRNE, PAULA, *Perdita: The Life of Mary Robinson* (London, 2004).

CAMERON, Sir C., *History of the Royal College of Surgeons in Ireland, and of the Irish Schools of Medicine* (Dublin, 1886).

CAMERON, H. C., *Mr Guy's Hospital, 1726–1948* (London, 1954).

CAMPBELL, R., *The London Tradesman* (London, 1747).

Canadian Dictionary of National Biography.

CANTLIE, SIR NEIL, *A History of the Army Medical Department*, 2 vols. (Edinburgh, 1974).

CARPUE, J., *A Description of the Muscles of the Human Body, as They Appear on Dissection* (London, 1801).

—— *A History of the High Operation of the Stone, by Incision above the Pubis; with Observations on the Advantages Attending it; and an Account of the Various Methods of Lithotomy, from the Earliest Periods to the Present Time* (London, 1819).

CARR-SAUNDERS, A. M., and WILSON, P. A., *The Professions* (Oxford, 1933).

A Catalogue of the Library of the Army Medical Department (London, 1833).

CHALMERS, PETER, *Historical and Statistical Account of Dunfermline*, vol. ii (Edinburgh, 1859).

CLARK, SIR GEORGE, *A History of the Royal College of Physicians of London*, 2 vols. (London, 1964).

CLARK-KENNEDY, A. E., *The London: A Study in the Voluntary Hospital System*, 2 vols. (London, 1962–3).

CLARKSON, L. A., and CRAWFORD, E. M., *The Ways to Wealth: The Cust Family of Eighteenth-Century Armagh* (Belfast, 1985).

COAKLEY, D., *Doctor Steevens's Hospital: A Brief History* (Dublin, 1992).

COLLEY, Linda, *Britons: Forging the Nation, 1707–1837* (London, 1992).

COLLIER, C., *Aristotle on the Vital Principle, Translated from the Original Text, with Notes* (London, 1855).

—— *An Essay on the Principles of Education, Physiologically Considered* (London, 1856).

—— *The History of the Plague of Athens: Translated from Thucydides, with Notes Explanatory of its Pathology* (London, 1857).

COLQUHOUN, PATRICK, *A Treatise on the Wealth, Power and Resources of the British Empire* (London, 1815).

The Commissioned Officers of the Royal Navy 1660–1815, (3 vols. n.p., 1954).

COMRIE, J. D., *History of Scottish Medicine*, 2 vols. (London, 1932),

CONSTANTINE, DAVID, *Fields of Fire: A Life of Sir William Hamilton* (London, 2001).

COOKSON, JOHN E., *The British Armed Nation, 1793–1815* (Oxford, 1997).

COPE, Z., *The Royal College of Surgeons of England: A History* (London, 1959).

CORFIELD, P. J., 'Concepts of the Urban Middle Class in Theory and Practice: England, 1750–1850', in B. Meier and H. Schultz (eds.), *Die Wiederkehr des Stadtbürgers: Stadtreformen im europäischen Vergleich, 1750–1850* (Berlin, 1994).

—— *Power and the Professions in Britain, 1700–1850* (London, 1995).

CORSI, PIETRO, *Genèse et enjeux du transformisme, 1770–1830* (Paris, 2001).

COUTTS, J., *A History of the University of Glasgow, from its Foundation in 1451 to 1909* (Glasgow, 1909).

COZENS-HARDY, B., *The Diary of Sylas Neville, 1767–1788* (London, 1950).

CRAIG, W. S., *History of the Royal College of Physicians of Edinburgh* (Oxford, 1976).

CRESWELL, C. H., *The Royal College of Surgeons of Edinburgh: Historical Notes from 1505–1905* (Edinburgh, 1926).

CROWE, KATE ELIZABETH, 'The Walcheren Expedition and the New Army Medical Board: A Reconsideration', *English Historical Review*, 88 (1973), 770–85.

CULLEN, M. J., *The Statistical Movement in Early Victorian Britain* (Hassocks, 1975).

CURRIE, ROBERT, *Methodism Divided: A Study of the Sociology of Ecumenicalism* (London, 1968).

DALRYMPLE, WILLIAM, *White Mughals: Love and Betrayal in Eighteenth-Century India* (London, 2004).

DALTON, CHARLES, *The Waterloo Roll Call*, 2nd edn. (London, 1971).

DAVIDOFF, L., and HALL, C., *Family Fortunes: Men and Women of the English Middle Class, 1780–1850* (London, 1987; rev. edn., London, 2002).

DAVIES, H., *The Young Wife's Guide during Pregnancy and Childbirth, and the Management of her Infant* (London, 1852).

DAVY, JOHN, *An Account of the Interior of Ceylon and its Inhabitants, with Travels in that Island* (London, 1831).

—— *Memoirs of the Life of Sir Humphry Davy*, 2 vols. (London, 1836).

—— *Notes and Observations on the Ionian Islands, with some Remarks on Constantinople and Turkey, and on the System of Quarantine as at Present Conducted* (London, 1842).

—— *Five Discourses Delivered before the General Agricultural Society of Barbados* (London, 1849).

—— *Introductions on the Present State of the West Indies, and on the Agricultural Societies of Barbados* (London, 1849).

—— *Lectures on the Study of Chemistry in Connection with the Atmosphere, the Earth and the Ocean* (London, 1849).

—— *The West Indies before and since Slave Emancipation, Comprising the Windward and Leeward Islands Military Command* (London, 1854).

—— *On some of the More Important Diseases of the Army, with Contributions to Pathology* (London, 1855).

—— *The Angler and his Friend, or, Piscatory Colloquies and Fishing Excursions* (London, 1855).

—— *Collected Works of Humphry Davy, Edited by his Brother, John Davy*, introd. David Knight (Durham, 2001).

DEAN, C. J. T., *The Royal Hospital Chelsea* (London, 1950).

DENT, W., *A Young Surgeon in Wellington's Army*, ed. L. W. Woodford (Old Woking, 1976).

Deputy Inspector General of Army Hospitals, C. Collier.... A Life Sketch by his Daughter, M. A. E. L. (London, 1870).

DES CILLEULS, J. et al., *Le Service de santé militaire dès ses origines à nos jours* (Paris, 1961).

DICKSON, SAMUEL, *On the Epidemic Cholera, and other Prevalent Diseases of India* (London, 1832).

—— *The Unity of Disease Analytically and Synthetically Proved, with Facts and Cases Subversive of the Received Practice of Physic* (London, 1839).

—— The Principles of the Chrono-Thermal System of Medicine, with the Fallacies of the Faculty (London, 1845).

—— *Revelations on Cholera* (London, 1848).

—— *The 'Destructive Art of Healing' or Facts for Families* (London, 1853).

—— *Memorable Events in the Life of a London Physician* (London, 1863).

—— *Fallacies of the Faculty, with the Principles of the Chrono-Thermal System of Medicine* (London, 1839; subsequent edns. 1841, 1843, 1845, 1853, 1865).

—— *The Forbidden Book: With New Fallacies of the Faculty: Being the Chrono-Thermalist, or People's Medical Enquirer*, 2 vols. (London, 1850–1).

DIGBY, ANNE, *Making a Medical Living: Doctors and Patients in the English Market for Medicine, 1720–1911* (Cambridge, 1994).

DOCKEY, MERRIAL, *The Trial between Mrs Docksey (Sister of the late David Garrick Esq.) Plaintiff and Stephen Panting of the City of Lichfield, Apothecary* (London, 1796).

DOUGLAS, J., *Diseases of the Army during the Campaign in Upper Canada, 1813–1815* (London, 1819).

DOUGLAS, ROBERT, with BROWN, SIR JAMES ROBERT, and MUIR, DR, *The Annals of Forres* (Forres, 1934).

DOW, D., and MOSS, M., 'The Medical Curriculum at Glasgow in the Early Nineteenth Century', *History of Universities*, 7 (1988), 227–57.

DREW, SIR R., *Commissioned Officers in the Medical Services of the British Army, 1660–1960*, 2 vols. (London, 1968).

Dublin University Magazine.

DUNCAN, A., *Memorials of the Faculty of Physicians and Surgeons of Glasgow, 1599–1850* (Glasgow, 1896).

DUNDAS, ROBERT, *Sketches of Brazil: Including New Views on Tropical and European Fever, with Remarks on a Premature Decay of the System Incident to Europeans on their Return from Hot Climates* (London, 1852).

EARLE, PETER, *The Making of the English Middle Class: Business, Society and Family Life in London, 1160–1730* (London, 1989).

Edinburgh Medical and Surgical Journal.

ELMER, PETER (ed.), *The Healing Arts: Health, Society and Disease in Europe 1500–1800* (Manchester, 2004).

ERICKSON, AMY LOUISE, *Women & Property in Early Modern England* (London, 1993).

ESTE, CHARLES, *My Own Life* (London, 1787).

—— *A Journey in the Year 1793 through Flanders, Brabant and Germany to Swizerland* (London, 1795).

ESTE, MICHAEL LAMBTON, *Remarks on Baths, Water, Swimming, Shampooing, Heat, Hot, Cold and Vapor Baths*, reprinted from the edition of 1812 (London, 1845).

EVANS, ERIC J., *The Forging of the Modern State: Early Industrial Britain 1783–1870* (London, 1983).

An Exposition of the state of the Medical Profession in the British Dominions; and of the Injurious Effects of the Monopoly, by Usurpation, of the Royal College of Physicians in London (London, 1826).

FARRELL, CHARLES, *Observations on Ophthalmia and its consequences* (London, 1810).

FERGUSON, WILLIAM, *Scotland 1689 to the Present* (Edinburgh, 1987).

FERGUSSON, WILLIAM, *Notes and Recollections of a Personal Life*, ed. James Fergusson (London, 1846).

Fifth Report of the Commissioners of Military Enquiry: Army Medical Department (London, 1808).

FISSELL, M. E., *Patients, Power and the Poor in Eighteenth-Century Bristol* (Cambridge, 1991).

FREIDSON, E., *Professional Powers: A Study of the Institutionalization of Formal Knowledge* (Chicago, 1986).

FLETCHER, ELIZA DAWSON, *Autobiography of Mrs. Fletcher of Edinburgh; With Letters and Other Family Memorials*, ed. Lady Mary Fletcher Richardson (Carlisle, 1875).

FOUCAULT, MICHEL, *The Birth of the Clinic: An Archaeology of Medical Perception*, trans. A. M. Sheridan Smith (New York, 1973).

FOWLER, SIMON, *Army Records for Family Historians*, Public Record Office Readers' Guide No. 2 (London, 1992).

—— and SPENCER, WILLIAM, *Army Records for Family Historians* (London, 2000).

FRASER, T. G., and JEFFREY, K. (eds.), *Men, Women and War* (Dublin, 1993).

FRASER, W., *A Letter Addressed to His Excellency the Right Honourable Earl of Chatham, K. G., Governor of Gibraltar . . . Relative to the Febrile Tempers of that Garrison* (London, 1826).

GALBRAITH, GEORGIANA (ed.), *The Journal of the Rev. William Bagshaw Steven* (Oxford, 1965).

GATENBY, P., *Dublin's Meath Hospital, 1753–1996* (Dublin, 1996).

Gentleman's Magazine.

GAY, PETER, *The Enlightenment: An Interpretation*, 2 vols. (London, 1966–70).

GEISON, G. (ed.), *Professions and the French State, 1700–1900* (Philadelphia, 1984).

GELFAND, TOBY, *Professionalizing Modern Medicine: Paris Surgeons and Medical Sciences and Institutions in the Eighteenth Century* (Westport, Conn., 1980).

GEYER-KORDESCH, J., *Physicians and Surgeons of Glasgow: The History of the Royal College of Physicians and Surgeons of Glasgow, 1599–1858* (London, 1999).

GIBNEY, WILLIAM, *De coeli caldi* (Edinburgh, 1813).

—— *A Medical Guide to the Cheltenham Waters, Containing Observations on their Nature and Properties; the Diseases in which they are Beneficial or Hurtful; the Rules to be Observed during their Use* (Cheltenham, 1821).

—— *Eighty Years Ago, or the Recollections of an Old Army Doctor; his Adventures on the Field of Quatre Bras and during the Occupation of Paris in 1815*, ed. Major R. D. Gibney (London, 1896).

GIBSON, TOM, *The Royal College of Physicians and Surgeons of Glasgow* (Glasgow, 1983).

[GILBERT, RICHARD,] *The Clerical Guide or Ecclesiastical Directory, Containing a Complete Register of the Dignitaries and Benefices of the Church of England* . . . (London, 1836).

GILLKREST, J., *Letters on the Cholera Morbus* (London, 1831).

GILLMAN, T., *A Short History of Sir Patrick Dun's Hospital* (Dublin, 1942).

GOLINSKI, Jan, *Science as Public Culture: Chemistry and Enlightenment in Britain 1760–1820* (Cambridge, 1999).

GOULD, TERRY, and UTTLEY, DAVID, *A Short History of St. George's Hospital and the Origins of its Ward Names* (London, 1996).

GRANT, SIR A., *The Story of the University of Edinburgh, during its First Three Hundred Years*, 2 vols. (London, 1884).

GRAY, SIMON, *The Happiness of States: or, an Inquiry Concerning Population, the Modes of Subsisting and Employing it, and the Effects of All on Human Happiness* (London, 1815).

GREGORY, GEORGE, *A Father's Legacy to his Daughter*, 1st edn. (1774).

—— *Elements of the Theory and Practice of Physic, Designed for the Use of Students* (London, 1825).

GRENHAM, JOHN, *Tracing your Irish Ancestors* (Dublin, 1992).

GUTHRIE, G. J., *A Treatise on Gun-Shot Wounds, on Inflammation, Erysipelas, and Mortification, on Injuries of Nerves, and on Wounds of the Extremities Requiring the Different Operations of Amputation* (London, 1815).

—— *Account of Two Successful Operations for Restoring a Lost Nose from the Integument of the Forehead in the Cases of Two Officers of his Majesty's Army* (London, 1816).

—— *History of the High Operation for the Stone, by Incision above the Pubis* (London, 1819).

—— *Treatise for an Operation for the Formation of an Artificial Pupil* (London, 1819).

—— *A Letter to the Right Hon. the Secretary of State for the Home Department, Containing Remarks on the Report of the Select Committee of the House of Commons on Anatomy* (London, 1829).

—— *Lectures on the Operative Surgery of the Eye: Being the Substance of that Part of the Author's Course of Lectures on the Principles and Practice of Surgery which Relates to the Diseases of that Organ: Published to the Purpose of Assisting in Bringing the Management of these Complaints within the Principles which Regulate the Practice of Surgery in General* (London, 1823, 1827, 1830 edns.).

—— *Remarks on the Anatomy Bill, in a Letter Addressed to Lord Althorp* (London, 1832).

—— *On the Operation for Extraction of a Cataract from the Eye* (London, 1834).

—— *On the Certainty and Safety with which the Operation of the Extraction of a Cataract may be Performed* (London, 1834).

—— *On Wounds and Injuries of the Arteries of the Human Body, with the Treatment and Operations Required for their Cure Illustrated by 130 Cases Selected from the Records of the Practice of the Most Celebrated Surgeons in Europe and America* (London, 1846).

—— *Commentaries on the Surgery of War in Portugal, Spain, France and the Netherlands, from the Battle of Roliça, in 1808, to that of Waterloo, in 1815*, 5th edn. (London, 1853).

HABAKKUK, JOHN, *Marriage, Debt, and the Estates System: English Landownership 1650–1950* (Oxford, 1994).

HALPIN, W., *Fact versus Assertion, or Critical and Explanatory Observations on some Erroneous Statements, Contained in Dr. Adam Neale's Pamphlet on the Nature and Properties of the Cheltenham Waters* (London, 1820).

HAMILTON, ROBERT, *The Duties of a Regimental Surgeon Considered*, 2 vols. (London, 1787).

HANNAH, L., *Inventing Retirement* (Cambridge, 1986).

HANNAWAY, CAROLINE, and LA BERGE, ANN (eds.), *Constructing Paris Medicine* (Amsterdam, 1998).

HARRIS, JOSE, *Private Lives, Public Spirit: Britain, 1870–1914* (Oxford, 1993).

HANS, NICHOLAS A., *New Trends in Education in the Eighteenth Century* (London, 1951).

HAYTHORNWHITE, PHILIP J., *Waterloo Men: The Experience of Battle, 16–18 June 1815* (Marlborough, 1999).

HEENEY, B., *A Different Kind of Gentleman: Parish Clergy as Professional Men in Early and Mid-Victorian England* (Hamden, Conn., 1975).

HELLER, SABINE, *Boerhaaves Schweizer Studenten: Ein Beitrag zur Geschichte des Medizinstudiums* (Zurich, 1984).

HENNEN, JOHN Snr., *Observations on some Important Points in the Practice of Military Surgery, and in the Arrangement and Police of Hospitals* (Dublin, 1818).

—— *Principles of Military Surgery, Comprising of Observations on the Arrangement, Police, and Practice of Hospitals, and on the History, Treatment and Anomalies of Variola and Syphilis* (London, 1829).

—— *Sketches of the Medical Topography of the Mediterranean, Comprising an Account of Gibraltar, the Ionian Islands, and Malta*, ed. John Hennen Jnr. (London, 1830).

HENSTOCK, ADRIAN (ed.), *The Diary of Abigail Gawthern of Nottingham, 1751–1810*, Thoroton Society of Nottinghamshire (Nottingham, 1980).

HEXTER, J. H., 'The Myth of the Middle Class in Tudor England', *Explorations in Entrepreneurial History*, 2/3 (1950), 128–40.

History of Hawick from 1832 (Hawick, 1902).

HOLMES, G., *Augustan England: Professions, State and Society, 1680–1730* (London, 1982).

HOLMES, RICHARD, *Wellington: The Iron Duke* (London, 2003).

HOPPEN, K. THEODORE, *The Mid-Victorian Generation 1846–1886* (Oxford, 1998).

HOSTETTLER, JOHN, *Thomas Wakley: An Improbable Radical* (Chichester, 1993).

HOWARD, MARTIN, *Wellington's Doctors: The British Army Medical Services in the Napoleonic Wars* (Staplehurst, 2000).

HUDSON, P., *The Industrial Revolution* (London, 1992).

HUGHES, EDWARD, 'Sir Charles Trevelyan and Civil Service Reform, 1853–5', *English Historical Review*, 64 (1949), 53–88, 206–34.

—— *North Country Life in the Eighteenth Century: The North East 1700–1750* (Oxford, 1952).

HUMBLE, J. G., and HANSELL, PETER, *Westminster Hospital, 1716–1966* (London, 1966).

HUTCHISON, JOHN, *History and Antiquities of the County of Dorset* (London, 1870).

Index of Irish Wills 1484–1858, Irish Record Index, vol. i (Dublin, 2003).

Instructions to Regimental Surgeons for Regulating the Concerns of the Sick and of the Hospital (London, 1803).

Les Invalides: trois siècles d'histoire (Paris, 1974).

JACKSON, ROBERT, *Remarks on the Constitution of the British Army with a Detail of Hospital Management* (London, 1803).

—— *A System of Arrangements and Discipline for the Medical Departments of Armies* (London, 1805).

—— *A Letter to Mr Keate, Surgeon General to the Forces* (London, 1808).

—— *A Letter to the Commissioners of Military Enquiry containing a Refutation of Some Statements made by Mr Keate* ... (London, 1808).

—— *A Letter to the Commissioners of Military Enquiry Explaining the True Constitution of a Medical Staff, the Best Form of Economy for Hospitals, etc.* (London, 1808).

—— *A View of the Formation, Discipline and Economy of Armies*, 3rd edn. (London, 1845).

JACYNA, L. S., *Philosophic Whigs: Medicine, Science and Citizenship in Edinburgh, 1789–1848* (London, 1994).

JENKYNS, RICHARD, *The Victorians and Ancient Greece* (London, 1980).

JERROLD, WALTER (ed.), *The Complete Poetical Works of Thomas Hood* (London, 1906).

The Journal of the Army Medical Corps.

KAUFMAN, MATTHEW H., *Surgeons at War: Medical Arrangements for the Treatment of the Sick and Wounded in the British Army during the Late Eighteenth and Nineteenth Centuries* (Westport, Conn., 2001).

—— *The Regius Chair of Military Surgery in the University of Edinburgh, 1806–55* (Amsterdam, 2003).

KEATE, THOMAS, *Observations on the Fifth Report of the Commissioners of Military Enquiry* ... (London, 1808).

KEATE, WILLIAM, *A Free Examination of Dr Price's and Dr Priestley's Sermons* (1790).

KELL, J., *On the Appearance of Cholera at Sunderland in 1831* (London, 1831).

KENNEDY, J., *Conversations on Religion with Lord Byron and Others, Held in Cephalonia, a Short Time Previous to his Lordship's Death* (London, 1830).

KENNEDY, PAUL, *The Rise and Decline of the Great Powers: Economic Change and Military Conflict from 1500–2000* (London, 1988).

KIRK, H., *Portrait of a Profession: A History of the Solicitors' Profession, 1100 to the Present Day* (London, 1976).

KIRKPATRICK, T. P. C., *The Book of the Rotunda Hospital: An Illustrated History of the Dublin Lying-in Hospital from its Foundation in 1745 to the Present Time* (London, 1913).

—— *The History of Dr. Steevens's Hospital, Dublin: 1720–1920* (Dublin, 1924).

KNIGHT, ROGER, *The Pursuit of Victory: The Life and Achievement of Horatio Nelson* (London, 2005).

KOPPERMAN, PAUL E., 'Medical Services in the British Army, 1742–1783', *Journal of the History of Medicine*, 34 (1979), 428–55.

Lancet.

LANE, JOAN, 'The Role of Apprenticeship in Eighteenth-Century Medical Education', in W. F. Bynum and R. Porter (eds.), *William Hunter and the Eighteenth-Century Medical World* (Cambridge, 1985), Ch. 3.

—— *Worcester Infirmary in the Eighteenth Century*, Worcester Historical Society Occasional Publications no. 6 (Worcester, 1992).

LANGDON-DAVIES, J., *Westminster Hospital: Two Centuries of Voluntary Service, 1719–1948* (London, 1952).

LANGFORD, PAUL, *A Polite and Commercial People: England, 1727–1783* (Oxford, 1989).

LANKFORD, NELSON D., 'The Victorian Medical Profession and Military Practice: Army Doctors and National Origins', *Bulletin of the History of Medicine*, 54 (1980), 511–28.

LARSON, M. S., *The Rise of Professionalism: A Sociological Analysis* (Berkeley, Calif., 1977).

LAWRENCE, C. J., 'The Edinburgh Medical School and the End of the "Old Thing" 1790–1830', *History of Universities*, 7 (1988), 259–86.

LAWRENCE, SUSAN C., 'Entrepreneurs and Private Enterprise: The Development of Medical Lecturing in London, 1775–1800', *Bulletin of the History of Medicine*, 63 (1988), 193–214.

—— *Charitable Knowledge: Hospital Pupils and Practitioners in Eighteenth-Century London* (Cambridge, 1996).

Laws of the Royal College and Corporation of Surgeons (Edinburgh, 1816).

LEADBETTER, CHARLES, *The Royal Gauger*, 3rd edn. (London, 1750).

LEMPRIERE, WILLIAM, *Practical Observations on the Diseases of the Army in Jamaica, as They Occurred between the Years 1792 and 1797* (London, 1799).

—— *A Report on the Medicinal Effects of an Alumnious Chalybeate Water, Lately Discovered at Sandrocks, in the Isle of Wight; Pointing out its Efficacy in the Walcheren and other Diseases Incident to Soldiers who have been Abroad, and More Particularly the Advantages to be Derived from its Introduction into Private Practice* (London, 1812).

—— *Popular Lectures on the Study of Natural History and the Sciences, as Delivered before the Isle of Wight Philosophical Society* (London, 1830).

LEWIS, R., and MAUDE, A., *The English Middle Classes*, 2nd edn. (London, 1953).

LLOYD, CHRISTOPHER, and COULTER, JACK L. S., *Medicine and the Navy 1200–1900*, iii: *1714–1815* (London, 1960).

LOUDON, IRVINE, *Medical Care and the General Practitioner, 1750–1850* (Oxford, 1986).

LUFFINGHAM, R. L., *John Alderson and his Family*, Centenary Monograph no. 21 (Hull, 1995).

—— *The Manuscript of Sir James Alderson*, Centenary Monograph no. 22 (Hull, 1995).

LUPTON, KENNETH, *Mungo Park: The African Traveller* (Oxford, 1975).

LYONS, J. B., *The Quality of Mercer's: The Story of Mercer's Hospital, 1734–1991* (Dublin, 1991).

MACAULEY, J., *Observations on Gymnastics, and the Gymnasium* (Dublin, 1828).

MACCARTHY, F., *Byron: Life and Legend* (London, 2002).

MCCLELLAND, C. E., *The German Experience of Professionalisation: Modern Learned Professions and their Organizations from the Early Nineteenth Century to the Hitler Era* (Cambridge, 1991).

MACDONAGH, OLIVER, *The Inspector General: Sir Jeremiah Fitzpatrick and the Problems of Social Reform, 1783–1802* (London, 1981).

MACDONALD, K. M., *The Sociology of the Professions* (London, 1995).

MCDOWELL, R. B., and WEBB, D. A., *Trinity College Dublin, 1592–1952: An Academic History* (Cambridge, 1982).

MCGRIGOR, SIR JAMES, *Medical Sketches of the Expedition to Egypt from India* (London, 1804).

—— 'Sketch of the Medical History of the British Armies in the Peninsula of Spain and Portugal', *Transactions of the Medico-Chirurgical Society*, 6 (1815), 381–449.

—— *Statistical Reports on the Sickness, Mortality and Invaliding among Troops in the West Indies, Prepared from the Boards of the Army Medical Department, and War Office Returns* (London, 1838).

MCGRIGOR, MARY (ed.), *Sir James McGrigor, The Scalpel and the Sword: The Autobiography of the Father of Army Medicine* (Dalkeith, 2000).

MCINNES, E. M., *St Thomas's Hospital* (London, 1963).

MACKERLIE, P. H., *History of the Lands and Their Owners in Galloway with Historical Sketches of the District, 5 vols.* (Edinburgh, 1870–9).

[MACLAGAN, DAVID], *Biographical Sketch of the Late John Alexander Schetky* (Edinburgh, 1825).

MACLEAN, DR CHARLES, *An Analytical View of the Medical Department of the British Army* (London, 1810).

MACLEOD, W., *Hydro-therapeutics or the Water Cure: Considered as a Branch of Medical Treatment* (London, 1855).

MAULITZ, RUSSELL, *Morbid Appearances: The Anatomy of Pathology in the Early Nineteenth Century* (Cambridge, 1987).

MAXTED, IAN, *The London Book Trades, 1775–1800: A Preliminary Check List of Members* (Folkestone, 1977).

Medical Directory for Scotland.

MEDVEI, V. C., and THORNTON, J. L. (eds.), *The Royal Hospital of St Bartholomew, 1123–1973* (London, 1974).

MILLAR, J., *A Guide to Botany, or, A Familiar Illustration of the Principles of Linnaean Classification* (London, 1821).

—— *Practical Observations on Warm and Cold Bathing, and Descriptive Notes of Watering Places in Britain* (London, 1821).

MITCHELL, ALISON (ed.), *Pre-1855 Gravestone Inscriptions and Index for the Stewarty of Kirkcudbright*, vol. v (Edinburgh, 1996).

MOISES, H., *An Inquiry into the Abuses of the Medical Department in the Militia of Great Britain with Some Amendments Proposed* (London, 1794).

MOKYR, J. (ed.), *The British Industrial Revolution: An Economic Perspective* (London, 1993).

MORAN, GERARD (ed.), *Galway History and Society: Interdisciplinary Essays on the History of an Irish County* (Dublin, 1996).

MORE, WENDY, *The Knife Man* (London, 2005).

MORGAN, NICHOLAS J., and MOSS, MICHAEL S., 'Listing the Wealthy in Scotland', *Bulletin of the Institute of Historical Research*, 59/140 (1986), 189–95.

MORRIS, W., *A History of the London Hospital* (London, 1926)

MUNRO, WILLIAM, *Records of Service and Campaigning in Many Lands*, 2 vols. (London, 1887).

NEALE, A., *Letters from Portugal and Spain; Comprising an Account of the Armies under their Excellencies Sir Arthur Wellesley and Sir John Moore, from the Landing of the Troops in Mondego Bay to the Battle at Coruna* (London, 1809).

—— *Travels through some Parts of Germany, Poland, Moldavia, and Turkey* (London, 1818).

NEALE, R. S., *Bath 1768–1850: A Social History, or, a Valley of Pleasure, yet a Sink of Iniquity* (London, 1981).

NEWELL, T., *A Letter to the Editor of the City Gazette upon the Misrepresentations Contained in a Pamphlet Recently Published by Dr. Neale, upon the Subject of the Cheltenham Waters by Thomas Newell, M.D., Surgeon Extraordinary to the King* (London, 1820).

NICOLAS, SIR NICHOLAS HARRIS (ed.), *Nelson's Dispatches*, 7 vols. (London, 1846).

Nineteenth Century Public Health and Epidemics: Some PRO Sources—Domestic Records Information 73 available at **http://catalogue.pro.gov.uk/** (July 2005).

Nomina eorum qui gradum medicinae doctoris in academia Jacobi sexti Scotorum regis quae Edinburgi est, adepti sunt (Edinburgh, 1846).

O'BRIEN, EOIN, CROOKSHANK, ANNE, and WOLSTENHOLME, GORDON, *A Portrait of Irish Medicine: An Illustrated History of Medicine in Ireland* (Dublin, 1984).

O'BRIEN, P. K., and QUINAULT, R. (eds.), *The Industrial Revolution and British Society* (Oxford, 1993).

O'DAY, R. *The Professions in Early Modern England, 1450–1800: Servants of the Commonwealth* (Harlow, 2000).

O'HALLORAN, T., *A Brief View of the Yellow Fever as it Appeared in Andalusia during the Epidemic in 1820* (London, 1821).

—— *Remarks on the Yellow Fever of the South and East of Spain; Comprehending Observations Made on the Spot, by Actual Survey of Localities, and Rigorous Examination of Fact at Original Sources of Information* (London, 1823).

OWEN, D., *English Philanthropy, 1660–1960* (Cambridge, Mass., 1965).

PAPPALARDO, BRUNO, *Tracing Your Naval Ancestors* (London 2003).

PARSONS, F. G., *The History of St Thomas's Hospital*, 3 vols. (London, 1932–6).

PARSONS, W. (ed.), *The Directory, Guide and Annals of Kingston-upon-Hull and the Parish of Sculcoates* (Leeds, 1826).

PEACHEY, G. C., *The History of St George's Hospital* (London, 1910–14).

PENCIER, HONOR de, *Posted to Canada: The Watercolours of George Russell Dartnell, 1835–1848* (Toronto, 1987).

PERKIN, H. J., *The Origins of Modern English Society 1780–1880* (London, 1969).

—— *The Rise of Professional Society: England since 1880* (London, 1989).

Perth Courant.

PETERSON, M. JEANNE, *The Medical Profession in Mid-Victorian London* (Berkeley and Los Angeles, 1978).

PETTIGREW, T. J., *Medical Portrait Gallery*, 4 vols. (London, 1838–40).

Piggot's Commercial Directory.

Piggot's Directory of Ireland.

PLARR, V. G., *Plarr's Lives of the Fellows of the Royal College of Surgeons of England*, 2 vols. (London, 1930).

PORTER, ROY, *Health for Sale: Quackery in England, 1660–1850* (Manchester, 1989).

—— *Enlightenment: Britain and the Creation of the Modern World* (London, 2000).

—— and TEICH, M. (eds.), *The Industrial Revolution in National Context* (Cambridge, 1996).

POWER, G. G., *An Attempt to Investigate the Cause of the Egyptian Ophthalmia, with Observations of its Nature and Different Modes of Cure* (London, 1803).

—— *The History of the Empire of the Musulmans in Spain and Portugal, from the First Invasion of the Moors to their Ultimate Expulsion from the Peninsula* (London, 1815).

PREST, W. (ed.), *The Professions in Early Modern England* (London, 1987).

—— *Albion Ascendant: English History, 1660–1815* (Oxford, 1998).

PRINGLE, SIR JOHN, *Observations on the Diseases of the Army* (London, 1753).

PROSSER, T., *A Treatise on the Strangles and Fevers of Horses: with a Plate Representing a Horse in the Staggers Slung* (London, 1790).

QUIST, GEORGE, *John Hunter 1728–93* (London, 1981).

Regulations for the Management of the General Hospitals in Great Britain (London, 1813).

Report of the Commission into Naval and Military Promotion (London, 1840).

Report of the Royal Westminster Ophthalmic Hospital, Charing Cross, Founded in 1816 for the Relief of Indigent Persons Afflicted with Diseases of the Eye, with a list of the Governors, Subscribers &c. to April 1856, and the Treasurer and Surgeon's Report to the End of the Year 1855 (London, 1856).

RICHARDSON, RUTH, *Death, Dissection and the Destitute* (London, 1987).

ROBBINS, KEITH, *Nineteenth-Century Britain: England, Scotland and Wales. The Making of a Nation* (Oxford, 1988).

ROBERTSON, H., *A Blast from the North in Vindication of the Medical Graduates of Edinburgh against the Invidious and Calumnious Aspersions Cast upon their Literary and Professional Education, through the Bye-laws of the London College of Physicians* (London, 1828).

ROBINSON, W., *The Story of the Royal Infirmary, Sunderland* (Sunderland, 1934).

ROSE, JUNE, *The Perfect Gentleman: The Remarkable Life of Dr James Miranda Barry, the Woman who Served as an Officer in the British Army from 1813 to 1859* (London, 1977).

ROSNER, LISA, 'Students and Apprentices: Medical Education at Edinburgh University, 1780–1810' (Ph.D. thesis, Johns Hopkins University, 1986) [Ann Arbor: University Microfilms Internations, 1988c1985].

——*Medical Education in the Age of Improvement: Edinburgh Students and Apprentices 1760–1828* (Edinburgh, 1991).

—— *The Most Beautiful Man in Existence: The Scandalous Life of Alexander Lesassier* (Philadelphia, 1999).

RUBINSTEIN, W. D., 'The Victorian Middle Class: Wealth, Occupation and Geography', *Economic History Review*, 2nd series, 30 (1977), 602–23.

——*Men of Property: The Very Wealthy in Britain since the Industrial Revolution* (London, 1981).

—— 'The Role of London in Britain's Wealth Structure, 1809–99: Further Evidence', in John Stobart and Alistair Owens (eds.), *Urban Fortunes, Property and Inheritance in the Town, 1700–1900* (Aldershot, 2000).

RULE, J., *Albion's People: English Society, 1714–1815* (Harlow, 1992).

Rules and Regulations of the Royal Westminster Ophthalmic Hospital . . . with a List of the Governors, Subscribers & c. to June 1851; and the Treasurer's and Surgeon's Report to the end of the Year 1850 (London, 1851).

Rules for the Government of the Royal Westminster Ophthalmic Hospital . . . with a list of the Governors and Subscribers and the Report of Receipt and Expenditure for the Year 1831, Corrected to July 1832 (London, 1832).

RUSSELL BARKER, G. F,. and STENNING, A. H., *The Record of Old Westminsters*, 2 vols. (London, 1928),

SAUNDERS, H. S., *The Middlesex Hospital, 1745–1948* (London, 1949).

SAVAGE, ROBERT BURKE, *Catherine McAuley: The First Sister of Mercy* (Dublin, 1949).

SCHAMA, S., *Patriots and Liberators: Revolution in the Netherlands 1780–1813* (London, 1977).

SCHOEMAN, KAREL, *The Bloemfontein Diary of Lieut W. J. St John* (Cape Town, 1988).

SCOTT, SHEILA, *My dear Cath . . . The Story of an Army Doctor's Wife in 1818–1819* (Peebles, 1976).

SCOTT, Sir WALTER, *The Surgeon's Daughter* (Edinburgh, 1827).

SHEAN, R., *Observations on the Most Prevalent Diseases of British Soldiers in the East Indies* (London, 1835).

SHERER, J., *Recollections of the Peninsula* (London, 1823).

SINCLAIR, CECIL, *Tracing Your Scottish Ancestors: A Guide to Research in the Scottish Record Office* (Edinburgh, 1990).

SINCLAIR, DAVID, *Sir Gregor MacGregor and the Land that Never Was* (London, 2003).

SINNOTT, NATHANIEL, *Observations Tending to Show the Management of the Medical Department of the Army* (London, 1796).

SMITH, C. MUNRO, MD, *A History of Bristol Royal Infirmary* (Bristol, 1917).

SMITH, F. B., *The People's Health, 1830–1910* (London, 1979).

SMITH, JOHN GORDON, *The Principles of Forensic Medicine* (London, 1821).

—— *An Analysis of Medical Evidence* (London, 1825).

—— *The Claims of Forensic Medicine* (London, 1829).

—— *Hints for the Examination of Medical Witnesses* (London, 1829).

—— *The English Army at Waterloo and in France* (London, 1830).

—— *Santarem; or, Sketches of Society and Manners in the Interior of Portugal* (London, 1832).

SONTAG, OTTO (ed.), *John Pringle's Correspondence with Albrecht von Haller*, Studia Halleriana, IV (Basel, 1999).

SOUTH, J. F., *Memorials of the Craft of Surgery in England* (London, 1886).

SPEER, T. C., *Thoughts on the Present Character and Constitution of the Medical Profession by T. C. Speer, M. D., M. R. I. A. Late Physician to the Dublin General Dispensary & c.* (Cambridge, 1823).

STILLE, ALEXANDER, *The Future of the Past: How the Information Age Threatens to Destroy our Cultural Heritage* (London, 2002).

STONE, L. (ed.), *An Imperial State at War: Britain from 1689 to 1815* (London, 1994).

—— and FAWTIER STONE, J. C., *An Open Elite? England, 1540–1880*, abridged edn. (Oxford, 1986).

Stowe Landscape Gardens (National Trust, 1997).

STRACHAN, HEW, *Wellington's Legacy: The Reform of the British Army, 1830–1854* (Manchester, 1984).

Sunderland Telegraph.

SURTEES, R. S., *Handley Cross* (London, 1854).

SWEET, R., *The English Town, 1680–1840: Government, Society and Culture* (Harlow, 1999).

THOMPSON, F. M. L. (ed.), *The Cambridge Social History of Britain, 1750–1950*, vol. iii (Cambridge, 1990).

THOMSON, A., *An Enquiry into the Nature, Causes and Methods of Cure of Nervous Disorders; in a Letter to a Friend* (London, 1782).

The Times.

Transactions of the Medico-Chirurgical Society.

The Trial of James Stuart Esq., Younger of Dunearn (Edinburgh, 1822).

TURNER, A. LOGAN, *Story of a Great Hospital: The Royal Infirmary of Edinburgh, 1729–1929* (Edinburgh, 1937).

TYTLER, H., *Works of Callimachus Translated into English Verse; the Hymns and Epigrams from the Greek, with the Coma Berenices from the Latin of Catullus; with the Original Text and Notes* (London, 1793).

University of Edinburgh Journal.

VAN MILLINGEN, J. G., *The Army Medical Officer's Manual upon Active Service* (London, 1819).

VOLDMAN, D., *Les Hôpitaux militaires dans l'espace sanitaire français, 1708–1789* (Paris, 1980).

VOLHARD, JACOB, *Justus von Liebig* (Leipzig, 1909).

WAHRMAN, DROR, *Imagining the Middle Class: The Political Representation of Class in Britain, c.1700–1840* (Cambridge, 1995).

WALKER, NORMAN L., *David Maclagan* (London, 1884).

WALL, CECIL, *The History of the Surgeons' Company 1745–1800* (London, 1937).

WALLACE, W., *Observations on Sulphureous Fumigations as a Powerful Remedy in Rheumatism and Diseases of the Skin* (Dublin, 1820).

WALLACE, W., *A Physiological Enquiry Respecting the Action of Moxa, and its Utility in Inveterate Cases of Sciatica, Lumbago, Paraplegia Epilepsy, and some other Painful, Paralytic and Spasmodic Diseases of the Nerves and Muscles* (Edinburgh, 1827).

WALLIS, PETER J. and WALLIS, RUTH, *Eighteenth-Century Medics: Subscriptions, Licences, Apprenticeships* (Newcastle, 1985).

WALSH, E., *Bagatelles or Poetical Sketches* (Dublin, 1793).

—— *A Narrative of the Late Expedition to Holland in the Autumn of the Year 1799* (London, 1800).

White's Directory of Bristol.

WIDDESS, J. D. H., *The Royal College of Surgeons in Ireland and its Medical School, 1784–1966* (Dublin, 1966).

—— *The Royal College of Surgeons in Ireland and its Medical School, 1784–1984* (Dublin, 1984).

WILKS, S., and BETTANY, G. T., *A Biographical History of Guy's Hospital* (London, 1892).

WILLIAMSON, J., *Medical and Miscellaneous Observations, Relative to the West Indian Islands*, 2 vols. (Edinburgh, 1817).

WILSON, CHARLES JOHN, 'Hawick and its People', *Transactions of the Hawick Archaeological Society* (1921).

WILSON, SIR W. J. E., *The History of the Middlesex Hospital during the First Century of its Existence* (London, 1845).

WOODFORDE, J., *The Diary of a Country Parson, 1758–1802*, ed. J. Beresford (Oxford, 1967).

WEBSITES

www.ancestry.com
www.a2a.org.uk
www.beattydna.org
www.burkes-peerage.net/sites/common/sitepages/page13i-dec.asp
http://catalogue.pro.gov.uk/.
www.cheshire.gov.uk/Recoff/eshop/Wills/home.htm
www.copac.ac.uk
www.eh.net/hmit/ppower/bp
www.familysearch.org
www.geolsoc.org.uk/template.cfm?name=medallistsfrom1831.
www.genuki.org.uk
www.gravesfa.org/gen228.htm
www.lambethpalacelibrary.org/holdings/Guides/clergyman.html,
www.medicalpioneers.com
www.naa.gov.au
www.nationalarchives.gov.uk/
www.national.archives.gov.2a
www.oxforddnb.com
http://members.tripod.com/~Glosters

www.royalsoc.ac.uk/page.asp?id=1727
www.scotlandspeople.gov.uk
www.scottishdocuments.com/
www.spaceless.com/fletcher/flet11.htm
www.theclergydatabase.org.uk
www.user.dccnet.com/s.brown/familytree/BROWNE-Janeville-Montague.htm
www.york.ac.uk/inst/bihr/probate%20.htm

Index